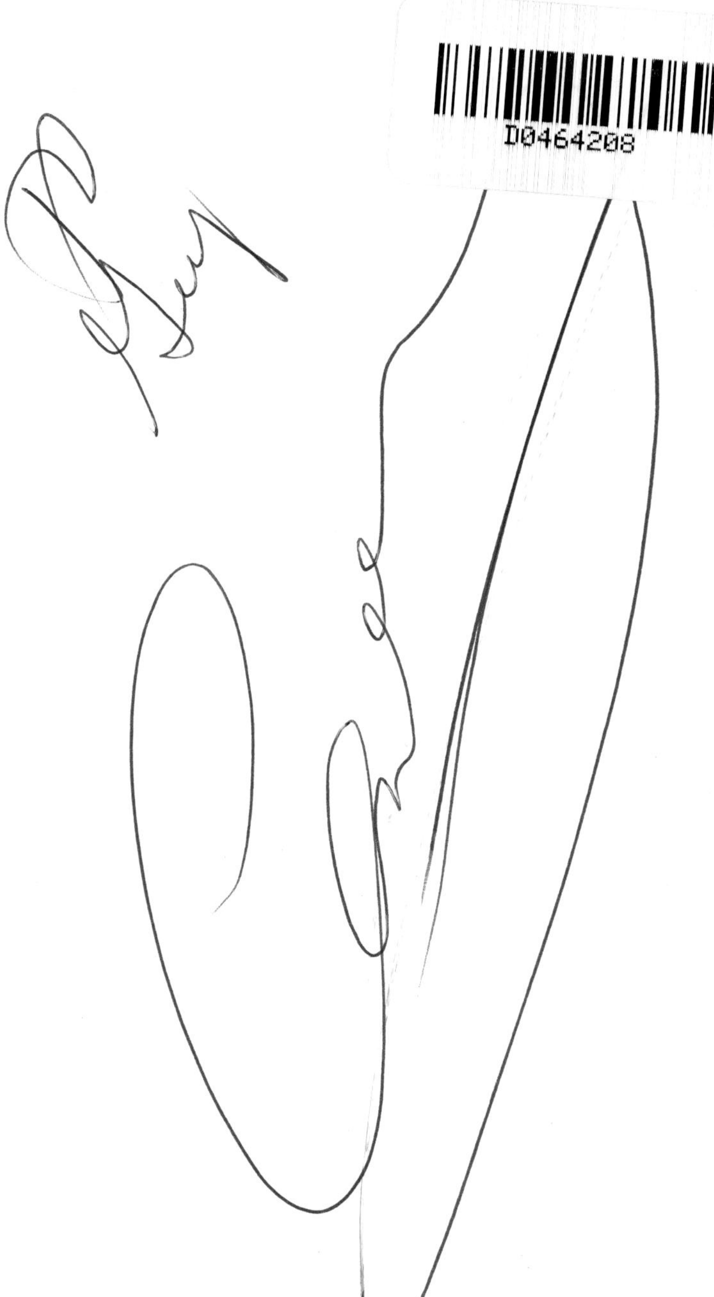

NATURE'S PAIN KILLERS

NATURE'S PAIN KILLERS

Proven New Alternative and Nutritional Therapies for Chronic Pain Relief

CARL GERMANO, R.D., C.N.S., L.D.N. and
WILLIAM CABOT, M.D., F.A.A.O.S., F.A.A.D.E.P.

Foreword by Prithvi Raj, M.D., F.A.C.P.M.
Editor-in-Chief, *Pain Digest*

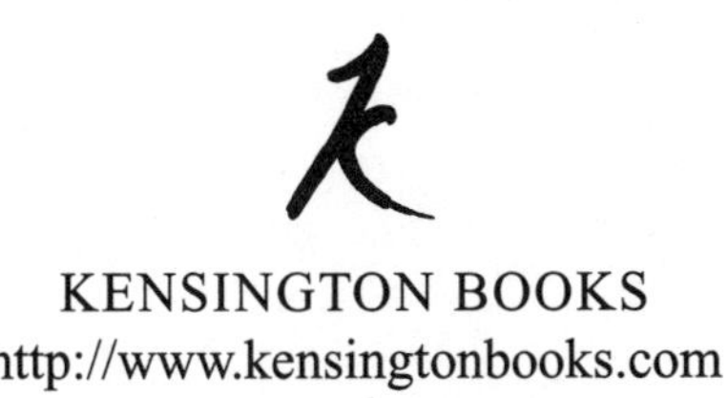

KENSINGTON BOOKS
http://www.kensingtonbooks.com

KENSINGTON BOOKS are published by

Kensington Publishing Corp.
850 Third Avenue
New York, NY 10022

Library of Congress Card Catalogue Number: 99-65996
ISBN 1-57566-502-6

First Printing: December, 1999
10 9 8 7 6 5 4 3 2 1

Printed in the United States of America

To my wife Alise, who has been a wellspring of love and support. To my son Grant and my daughter Samantha, who have been my source of life, joy, happiness. To my mother Frances and stepfather Vincent—thanks for the endless love and guidance. All of you have provided me the strength, love, support and insanity so necessary for my existence.

—Carl Germano, R.D., C.N.S., L.D.N.

For Susie, whom I love so much—I could never have done it without you.

For Adam and Brandy—I am so proud of you. You are such a source of joy.

—William Cabot

CONTENTS

ACKNOWLEDGMENTS

A very special thanks to Neenyah Ostrum, whose special editing and writing has made this book a great success. You were wonderful at taking the sterile medical information we provided and turning it into an orchestral movement. Your touch is felt on every page.

We are also grateful for the medical artwork provided by Myrna Plymire, President of Myrna Plymire Associates, an interior design firm in Atlanta.

CONTRIBUTORS

This book could not be possible without the contribution of the following key individuals who have provided their wisdom and expertise.

Prithvi Raj, M.D., F.A.C.P.M., is professor of anesthesia, department of anesthesiology at Texas Tech University Health Sciences Center and is presently the chief editor of *Pain Digest*. Dr. Raj is a renowned specialist in the field of pain management known for his contributions in pain control for reflex sympathetic dystrophy and failed back syndrome.

Jeffrey Jacob, L.Ac., O.M.D., is a licensed acupuncturist and doctor of Oriental medicine who presently practices at the Chinese Acupuncture Clinic in Asheville, North Carolina. A former director of The New York Center for Pain Management, the largest pain clinic in the United States integrating Eastern and Western medicine, Jeff also practices

Herbology, Tui Na, Shiatsu, Craniosacral Therapy, Deep Tissue and Polarity Therapy. He has taught throughout the United States and Japan and is the author of *The Acupuncturist's Clinical Handbook.*

Jennifer Kelly, Ph.D., is a practicing clinical psychologist in Atlanta, Georgia, where she is president of Atlanta Behavioral Medicine. She also serves as the current president of the Georgia Psychological Association and is an active member of the editorial staff of the journal *Pain Digest*. In addition to her clinical practice Dr. Kelly works actively with Rosalynn Carter on the executive committee of Project Interconnection, an organization devoted to finding housing for individuals with mental illness.

Phillip Klein, a graduate of Life Chiropractic College, is a chiropractor in private practice in New Hempstead, New York. His practice's primary focus is on wellness, and prevention. Dr. Klein has completed post-doctoral training becoming board certified as a Diplomate in Applied Chiropractic Sciences. Dr. Klein is a member of the New York Chiropractic Council.

Jay Lombard, M.D., is Chief of Neurology at Westchester Square Medical Center and Assistant Clinical Professor of Neurology at New York Hospital, Cornell Medical School. He is certified in neurology by the American Board of Psychiatry and Neurology. As a private practitioner in New York City, he specializes in neurodegenerative diseases using conventional and complementary approaches. Dr. Lombard is also co-author with Carl Germano, of the best selling book, *The Brain Wellness Plan.*

Brian Appell received his Bachelor of Science in Nutrition from Rutgers University. He is a senior technical writer in nutriceutical research and development with a major dietary supplement company and has significantly contributed to several major books on nutritional therapy in health and disease. Additionally, he was a former editor for *The Ankh: Perspectives in Health and Well-Being.*

FOREWORD

Pain treatment has come of age. It was only a few short years ago (1974) that we first gave serious consideration to patients suffering from acute and chronic pain, and a society composed of multiple medical disciplines was formed to study pain. This society, the International Association for the Study of Pain (IASP), took the challenge seriously and encouraged clinicians and basic scientists alike to determine whether pain is only a symptom of another disease, or a significant disease itself.

We have accomplished a lot in the twenty-five years. We better understand the mechanism of commonly seen pain syndromes, the site of action of analgesics, and the numerous options available to us, the clinicians, to manage chronic pain.

In spite of these achievements, the knowledge is not universal to all and is confusing to many, especially to those who do not specialize in pain management. Patients who suffer from chronic pain are also at a disadvantage, since they do not usually get a well-balanced, multidisciplinary, and effective pain management regimen. Furthermore, it is no surprise that medical and even behavioral models of pain management have failed to produce a reliable, effective treatment.

Due to the failure of Western medicine, many patients have turned to alternative medicine for answers. Today, we have revealed a great arsenal of natural remedies for pain. Standardized herbs and nutritional supplements, acupuncture, chiropractic, and psychological intervention are slowly becoming important adjuncts to medical plans directed at treating chronic pain.

Dr. Cabot and his colleague, Carl Germano, have embarked on a mission to educate patients and their caregivers about our current understanding of the physiology of pain, common pain syndromes, and the scientific basis of alternative therapies. They place special emphasis on nutritional therapy in their fascinating new book, *Nature's Pain Killers*.

I wish them great success and hope chronic pain patients derive knowledge and empowerment from this book.

—Prithvi Raj, M.D., F.A.C.P.M.
Editor-in-Chief, *Pain Digest*
Professor of Anesthesia, Department of Anesthesiology
Texas Tech University Health Sciences Center

INTRODUCTION

Pain is a fact of modern life. Our jobs cause us pain. People whose jobs require physical activity—construction workers, truck drivers, high school athletic coaches—strain muscles and tendons, throw their backs out, and sometimes endure even worse injuries. Those of us in sedentary jobs also encounter pain as part of daily living, caused by stress, anxiety, or even just sitting motionless at our computers hour after hour. Even having fun produces pains! Jogging, in-line skating, friendly basketball or softball games all result in sprained ankles, strained muscles, the occasional torn ligament, or even a broken bone.

Like stress, we must learn to cope with pain in ways that don't damage the other parts of our lives. In *Nature's Pain Killers*, you'll learn methods of coping with pain that actually make you healthier and happier, and more in control of your own life. You no longer have to rely on medications, with their many side effects and the potential for addiction, or be frightened into having surgery that may leave you in worse pain than you're feeling. We're going to introduce you to a whole range of natural substances—foods, herbs, and supplements—that can help you better control your pain and your entire life.

THE PROBLEM OF CHRONIC PAIN

While acute pain—like that from a sprained ankle or broken bone—warns us that something is very wrong, *chronic* pain is entirely different. In fact, researchers now suspect that chronic pain is a completely separate disease state, a nonending feedback loop of chemicals produced inside our own bodies, that is *not* a helpful response to our environment.

To stop chronic pain, we have to learn how to interrupt that misery-producing feedback loop.

Modern Western medicine is incredibly good at solving acute health situations, including those that produce acute pain. Our medical system has been a dismal failure, however, in treating chronic pain. Our repertoire is extremely limited, and focuses on drugs that have many serious, negative side effects. Far too many people who suffer from chronic pain also suffer from its treatment, in the form of addiction to narcotic pain killers. Along with addiction comes the problem of tolerance: the more pain killer you take, the more you require to ameliorate your pain. And if a narcotic-addicted person attempts to stop taking them abruptly, he or she experiences the agony of withdrawal.

Did you know that not only the brain, but also the immune system, contributes to causing chronic pain? *Nature's Pain Killers* is the first book to reveal that the immune system is, in fact, just as important as the nervous system in creating and perpetuating chronic pain.

Immune system cells make "pro-inflammatory" chemicals that not only cause inflammation (like we feel in arthritic joints or when we sprain an ankle), but are also integral in causing pain. These stunning new discoveries help us understand how pain begins and how to stop it, and provide clues about the natural substances and foods we can use to stop the vicious cycle of chronic pain.

It's probably no surprise to you that the nervous system—our brains, spinal cord, and peripheral nerves—is central in generating and stopping pain. You probably didn't know, however, that the nervous system acts *with* the immune system to generate certain chemicals that cause pain, and other chemicals that are pain killers as powerful as morphine. We make these chemicals—the pain causers as well as the pain killers—in our bodies. Therefore, we can influence how much of which kinds of these chemicals we make by changing what we eat, and the supplements we take. In *Nature's Pain Killers*, you'll learn about the foods and supplements that assist the nervous system in making our "natural morphine" and other chemicals that lessen pain. We'll also tell you about the foods that can contribute to making your pain worse, so you can avoid them.

We'll also examine safe, natural methods of controlling the depression that often accompanies chronic pain. Antidepressant medications not only alleviate depression, they can also act as mild pain killers. Fortunately, it's not absolutely necessary to resort to antidepressant medications in all cases. Did you know that the very same foods and nutrient supplements that help us combat depression also alleviate pain? In *Nature's Pain Killers*, you'll learn about foods, herbs, and supplements that simultaneously combat pain and depression.

Much of the pain we deal with every day originates in the musculoskeletal system—our bones, muscles, ligaments, and tendons. Let's examine one of the commonest—and costliest—chronic pains in the United States today: low back pain.

Low back pain is the second leading cause of absenteeism from work, behind only the common cold. It is the third-most-common reason that people go to see their physicians. In fact, data from the National Center for Health Statistics show that 14.3 percent of new patient visits to physicians are for low back pain. Approximately 2.4 million Americans are permanently disabled from chronic low back pain, and an additional 2.4 million are temporarily disabled.

Society as a whole feels the impact of low back pain. It is the most frequent cause of limitation of activities in people younger than forty-five. It's also the third-most-common reason that people undergo surgery. Unfortunately, many of them are worse off after the surgical intervention than they were before the surgery. Back surgery's track record has been disappointing, to say the least.

The vast majority of people who suffer from low back pain recover by themselves, without any help from a physician. A Swedish study provides insight into the typical "natural history" of low back disorders: 57 percent of patients recover in one week, 90 percent in six weeks, and 95 percent after twelve weeks.

Sometimes, however, the condition causing low back pain is serious and requires medical treatment. A herniated, or slipped, disk usually causes low back pain that also "radiates" down the leg. This leg pain, called sciatica, is present in about 25 percent of the people with back problems.

Sciatica usually gets better by itself without any surgery; only a minority of people requires surgery for this condition. *The worst thing you can do is to rush into surgery for low back pain without having properly assessed your problem.* Most episodes of low back pain, and even sciatica, will disappear spontaneously within about twelve weeks. Only 1 to 2 percent requires evaluation for surgery.

If you are having severe neurological problems, then surgery is mandatory, and time is of the essence. Unless you have a significant neurological deficit, like bowel or bladder incontinence or muscle weakness, you are much better off pursuing any of the numerous conservative treatments we'll discuss in later chapters before resorting to surgery.

Among those treatments (which we'll discuss in detail in Chapter 1) are nonsteroidal anti-inflammatory drugs (NSAIDs), a class of drugs that includes the popular Motrin. Inflammation causes most low back pain, at least in part, and controlling the inflammation will, in most cases, lessen the pain significantly.

The problem with NSAIDs, however, lies not in their use but in their overuse. Many people feel they cannot live without them. Statistics show that the vast majority of the human population uses over-the-counter NSAIDs on a regular basis.

Why is that so bad? Like all potent drugs, NSAIDs can produce serious side effects, especially if used excessively. Stomach problems like nausea, heartburn, diarrhea, vomiting, ulceration, and bleeding; skin rash and itching; and even kidney failure and liver damage can result from the excessive use of NSAIDs over time.

Aspirin and other NSAIDs have been the cornerstones of treatment for inflammation and pain for many years, and their effectiveness is not without merit, particularly in the short term. More often than not, however, people looking for relief from pain rely on a daily intake of NSAIDs sometimes for weeks, months, or even years. When used for so long, the therapeutic value of these drugs *ceases*. In addition to the deleterious effects of NSAIDs on the gastrointestinal tract, liver, and kidneys, their effect on inflamed joints (in arthritic patients, for example) may only be palliative. Over extended periods of time, NSAIDs may actually contribute to joint degradation *despite* their anti-inflammatory activity. Are NSAIDs the only remedy?

For these and many other reasons, the answer must be "No." It's critical that we develop anti-inflammatory medications that are less harmful than those we now have. We simply can't afford the financial and human suffering associated with the side effects of existing NSAIDs.

Your best approach is learning how to cope with the pain by increasing your activities, by relying less on medication and the traditional medical establishment, and by taking more responsibility for your clinical predicament. To start down this path, it's necessary for you to know as much as possible about the nature of the pain you're experiencing, so you can discuss it intelligently with your doctor as well as more fully understand it yourself.

You, like many people with chronic pain, are probably tired of getting the same old choices from your doctor—narcotics, NSAIDs, or surgery, treatments that have not produced a high percentage of good results in the past. Increasing numbers of Americans are refusing to accept these limited choices. Instead, they are gradually taking charge of their own health and seeking gentler, less invasive methods to ease their debilitating chronic pain.

In *Nature's Pain Killers*, we're going to present a revolutionary breakthrough: Using nutritional medicine and alternative therapies, you can treat chronic pain safely and naturally with greater success than you've previously achieved with prescription pain medications.

TWENTY-FIRST-CENTURY PAIN RELIEF

Over the last few years, nutritional scientists have gained extraordinary insight into how natural plant compounds can affect the underlying biochemistry of pain. The most exciting news comes from our emerging scientific understanding of how to use herbal medicine, acupuncture, chiropractic, massage, and psychological techniques to treat chronic pain safely. Greater knowledge about the chemistry of herbs and other nutrients has led to the development of a new class of dietary supplements called phytoanalgesics to control chronic pain safely and effectively. Today, you have new choices.

We'll introduce you to the latest developments in chronic pain management and nutritional therapies. You'll learn about the phytoanalgesic herbs that treat pain, and identify the foods that fight—or cause—pain.

Americans have used supplements significantly more over the past few years. Both physicians and patients looking for more natural methods of healing have sought herbal and nutritional therapies. These natural therapies are especially suitable for treating chronic diseases because of their lack of side effects. Unlike pharmaceutical drugs, which are singular in their purpose, herbal and nutritional supplements have many effects and interact with numerous biochemical pathways. Their combination of ingredients generates their therapeutic benefits.

For example, we used to prescribe vitamins and minerals only to prevent deficiencies (in other words, at very low levels). We now use them as "dietary supplements," in dosages that far exceed minimal requirements.

As we learn more about the clinical benefits of herbal and nutritional therapy, we'll be able to segregate useless and occasionally dangerous practices from scientifically viable approaches. Nowhere will this be more important than in pain and inflammation management.

For example, a new class of herbs and nutrients, called phyto-anti-inflammatory drugs (PAIDs), are no longer untested remedies. We've learned that some PAIDs inhibit arachidonic acid metabolism, while others inhibit the release of cytokines and prostaglandins. Others directly relieve pain, and you'll learn about all of them in *Nature's Pain Killers*.

We'll explore the latest information on alternative therapies, from acupuncture to chiropractic. You'll discover common herbs—like boswellia, devil's claw, and stinging nettle—that can help you conquer pain. *Nature's Pain Killers* will also reveal how to use supplements like perilla seeds, devil's claw, stinging nettle, Pycnogenol®, glucosamine, and chondroitin sulfate to halt the cycle of inflammation that keeps chronic pain returning, over and over, causing misery that can last a lifetime.

Believe it or not, even changing your diet can help alleviate chronic pain. We'll identify ordinary foods that intensify your pain and inflammation, and those that relieve it, and help you plan your diet accordingly. Additionally, you'll learn how simply adding ordinary spices like curcumin, healthy oils containing omega-3 essential fatty acids, and sea vegetables to your everyday diet can help ameliorate chronic pain.

You can stop the cycle of chronic inflammation and pain. We'll provide you with the tools and the information you need to treat chronic pain safely and effectively without narcotics or even common pain medications. Medical practitioners have known for years that patients only begin to improve rapidly when they become active participants in their own care and recovery. How well you recover from chronic pain can depend upon how well you educate yourself. Using *Nature's Pain Killers*, you will be able to take charge of your pain, and improve the quality of your life and the lives of those you love.

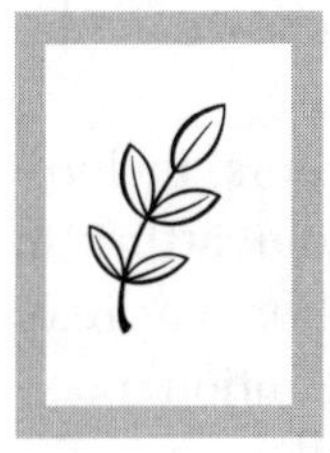

Chapter 1 THE SCOPE OF THE PROBLEM

PAIN IN OUR SOCIETY

You probably picked up this book because you are in pain. You may have sharp, short-term pain (also called acute pain), or you may be unfortunate enough to have chronic pain. If you are a victim of chronic pain, you may also know that we've recently made fantastic scientific advances in understanding pain and how to treat it. New, powerful drugs are available, but the relief they provide comes at a price with a slew of serious side effects. In *Nature's Pain Killers*, you'll gain knowledge to help you achieve pain relief without enduring side effects from the medications now available and those to come.

Of the painful conditions that people deal with on a day-to-day basis many originate in the musculoskeletal system—bones, joints, tendons, ligaments, and muscles. Although most stem from back injuries, a host of other conditions, which also affects our joints, can cause us significant grief almost as soon as they develop.

If you suffer from chronic pain, you know all too well how quickly pain can become the center of your entire life. It can damage relationships with family, friends, and coworkers. Indeed, pain sufferers sometimes find that, although they were once friendly and outgoing, they've gradually become reclusive, not interacting well with other people as they once did. Many chronic pain patients become socially isolated, experiencing depression and a downward spiral in their lives. If these gloomy statements describe you—or you're afraid they soon will—take heart! We're going to explain how to treat your pain with natural substances that *don't* have the serious side effects of your current medicines.

Western medicine uses drugs to treat all kinds of disorders, including, of course, pain. Musculoskeletal pain—whether from arthritis, strains, or tendinitis—usually results from inflammation. For that reason, we use anti-inflammatory medications to treat it. In addition, people often take narcotics or analgesics, despite their unpleasant side effects, which include addiction and tolerance. The drug simply stops working if you use it on a regular basis. Then, not only are you in pain, you can become depressed and addicted as well. Although you may take one or many pain killers every day, plus anti-inflammatory medicine, you may still suffer. And if you try to stop taking the pain killers abruptly, you'll experience the misery of withdrawal, which can be dangerous to your overall health.

Is there an answer to this problem? Yes! Herbs, nutrients, and plant-based analgesics provide pain relief without the many side effects produced by prescription and over-the-counter medications. Research has consistently demonstrated that many of these natural substances not only control pain but also accelerate healing—so you get well faster, with less pain.

Common Inflammatory Conditions That Can Lead to Chronic Pain

- arthritis
- asthma
- sprains
- carpal tunnel syndrome
- bursitis
- myositis
- fibromyalgia and fibrositis
- gout
- cumulative trauma disorders

Another reason to use natural substances to treat pain is that many inflammatory conditions—particularly those that affect our joints—don't respond to the "quick-fix" approach of traditional Western medicine. Herbs and plant-based analgesics are also, in many cases, more effective and less toxic than traditional medicines. Plant-based treatments like perilla seed, boswellia, devil's claw, stinging nettle, willow bark, curcumin, and many others may provide the help you need, and we'll describe them in detail in the following chapters.

How many people in the world suffer pain on a regular basis? Too many! You are not as alone as you may have thought. A study in the United Kingdom, for example, showed that almost one-eighth of the population suffers chronic pain, defined there as pain that occurs every day for at least twelve weeks. Much of this pain comes from the inflammation that accompanies conditions like arthritis.

Statistics in the United States are equally distressing. Some studies reveal that as many as 20 percent of Americans suffer chronic pain, or are partially (or completely) disabled by pain for at least a few days every month. A considerable amount of this pain results from workplace injuries, and the costs in that arena are astronomical.

What is causing all this pain? Often, problems like rheumatism or arthritis. These terms loosely describe painful, swollen, stiff joints that you can't move normally. Additionally, 80 percent of the adult population in the United States will suffer back pain at some point in their lives. This back pain may arise from a herniated disk with bad surgical results, from straightforward muscle strain, or from wear-and-tear arthritis of the spine. These conditions, however, all have one thing in common: inflammation. So let's take a closer look at the inflammation that's causing all this pain.

THE INFLAMMATORY PROCESS AND HOW CONNECTIVE TISSUES HEAL

Did you ever sprain your ankle or wrist while playing sports? Remember how it swelled? That swelling is part of the body's defense response to injury. When we damage our joints, tendons, or muscles by stretching, tearing, or overusing them, an inflammatory process begins. Inflammation has many symptoms, of which swelling is only one.

The four "cardinal symptoms" that accompany inflammation of joints and other musculoskeletal structures are redness, pain, heat, and swelling. Researchers recently added a fifth symptom, loss of function of the injured area, to the list, but its presence depends on the location and degree of your injury.

Injury causes inflammation, which causes pain. For that reason, we treat pain with anti-inflammatory medications, usually nonsteroidal anti-inflammatory drugs (NSAIDs). Orthopedists use NSAIDs more than any other medication. Unfortunately, these drugs produce many undesirable side effects, including gastrointestinal disturbances, peptic ulcer disease, and even kidney or liver damage. This is why researchers are working to develop new anti-inflammatory medications that decrease inflammation and, therefore, pain, without the NSAIDs' many harmful side effects.

Symptoms of Inflammation

The five "cardinal symptoms" of inflammation:

- redness
- pain
- heat
- swelling
- loss of function of the injured area

Inflamed, injured tissue releases chemicals that irritate your nerves and cause pain. Histamine, found in many cells in the body, is one of those chemicals. It dilates, or opens, and increases the permeability of blood vessels. That, in turn, causes bothersome symptoms like a runny nose. What medication do you usually take for a runny nose? An antihistamine, of course, to stop your cells from releasing histamine. Antihistamines have directly opposite effects to histamine: Antihistamines constrict, or narrow, and decrease the permeability of blood vessels. They usually stop the runny nose and make us feel better.

Most substances in our bodies perform positive functions, and histamine is no exception, runny noses aside. When we injure ourselves, histamine helps to start the inflammatory process so we can repair the injury. During inflammation, the body produces many soldiers like histamine that rally to our defense, including antibodies, white blood cells, and chemicals that help blood clot (see Table 1-1).

In Chapter 4, we'll discuss the parts of the musculoskeletal system, our "connective tissues," in detail. They include the muscles, tendons, ligaments, and fascia, as well as the bones. They can all be injured and, subsequently, develop inflammation.

Table 1-1 CHEMICALS THAT CONTRIBUTE TO INFLAMMATION
1. Histamine A chemical found in the blood, platelets, and white blood cells called basophils. Also found in connective tissue (in mast cells). Released in response to injury, histamine dilates (widens) the blood vessels and increases their permeability.
2. Kinins Proteins found in the blood that dilate the blood vessels and increase their permeability. These proteins attract white blood cells to the site of inflammation.
3. Prostaglandins When arachidonic acid (a fatty acid) breaks down, the Cox-1 and Cox-2 enzymes form these lipid substances. Those formed by Cox-2 contribute to inflammation by intensifying the effects of histamine and kinins. Those formed by Cox-1 are beneficial and protective.
4. Leukotrienes Chemicals produced by white blood cells (basophils) and connective tissue mast cells. Besides increasing the permeability of blood vessels, they also attract white blood cells to the site of inflammation and help destroy any bacteria present.
5. Complement Proteins in the blood that are active during inflammation by stimulating histamine release and helping to destroy any bacteria present.

THE CHEMICALS THAT CONTROL INFLAMMATION

Say you've injured a piece of connective tissue—you've torn your Achilles tendon playing basketball, for example, or suffered a repetitive trauma injury, like tennis elbow. As soon as you sustain an injury, the body starts to heal itself. There are three phases in the healing process: *inflammation, repair,* and *remodeling.*

Inflammation has a distinct purpose: It protects us. It helps the body dispose of toxins, bacteria, and any other foreign material at the site of the injury, which prevents their spread to our other organ systems. In addition, inflammation helps prepare the site of injury (or repetitive trauma) for tissue repair.

Immediately after a tissue is damaged, the blood vessels in that area dilate and, as a result, become more permeable (i.e., substances move more easily in and out of the blood vessel walls). This vasodilation allows more blood to flow through the damaged area, and the vessels' increased permeability allows our defense materials to enter the injured area and go to work. Vasodilation also results in heat, redness (erythema), and swelling (edema) in the affected area. The rise in local temperature—heat—around the injured area prompts all chemical reactions to occur more rapidly, and this increased metabolism creates even more heat. Have you ever noticed how a badly cut finger, for example, not only swells, but feels hot, as well as hurts? Vasodilation produces the heat you feel in the cut finger.

The Healing Process

- Inflammation protects us by removing toxins, bacteria, or other foreign matter from the site of the injury so they won't spread throughout the body. Inflammation also helps prepare the injured site for repair. In the process, however, it causes increased blood flow (vasodilation), which results in swelling, heat, redness, and pain.
- Repair begins when we generate new connective tissue, the major components of which are collagen, proteoglycans, and cells.
- Remodeling occurs after repair is largely complete; it "smoothes out" the rough edges that can remain after a broken bone, for instance, knits itself back together.

More than swelling and heat though, we feel pain the most. Pain is the red flag that tells us we have an injury and inflammation. Pain can begin immediately, or it may not start until several days after an injury. A variety of factors cause pain: First, pain can result from actual injury to the nerve fibers in the damaged area. Second, toxic chemicals produced by bacteria in that area can irritate nerve fibers. Third, small proteins called "kinins" are present at the site of inflammation, and they also contribute to pain. Inflammation "turns on" kinins and, once activated, they affect the nerves, so we feel increased pain. An especially powerful kinin, bradykinin, is a potent vasodilator—and vasodilation, as we just discussed, also causes pain. Other chemicals that cause pain when we're injured include substance P, the eicosanoids (the prostaglandins, leukotrienes, and thromboxanes), and platelet activating factor. So get ready: here comes a lesson on the pain-causing chemicals that cause us so much grief.

CHEMICAL PATHWAYS THAT CONTRIBUTE TO PAIN

The Eicosanoids

Now that you know our bodies produce numerous chemicals that cause pain, let's learn a little about how and when we make them, so we can decide how to stop them and the pain they cause.

A scientist named J.R. Vane discovered that arachidonic acid, a fat found naturally in most human cells, produces chemicals called eicosanoids when it breaks down. There are three types of eicosanoids: the prostaglandins, the leukotrienes, and the thromboxanes (which are modified prostaglandins). The thromboxanes differ from prostaglandins and leukotrienes, and are more beneficial.

Eicosanoids first became popular research subjects in the 1930s among scientists studying the hormones that control growth and wound healing. The eicosanoids play major roles in inflammation and other bodily functions. Anti-inflammatory drugs—both nonsteroidals and the steroids—work by inhibiting both the eicosanoids and the synthesis of platelet aggregating factor, which will be discussed a little later in this chapter.

The eicosanoids are intriguing, because they may have great medicinal potential. Their many effects include raising or lowering blood pressure, reducing stomach acid production, dilating or constricting airways in the lungs, stimulating or inhibiting blood platelet aggregation (blood clotting), contracting or relaxing intestinal and uterine smooth muscle, and stimulating steroid production.

Damaged cells break down arachidonic acid to release the eicosanoids called prostaglandins, which are fatty substances (lipids). There are many different prostaglandins, but the breakdown of arachidonic acid creates them all. Both prostaglandins and leukotrienes (which the breakdown of arachidonic acid also produce) act as hormones in most tissues, but they also induce inflammation (see Table 1-2).

Prostaglandins *always* accompany inflammation. At the injured site, as you now know, they act as powerful vasodilators, expanding blood vessels. The chemicals histamine and bradykinin (another powerful pain producer) help in this task. The combined actions of prostaglandins, histamine, and bradykinin produce the redness and swelling you see at injured areas of your body.

A specialized prostaglandin helps to produce the fever that sometimes accompanies inflammation. Some NSAIDs inhibit this prostaglandin, lowering fever.

The Eicosanoids

These natural chemicals play major roles in the inflammatory reaction. Prostaglandins, leukotrienes, and the thromboxanes are all eicosanoids. In addition to influencing inflammation, they

- raise blood pressure;
- lower blood pressure;
- reduce stomach acid;
- dilate (open) airways in the lungs;
- constrict (close) airways in the lungs
- stimulate blood platelet aggregation (make blood clot);
- inhibit blood platelet aggregation (stop blood clotting);
- contract intestinal and uterine muscle;
- relax intestinal and uterine muscle; and
- stimulate steroid production.

In 1971, scientists discovered a critical fact about aspirin and NSAIDs: These pain relievers inhibit a key enzyme in prostaglandin synthesis. The enzyme is cyclooxygenase, or "Cox," for short. In 1990, another key discovery revealed that two Cox enzymes exist, so scientists named them Cox-1 and Cox-2.

Cox-1 is present in our tissues under everyday conditions. It produces the prostaglandins that regulate our normal bodily functions.

Cox-2, on the other hand, is *not* present under normal conditions. We produce Cox-2 only at sites of inflammation, where it helps make prostaglandins that increase inflammation. In other words, the Cox-2 enzyme plays a major role in causing the pain and inflammation common to many musculoskeletal problems.

Although researchers developed NSAIDs in the 1970s, until just recently, all available NSAIDs inhibited both Cox-1 and Cox-2. They control pain by inhibiting Cox-2 and, therefore, inflammation, which is their beneficial action. However, these NSAIDs also inhibit Cox-1, which means that we stop making the good prostaglandins that protect the stomach's lining and help blood to clot.

So scientists began searching for drugs and natural substances that inhibit *only* Cox-2 enzymes. Using such substances, we can halt the pain caused by Cox-2, but still allow Cox-1 to work normally so we continue to make the good prostaglandins.

Leukotrienes, another type of eicosanoids, are also active in inflammation. Clinical studies have shown that leukotrienes actively contribute to mucous secretion in our bronchial tubes, and so play a significant role in allergies.

Platelet-Aggregating Factor (PAF)

Platelet-aggregating factor is a fatty substance (a lipid) that is extremely active in all kinds of allergies and inflammations. White blood cells make PAF. It causes vasodilation of the blood vessels, redness and, increases blood vessel permeability. Platelets are the cells that help to form blood clots. PAF, as its name signifies, induces local aggregation of platelets—that is, a blood clot—as well as white blood cell accumulation.

Platelet-Aggregating Factor (PAF)

This important mediator of inflammation and allergy also

- induces platelet aggregation (blot clot formation);
- causes redness;
- induces vasodilation;
- increases blood vessel permeability; and
- activates enzymes that produce eicosanoids.

PAF is very important in asthma's inflammatory process. Research shows that PAF is effective in bringing eosinophils, one of the cells the body rushes to the site of an asthma attack, into the lining of the bronchial tubes in the lungs, where they combat the effects of histamine. Eosinophils also ingest and destroy the foreign matter and cell debris produced by asthma's allergic reaction. Additionally, PAF helps activate various enzymes that generate eicosanoids. PAF, therefore, is a significant player in inflammation. This is why substances that antago-

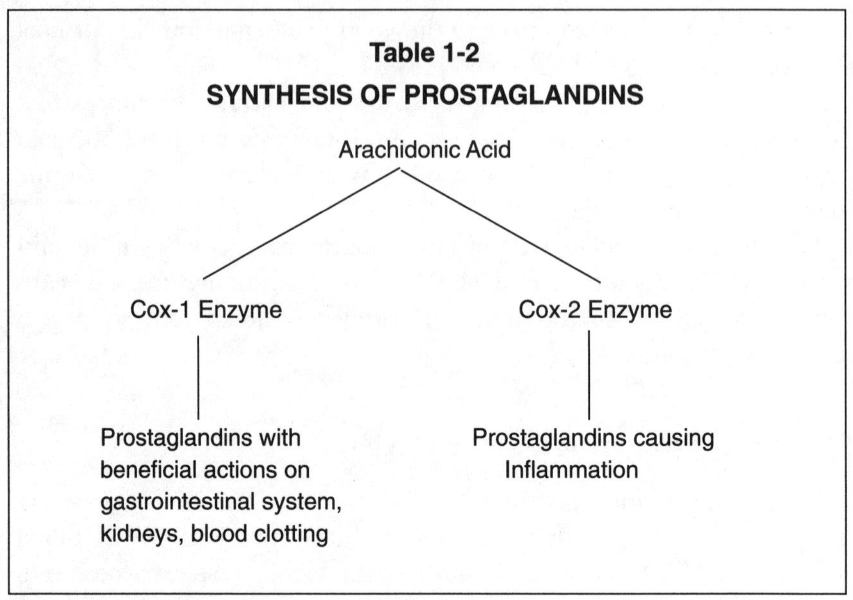

Table 1-2
SYNTHESIS OF PROSTAGLANDINS

nize, or try to stop, the actions of PAF are useful anti-inflammatory drugs.

Now that you're injured, swollen, red, feverish, in pain, and understand precisely why, let's see how the body cures all this misery.

REPAIR OF CONNECTIVE TISSUES

Repair is the second phase of connective tissue healing. It follows inflammation, and starts approximately two days after an injury. Even while our tissues are enduring inflammation, they start to repair themselves by generating new connective tissue. Collagen, proteoglycans, and cells act together to form the connective tissue that allows us to heal.

Collagen is the essential building block of connective tissue, and we cannot recover without it. It is a stringy substance made from amino acids (the building blocks of all proteins). Collagen is the active substance in wound healing and scar formation.

Imagine proteoglycans as protein-and-sugar gels.

Many different kinds of cells contribute to repair. Fibroblast cells synthesize collagen and osteoblast cells synthesize new bone. Osteoclast cells destroy bone during remodeling (the third phase of healing), and when the body needs calcium. Chondrocyte cells manufacture the smooth cartilage in our joints (hyaline cartilage), as well as producing collagen and proteoglycans.

How badly you injure your connective tissues determines exactly how long they will take to heal. When you strain your back, for instance, you may cause either a small (microscopic) or a large (macroscopic) tearing of muscle tissues or ligaments. The repair phase may last only six weeks or could continue for several months, depending on the extent of the injury. The good news is that, in most cases, our bodies can repair important structures so that they're almost as good as new.

Scar tissue, of course, repairs the defects created by trauma—not just trauma from a ligament or muscle tear, but also from surgery. That's good news, too. On the negative side, however, when rigid scar tissue takes the place of a flexible tissue like muscle, there may be lingering pain and disability. Normal muscle fibers can expand and contract, but scar tissue can't.

Additionally, scar tissue doesn't always bind structures together as tightly as ligaments and tendons. If you tear a ligament that connects two bones and scar tissue replaces it, the ligament usually functions well. In other cases, however, the scar tissue does not hold the bones together as tightly as necessary, and instability results. This is why some people have chronic, recurring ankle sprains—their ligament never heal tightly enough to return to normal.

REMODELING OF CONNECTIVE TISSUES

The third step in healing involves a gradual process of remodeling. How does remodeling differ from repair? Where repair does most of the work, remodeling supplies the finishing touches. For example, after you break a bone and it heals, you may be able to feel bumps on its surface under the skin. Over time, as remodeling occurs, the bone becomes smoother: It grows in places where it is too thin, and narrows somewhat where extra bone grew after the injury. This remodeling occurs in all healing structures, not just bone, but muscle and ligament also. You never wind up with exactly what you had before the injury but, in many cases, the structures heal and function very well.

Now you know the three steps in wound healing: inflammation, tissue repair, and remodeling. Although it all may proceed according to a divine plan, this doesn't mean that the pain necessarily stops at the end of the process.

A multitude of factors affects how long it takes you to heal from, for instance, a ligament you tore playing tennis. In the best situation, the inflammatory process ends in about a week, in which case it's called acute inflammation.

We don't always have acute inflammation following an injury, however; sometimes the inflammation is less intense but longer lasting. This is chronic inflammation. Can you predict how long inflammation will last after an injury? No, you can't. Several factors, including poor nutrition, immobilization, age, hormonal changes, and overall health status play roles in how quickly we heal inflammation.

One thing we know for sure: We can prevent an acute injury from becoming chronic by reducing inflammation as soon as possible. Obviously, as we've discussed, inflammation is necessary to heal tissues. If we totally eliminate inflammation while trying to treat the pain it causes, we run the risk of preventing the body from being able to heal itself properly. Excessive use of the strongest anti-inflammatory substances, steroids, can create this unhealthy situation.

Many traditional medications for inflammation and pain that aren't as strong or as dangerous as steroids are readily available. Unfortunately, none is ideal. The widely used NSAIDs aren't as powerful as steroids but they, too, are far from perfect, as Table 1-3 reveals. While the newer NSAIDs have significantly fewer side effects, many patients report they are not as effective as the older ones.

The simplest analgesics, such as Tylenol (acetaminophen), and even simple anti-inflammatories like aspirin can also cause a host of side effects, including rather significant liver and/or kidney damage.

Let's sort out the pros and cons of the medications that we commonly use to treat pain today.

Table 1-3 SIDE EFFECTS OF NSAIDs	
Gastrointestinal Nausea Heartburn Diarrhea Vomiting Ulcer disease and bleeding	***Renal*** Kidney failure
Skin Itching Rash	***Miscellaneous*** Headache Dizziness Dry eyes and mouth Anemia

THE COMMON TREATMENTS FOR CHRONIC PAIN

The NSAIDs

The cornerstones in arthritis treatment for many years and the mainstays in treating other painful inflammations in the musculoskeletal system are the NSAIDs. Today, however, NSAIDs, because of their many side effects (see Table 1-3), concern the medical community and consumers alike. This is why researchers are now developing new medications that can control inflammation and pain without known side effects.

Nonetheless, at present count, more than fifty NSAIDs are on the market (see Table 1-4), with more in development as we write this book. None of them has proved ideal for controlling the symptoms of inflammation, particularly in arthritis. Additionally, the NSAIDs' side effects, which create problems enough for younger people, can be deadly in the elderly. While NSAIDs reduce inflammation and pain, they can seriously damage the liver, kidneys, and central nervous system. Holes in the stomach from excessive NSAIDs use can lead to significant ulcers and even bleeding. NSAIDs can also stop blood from clotting properly.

From a surgical standpoint, this last problem is very significant. You must delay surgery until NSAIDs are discontinued, or else risk excessive bleeding. Anti-inflammatory substances that don't cause blood clotting problems are superior to NSAIDs because they enable us to proceed with the rest of our treatment plan, including surgery, if necessary.

All of these problems have motivated a search for alternatives to NSAIDs. Is it possible that nutritional supplements, alterations in our diet, and lifestyle changes can interrupt the vicious cycle of inflammatory pain? Yes, it is, as you'll learn in later chapters. And, if we can be even more optimistic for a moment, it's possible that we may discover new, natural anti-inflammatory substances that will decrease pain and inflammation with even fewer side effects than any now on the market.

The Steroids

No discussion of inflammation and its treatment is complete without considering steroids. If you are a baby boomer and ask your parents about the regular medications their family physicians used to prescribe, they will probably tell you about cortisone. In fact, cortisone worked miraculously, curing the vast majority of ailments—particularly muscle aches—so doctors prescribed it often. Today, of course, because of the serious side effects associated with cortisone use, we're much more cautious about prescribing it (see Table 1-5).

Cortisone is an artificially produced drug. It mimics the action of natural chemicals made by the adrenal gland (a small endocrine gland that sits on top of each kidney). The adrenals make several steroids: Some are the sex hormones, mainly androgens (male hormones you've probably heard of); others are the glucocorticoids, the natural counterparts to cortisone. You may know them as hydrocortisone or corticosterone. Our bodies need the corticosterones for many everyday functions, like regulating metabolism, maintaining the correct salt and water balance, and controlling our response to stress.

A deficiency in streroid production called Addison's disease does affect some people. (President John F. Kennedy had this disease). Its symptoms include muscle weakness, low blood pressure, depression, loss of appetite and weight, and low blood sugar. Addison's disease can also result from taking cortisone (or prednisone) for prolonged periods of time to cure a chronic inflammation. The body detects the extra steroids, and the adrenal glands stop making their own. This is why, when treating a disorder with steroids, it's necessary to stop taking them *gradually*. That way, the adrenal glands can start making the proper amount of natural steroids once we stop taking the artificial variety.

Table 1-4
COMMONLY USED ANTI-INFLAMMATORY MEDICATIONS

Bayer	Ansaid
Ecotrin	Celebrex
Dolobid	Relafen
Disalcid	Toradol
Trilisate	Meclomen
Arthropan	Lodine
Motrin	Feldene
Rufen	Cataflam
Advil	Voltaren
Medipren	Tolectin
Nuprin	Indocin
Naprosyn	Clinoril
Anaprox	Daypro
Nalfon	Oruvail
Orudis	

Steroids are sometimes required to treat serious conditions like septic shock from a severe infection, as well as autoimmune diseases like lupus and rheumatoid arthritis. Steroids are also immensely valuable in treating inflammatory conditions like anaphylactic shock, which can be life threatening.

Steroids inhibit both the early and late stages of inflammation. They reduce vasodilation and, therefore, swelling and redness (erythema). Steroids also decrease the accumulation of white blood cells at the site of inflammation.

Steroids are so strong that they can stop the formation of certain eicosanoids, including the prostaglandins. In addition, they actually stop histamine release. Because they work so rapidly to stop inflammation, people taking them generally feel much better at first.

Don't forget—it's necessary to form new tissue to heal any severe inflammation, and steroids can stop this process, slowing healing. Fibroblasts, the cells that make collagen, are less active in the presence of steroids. Steroids also inhibit osteoblasts, which is why taking them for a long time can cause us to develop osteoporosis (thin bones).

If you take too much cortisone or your body produces excessive amounts of glucocorticoids, you run the risk of developing Cushing's syndrome. Its symptoms resemble steroid side effects (see Table 1-5).

Prolonged steroid use can cause avascular necrosis, in which the bone that forms the ball of the hip joint dies. People who have organ transplants often must take steroids for long periods of time and, unfortunately, significant percentages of them develop avascular necrosis of the hip and require hip replacement surgery.

A host of other undesirable side effects occurs with prolonged steroid use. Your immune system can suffer, decreasing your response to infection or injury; stomach ulcers and osteoporosis can develop; and, over time, diabetes and cataracts can appear.

We've also learned over the years that even small doses of steroids can induce many of these severe side effects. That's why the medical community welcomed the discovery of NSAIDs. By using NSAIDs instead of steroids, we can decrease inflammation with far fewer side effects. Don't forget, however, that NSAIDs possess significant side effects of their own (see Table 1-3).

Nonetheless, we need steroids to treat many serious medical conditions, including anaphylactic shock and autoimmune disorders. Additionally, it's appropriate to treat severe inflammations with either a very short course of oral steroids or a direct injection into the site. This is frequently very helpful and sometimes curative. If we use small doses over a short period of time, we obtain the beneficial effects of steroids without the side effects associated with their prolonged use.

In other words, never using steroids is no wiser than overusing them. The best course of action is to *use steroids only when absolutely necessary and then for short periods of time*.

THE SEARCH FOR GOOD ALTERNATIVES

After reading about pain and inflammation, you may think them tremendously complicated. The most important lesson to learn from this chapter, however, is that new medications and nutritional substances that safely stop inflammation and pain already exist. And scientists continue to search for even better, safer, natural alternatives for stopping pain and inflammation.

More and more people, not only in the United States but in Europe and elsewhere, are turning to alternative medicine to treat illness and

Table 1-5 SIDE EFFECTS OF STEROIDS	
Fluid and Electrolyte Imbalance Sodium retention Fluid retention Congestive heart failure Loss of potassium High blood pressure	**Nervous System** Convulsions Vertigo Headache
Musculoskeletal System Muscle weakness Muscle atrophy Osteoporosis Avascular necrosis of hip and shoulder ball joint	**Glandular** Cushing's syndrome Menstrual irregularities Suppressed growth in children Diabetes mellitus
Gastrointestinal Peptic ulcer Pancreatitis Inflammation of the esophagus	**Eyes** Cataracts Glaucoma
Skin Disorders Impaired wound healing Thin, fragile skin Black and blue marks Increase in sweating	

injury. Many physicians now make alternative medicine a significant part of their practices. In many instances, the best treatment combines both traditional and alternative therapies, a type of practice called "complementary" or "integrative" medicine.

The total number of visits to physicians providing alternative medicine increased 47 percent from 1990 to 1997 (from 427 million to 629 million visits). Alternative medicine is clearly growing in popularity, and statistics indicate that the end of this trend is nowhere in sight.

Likewise, the number of people seeking natural alternatives to traditional anti-inflammatory medications is also growing. As you now know, inflammation is a normal part of everyday life for the average active person, and it certainly occurs even in an inactive individual. Since most of us suffer from pain and inflammation, doesn't it seem reasonable to deal with these conditions by using natural, nontoxic treatments?

Natural and nutritional alternatives to traditional anti-inflammatory medications already exist and, in later chapters, we'll discuss them in detail. Acupuncture, chiropractic, physical therapy, and targeted exercises are all effective in controlling pain as well. You have already made the right choice by deciding to educate yourself about natural alternatives to traditional pain medications—so you are well on your way to becoming an effective partner with your doctor in choosing the best therapeutic approach for you.

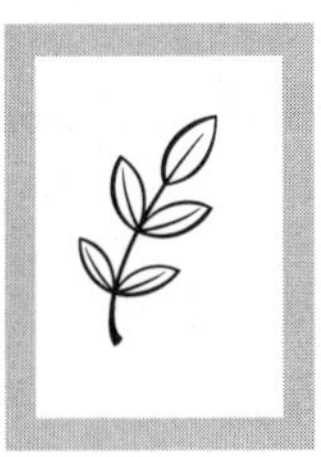

Chapter 2 THE PHYSICAL CAUSES OF PAIN

Pain is a fact of life. You may be in pain right now. Those of us writing this book spend the vast majority of our professional lives dealing with people whose chief problem is pain. We now realize that both patients and health-care professionals must understand the root causes of pain to discover natural, safer ways to treat it. This is especially important when dealing with back pain (which we'll discuss in detail in Chapter 4).

If you look around your neighborhood, you'll see that Americans are much more active than they were twenty years ago. Today, many people jog, play tennis, in-line skate, or bicycle for exercise and enjoyment. As you surely know if you've ever tried to "get into shape" in a hurry, many people weren't totally prepared for these activities when they started; they were vulnerable to injuries that caused inflammation and pain. The increased number of sports-related injuries Americans experience is one reason anti-inflammatory medications are selling better than ever. Gastroenterologists are also busy, because many people who take too many anti-inflammatory medications end up with the gastrointestinal problems described in Chapter 1, including stomach pain, ulcers, and even bleeding.

In reality, pain is a common experience for most people. Happily, most of the pain we experience on a daily basis comes from mild inflammations like strains, sprains, and tendinitis, and it doesn't last very long. Still, far too many pain experiences are severe and constant, eventually dominating every aspect of a person's life. Orthopedic problems, like scarring of the nerves in the lower back, frequently cause severe pain. Chronic and debilitating arthritis, which often occurs in numerous joints, also produces severe pain.

A bright light shone on the horizon in the mid-1970s when researchers developed new techniques, including patient controlled analgesia (PCA) and epidural injections, to help arthritis patients deal with their incapacitating pain. PCA, for example, is excellent for controlling pain after surgery. The doctor inserts a catheter either into the vein or into the epidural space (around the spinal cord) to deliver narcotics. It's effective, because the patient controls when he or she takes a dose, and it's very safe, because a computer controls the total amount of medication taken, so it's not possible to overdose. Despite the advent of these new techniques, as well as the use of plain old anesthesia, too many people continue to suffer. We obviously still have a lot to learn.

The New Paradigm

The partnership between doctor and patient is important in areas other than pain management. Every issue—including activity levels, type of therapy selected, and positions for sexual intercourse—should be open for discussion between doctor and patient. The final decision about treatment should be the patient's, after receiving good advice from his or her physician, but together they must form a partnership to create a treatment plan that will be more effective than either could devise alone.

Health-care professionals must educate themselves about new methods of treating chronic pain, and patients must learn to avoid the pitfalls of overmedication and dependence on pain killers. Because drug dependence is such a problem in our culture, it's crucial that we turn to natural substances to control inflammation and pain.

A NEW PARADIGM

Today more than ever before, people accept responsibility for their own health. Patients question their treatment, as well as their doctors' decision-making. Control is shifting from the physician to the physician-patient partnership, a trend stimulated, in part, by the plethora of self-help books available. This new paradigm shows us the future of pain control, because we know that people's quality of life really improves only when they take control of their pain.

This partnership between patient and doctor is important in areas other than pain management. Every issue—including activity levels, type of therapy selected, and positions for sexual intercourse—should be open for discussion between doctor and patient. The final treatment decision should be the patient's, after receiving good advice from his or her physician, but together they must form a partnership to create a treatment plan that will be more effective than either could devise alone. Although some people will probably continue to believe that the physician should remain in total control, that old paradigm simply does not work.

THE REALITY OF PAIN

All pain is real. You probably see this as an obvious statement. The medical establishment, however, has probably treated many of you as if your pain were imaginary or exaggerated. A doctor may even have told you that it's "all in your head"—an insensitive statement guaranteed to produce anger and frustration.

Medical education trains physicians to assume that a pain is "real" only when they can see it on an X ray or another test such as magnetic resonance imaging (MRI). Consequently, physicians often assume that pain without an identifiable physical problem (like a broken bone) is all in the mind. Psychological pain, of course, is just as real as physical pain, but its treatments are not the same. Although we are learning that most pain has both a psychological *and* a physical basis, it is still important to determine whether a particular pain is physical or psychological in origin, so it can be treated properly.

It's especially difficult to determine the origin of back pain because, in many cases, there is nothing to see on an X ray that explains why you hurt. This *doesn't* mean there is no pain.

First, Do No Harm

Most people with back pain and other musculoskeletal problems improve all by themselves, without ever consulting a physician. The best orthopedists know they should heed the Hippocratic Oath's instruction: "First, do no harm." Many orthopedic specialists practice "benign neglect," allowing the body to heal itself if it can, before resorting to drugs or surgery.

Let's examine what could happen if you develop a physical problem that may require surgery, like a herniated disk in the lower back or spinal stenosis (when the space around the spinal cord narrows and pinches nerves). Your doctor might suggest that you have a "simple operation" to resolve the problem. If the operation does not work out as planned, however, which occurs all too often, you can wind up just as you began, with ongoing, chronic pain.

In fact, many patients in this situation have multiple surgeries, none of which are completely successful, resulting finally in failed back syndrome. Not only do these people suffer chronic, even incapaciting pain, but they become psychologically disabled from it. Their personalities often change dramatically: an outgoing, friendly person can become hostile, withdrawn, and severely depressed.

Fortunately, most patients with musculoskeletal problems get better by themselves within about two months without any help from a physician—exemplifying one of the most important parts of the Hippocratic Oath: "Do no harm." The best orthopedic surgeons know this. According to a well-known orthopedic surgeon at a prestigious center in Memphis, Tennessee, "benign neglect," in fact, is the best way to treat many orthopedic patients. If we allow nature to take its course, the body will heal itself!

We feel different types of pain, depending on what stimulates which nerves. To stop pain, we have to understand a bit about the nerves that transmit it. So get ready—here comes a lesson on how the nervous system works, and how we can make it work *for* us, instead of *against* us.

TYPES OF PAIN

We've all experienced different kinds of pain, even in the same parts of our bodies—the dull pain of a minor toothache, for instance, compared to the yelping pain we feel when the dentist hits an exposed nerve with his drill. We describe pain in many different ways but, as that example shows, we probably most often characterize it as acute or chronic. Acute pain lasts three months or less. Definite tissue damage, like a fall on your head or a severe cut, usually causes it. Chronic pain, on the other hand, persists longer than three months, past the time it usually takes for tissues to heal.

Unfortunately, we can't always find a damaged tissue to blame for chronic pain. Furthermore, we're learning that psychological factors play a significant role in our perception of chronic pain.

We also describe pain as fast or slow. We feel fast pain within a tenth of a second after the painful stimulus occurs. An example of a fast pain is a knife cut or a burn from a hot stove. Slow pain begins at least one second or more after the stimulus, and sometimes increases in intensity over time. Tissue destruction, like cancer, usually causes slow pain. We often describe it as aching, throbbing, or chronic (see Table 2-1).

Different pathways conduct these two types of pain sensations. Small, "type A pain fibers" transmit fast, sharp pain signals. Larger, "type C pain fibers" transmit slow, chronic pain.

We further classify pain by which receptors are stimulated. Superficial somatic pain originates in nerves in the skin. ("Somatic" means "pertaining to the body," as opposed to "psychological," which pertains to the mind.) Pain from deeper structures—like skeletal muscle, joints, and tendons—is deep somatic pain. Pain from our organs is visceral pain.

Referred pain is a rather mysterious phenomenon: We injure one structure, but feel the pain elsewhere. Pain from a heart attack, for example, may be felt not only in the chest, but also along the left arm. Some people who have heart attacks experience only neck or shoulder pain—or even just pain in their teeth, believe it or not—and have no pain whatsoever in the their chests! This is typical of referred pain, which we don't entirely understand.

With referred pain, the same section of the spinal cord serves all the areas involved. When we injure or irritate one area, it produces painful sensations in another.

Table 2-1
TYPES OF PAIN

Type of Pain	What It Is
Acute pain	Lasts less than three months and is associated with an injury or trauma, like a broken bone. Acute pain is a warning to us that we're doing something dangerous.
Chronic pain	Lasts longer than three months, past the time when an injury should have healed. The organic source of chronic pain can be elusive.
Fast pain	Is felt immediately, like when we're cut or burned.
Slow pain	Is delayed by one second or longer, and can increase over time. An example is pain from cancer.
Superficial somatic pain	Arises from pain receptors in the skin.
Deep somatic pain	Arises from muscles, joints, and tendons.
Visceral pain	Arises from our internal organs (the viscera).
Referred pain	Occurs when one tissue is damaged, but we feel the pain elsewhere. For instance, a heart attack can produce pain in the arm.
Phantom limb pain	Occurs when a limb has been amputated, but the patient still feels pain that seems to come from the missing limb.

Phantom limb pain affects patients who have had a limb amputated. Many such patients still experience sensations like pain or itching, as if the limb were still there. There is a scientific explanation for phantom limb pain: Nerve impulses still start in the nerve fibers that served the amputated limb. A series of connections transfers these impulses to the brain. The brain interprets them as coming from a limb that is no longer there because, although the arm or leg is gone, the nerves that once served it remain.

Acute pain signals your body that something is wrong, so you can take appropriate protective measures. If you strained your back moving a heavy piano, you obviously know where the pain is coming from. Certainly you would avoid moving another piano anytime soon, and limit your movement of the injured area so you don't make it any worse.

Acute pain, then, enables us to act. If you have a toothache and know that it's due to an infection, you would see your dentist and start taking antibiotics.

Chronic pain is different. When it continues for months or even years, it doesn't serve any useful purpose and, in fact, there is often no organic reason for the pain. For instance, you may have had a "perfect" operation, with all X rays, MRIs, and other tests revealing that everything looks normal afterward. But looks can be deceiving, especially when you continue to have pain.

Stress frequently plays a part in this type of chronic pain, which we label "psychogenic pain." There is a physical basis to much psychogenic pain that the doctor just can't explain. Nevertheless, its cause can be extremely elusive and, in many cases, impossible to find. This situation often causes fear, anxiety, or depression—quite normal reactions, under the circumstances.

In addition, individuals have different pain thresholds, or tolerance for pain. The psychological aspects of pain play an extremely large role in a person's pain threshold. Pain tolerance not only differs from person to person, but can vary within the same person depending on how he or she feels at a particular time. When you feel depressed and unable to cope, more pain messages pass through to your brain.

PAIN RECEPTORS AND MUSCLE SPASM

Now you know why we feel pain: It is a warning that something is wrong in our bodies, a signal to act. But *how*, exactly, do we feel pain?

We feel pain through our pain receptors, called nociceptors, which are simply free nerve endings all over our bodies. Although we may curse them when we're in pain, nociceptors protect us by responding to anything powerful enough to damage our bodies.

Many different chemicals contribute to causing pain, and we'll discuss them in detail in Chapter 3. Some of them increase the pain sensations we feel. Prostaglandins and substance P, in particular, enhance the sensitivity of pain endings and, therefore, our perception of pain. Bradykinin, serotonin, and histamine also play important parts in pain transmission.

When we irritate or injure a tissue, we release chemicals like prostaglandins and kinins, and they stimulate the nociceptors. Pain frequently persists even after the injury is healed, because prostaglandins and kinins are still in the area, continuing to stimulate the nociceptor.

Our bodies have many other receptors that contribute to pain perception. Thermoreceptors detect changes in temperature, photoreceptors detect light striking the retina of the eye, and chemoreceptors detect the chemicals intimately involved in taste and smell (see Table 2-2).

Besides all of these, the musculoskeletal system has two additional receptors that help us avoid injuring ourselves. Tendons possess golgi tendon organs, found where a tendon joins a muscle. When we apply tension to the tendon because a muscle contracts, we stimulate the golgi tendon organs, and nerve impulses rush to the brain. These nerve impulses tell us how much pressure the muscular-tendon junction is under and, if necessary, we can relax the muscle before it tears.

Our joints have joint kinesthetic receptors around the lining of the joint (called the capsule) that respond to pressure. Joint kinesthetic receptors detect when we are putting too much strain on a joint, and they stimulate pain nerve fibers that communicate with the brain. We can then decide if we're stretching our ligaments too much, and move our leg or arm to decrease the strain on the joint before we hurt ourselves.

Most musculoskeletal injuries involve sprained or torn ligaments or damaged joints. When we injure tendons or joints, the muscle that surrounds them usually spasms, causing even more pain. Muscle spasm can be localized or widespread. You can have a local muscle spasm around a solitary injured joint in your back, for example. Other conditions that affect many muscles, like fibromyalgia and myofascial pain syndrome, produce widespread muscle spasm.

Muscle spasm stimulates pain receptors known as mechanoreceptors. They detect mechanical pressure and stretching, as well as sensations like touch, pressure, and vibration.

Muscle spasm also compresses blood vessels in the area. This leads to ischemia, the medical term for decreased blood flow. When less blood

Table 2-2
TYPES OF PAIN RECPTORS

Type of Pain Receptor	**What It Does**
Nociceptor	A pain receptor that is stimulated by pain-producing chemicals
Thermoreceptor	The receptor that detects temperature change
Photoreceptor	Receptors in the eye that detect light
Chemoreceptor	Receptors that detect the presence of chemicals involved in taste and smell
Mechanoreceptor	Receptors that detect touch, pressure, and vibration
Golgi tendon organs	Receptors that detect when a tendon is stressed
Joint kinesthetic receptors	Receptors that detect when a joint is stressed

flows into an area, lactic acid accumulates in the tissues, stimulates pain nerve endings, and causes pain.

THE SPECIFICITY THEORY OF PAIN

Believe it or not, your personal approach to pain varies with your social circumstances. For example, we've found that people can tolerate more pain if their friends are watching or if there is some kind of reward. This observation contradicts the Specificity Theory of Pain, once held by doctors, and described by French philosopher and mathematician René Descartes (1596–1650) more than three hundred years ago.

Descartes proposed a direct relationship between the amount of damage sustained and the pain experienced. In other words, his theory assumed that the intensity of the pain is directly proportional to the severity of the injury. If this theory were completely correct, we could eliminate pain with surgery or medication if we knew its cause, but this has not proved to be true.

Dr. Henry Beecher performed a tremendous amount of pain research while working with severely wounded soldiers during World War II. Approximately one-third of them complained of pain severe enough to require morphine injections. This was in direct opposition to his experience in private practice, where the vast majority of his patients with similar wounds required morphine to control their pain. Dr. Beecher quite correctly concluded that there is really no simple relationship between the severity of a wound and the pain experienced by the patient, but that many other factors come into play. For instance, a seriously injured soldier may have been extremely thankful that he escaped from the battle alive, and so was euphoric. We now know that this euphoria can cause the release of substances called endorphins, natural morphine-like chemicals produced in the brain.

Physicians also have a problem explaining phantom limb pain (in which, as we discussed, a patient continues to feel pain from a missing arm or leg) by using the Specificity Theory of Pain. Both phantom limb pain and the experiences of Dr. Beecher show quite conclusively that the Specificity Theory of Pain does not explain a great deal of what we see in real life.

THE GATE CONTROL THEORY OF PAIN

Dr. Ronald Melzack in Canada and Dr. Patrick Wall in Britain made tremendous strides in explaining how pain occurs. They described the Gate Control Theory of Pain, which much more readily explains what physicians and patients experience on a regular basis.

Melzack and Wall proposed that hypothetical gates exist between the spinal cord and the brain. When these gates are open, the pain impulses can move freely to the brain. When the gates close, the impulses simply don't reach the brain, so we don't perceive pain.

Two Theories of Pain

French philosopher René Descartes described the Specificity Theory of Pain in the 1600s. According to Descartes' theory, the severity of an injury correlates directly to the amount of pain produced.

Melzack and Wall, in the twentieth century, formulated a theory called the Gate Control Theory of Pain. According to this theory, it's not the severity of an injury but the number of pain impulses that reach the brain through various "gates" that governs how much pain we feel. If we close the gates (by inducing our natural pain-controlling substances through meditation or other means), fewer pain impulses reach the brain, so we feel less pain.

For example, just because you experience a certain amount of trauma doesn't mean you feel an exact amount of pain. Depending on the circumstances, your brain may perceive more pain on one occasion than it does on another. Why does this happen?

Our nervous systems are complex, even if you just look at their biology. But when you add in our ability to *think* about the signals our nervous systems process, you add another layer of complexity. Let's examine how the body and mind work together when we experience pain.

How Pain Signals Reach the Brain

Pain, as we've discussed, travels along nerve fibers to the brain. Nerve fibers are made up of nerve cells (neurons), which are amazing and complex creations. A neuron looks a little like a starfish. Neurons have a nerve body and its associated branches, the axons. Chemicals called neurotransmitters assist neurons in transmitting pain, which we'll discuss in Chapter 3.

Three kinds of neurons form the pathways along which pain travels: first order neurons, second order neurons, and third order neurons. Nerve pathways start at the receptors and end in the brain's cerebral cortex.

First order neurons carry signals from the receptor into either the spinal cord or the brain stem, the portion of the brain directly above the spinal cord. Sensations from the face, mouth, teeth, and eyes proceed directly to the brain stem; others go to the spinal cord first.

Second order neurons pick up the signal in the spinal cord or brain and send it to the area of the brain known as the thalamus, where we actually perceive pain.

Third order neurons go from the thalamus to the cerebral cortex, a more complex part of the brain where our conscious mind processes pain. In the cerebral cortex, factors like emotions are added to the pain message, which can alter our perception of the pain we're experiencing. This alteration plays a significant role in the pain gate theory.

The cerebral cortex is a large structure, and only one part of it, the somatosensory cortex, deals with pain. It has actually been "mapped" by scientists so that we know exactly what part of the somatosensory cortex receives sensation from the lips, legs, arms, and every other part of the body.

Let's follow a pain signal all along the nerve pathways from a hurt finger to the brain. Imagine that, as you were slicing your grapefruit this morning, the knife slipped, and you cut your finger instead of the fruit. This trauma initiates a pain message, which travels along nerve fibers from your finger to an area in the spinal cord known as the dorsal horn, which runs up and down its entire length. The pain message then encounters a synapse, the gap between two nerves. How does it bridge this gap? By relying on neurotransmitters, chemicals that ferry the message across the synapse from one nerve fiber to the next.

The pain message then travels up the spinal cord to the thalamus (the base of the brain), where it encounters a second synapse. After crossing it, the message finally arrives in the brain's cerebral cortex.

As you now know, the thalamus and cerebral cortex both play very important roles in dealing with pain. Our reflexes originate in the thalamus; it makes us immediately draw back from a painful stimulus. If you've ever picked up a steaming hot vegetable and then instantly dropped it, you've observed your thalamus in action. You don't think about reflex actions—your body performs them automatically, to protect you.

How Pain Signals Reach the Brain

When we are injured, pain signals travel along nerve fibers to the brain. The first order neurons take signals directly from the injured spot to the spinal cord. Second order neurons pick up the signal in the spinal cord and send it to the base of the brain, the thalamus. Third order neurons then take the signal further into the brain, to the cerebral cortex, where we make conscious decisions about how to respond—by screaming, jumping, or meditating.

The cerebral cortex, on the other hand, can modify the painful experience, either minimizing or intensifying it in the mind. When pain reaches the cerebral cortex, we decide how to react to it—by beating our heads against the wall, screaming, or starting to meditate.

In recent years, we've learned that positive thoughts and emotions can actually decrease the amount of pain we perceive. In the Gate Theory of Pain, that's called "opening and closing the gates."

Opening and Closing the Gates

Several factors influence the opening and closing of pain gates, including the extent of the injury itself, inactivity, debilitation, long-term narcotic use, poor body mechanics, and physical conditioning. Negative factors, like drug use and inactivity, open the pain gates, so more pain messages pass through. Therefore, we perceive more pain if our bodies are run-down or already unhealthy.

Emotional factors also play a significant part in the perception of pain. Research has shown that emotions like sadness and anger, and the causative or resulting anxiety, depression and stress can open the pain gates. In other words, our thoughts can allow more pain impulses to reach the brain, which makes the pain we feel more intense. This is why some researchers argue that it's possible to use the mind to control the amount of pain you feel. Studies show that replacing negative with positive thoughts really can decrease pain.

Therefore, we can limit pain by controlling the gates that allow the impulses to pass through to the brain. We can gradually increase activity, use less addictive pain medication, and practice relaxation therapies to close the pain gates. You can also decrease pain by maintaining a positive attitude and by doing everything you possibly can to limit the depressing episodes in your life. In this regard, stress management is critical to controlling the amount of pain that we live with.

Yes, we are placing the burden exactly where it belongs—on ourselves. To a great extent, we really can control our lives, both the negative and positive aspects, by our thoughts alone—and the same goes for the pain we feel.

Here's a good example of the Gate Control Theory in action. Try to imagine that you have a clothespin attached to your arm, and you try to keep it there for an entire day. Obviously, it is going to hurt quite a bit, pinching your skin and the soft tissue beneath it. Pain receptors do their job and transmit the pain message up the spinal cord to your brain. However, the ability to reason separates humans from other species. After a while, you may realize that although the pressure is painful, you're not sustaining any terrible damage. Although your thalamus perceives pain from the clothespin, your cerebral cortex pays less attention to this pain message and, in fact, closes the pain gates to a certain degree, so that your arm no longer transmits pain impulses to the brain. Therefore, you actually feel less pain from the clothespin attached to your arm.

HOW DO MEDICATIONS AND SURGERY ALTER PAIN?

Perhaps you need some help in closing the pain gates, so let's look at how medications and surgery interrupt pain messages.

Nonsteroidal anti-inflammatory drugs (NSAIDs), the simplest of which is aspirin, affect pain by blocking the formation of prostaglandins. These chemicals (which we'll discuss in Chapter 3 along with many other pain chemicals) stimulate nociceptors, those free nerve endings all over our bodies. As aspirin blocks prostaglandin production, we notice a decrease in pain. In addition, aspirin decreases inflammation (see Table 2-3).

Local anesthetics such as xylocaine and Novocain provide pain relief by blocking nerve impulses from traveling along the nerve fibers. Obvi-

Table 2-3
INTERRUPTING PAIN

The Pain Interrupter	How It Blocks Pain
Acetaminophen: Tylenol	Inhibits prostaglandin production in the central nervous system. Works as painkiller, not anti-inflammatory.
NSAIDs: aspirin, ibuprofen, and so forth	Block the formation of prostaglandins. This action decreases inflammation and pain.
Steroids	Inhibit early and late manifestation of inflammation and therefore decreases pain.
Local anesthetics: Novocaine, xylocaine	Interrupt the path that the pain signal travels from the site of the injury to the brain.
Opiates: Morphine	Alter the quality of pain perception. Binds to pain receptors in the brain.
Natural pain killers: endorphins, enkephalins	We produce these opiate-like susbtances in our bodies. We stimulate their production by exercise and even by positive thinking.
Surgery: rthizotomy	Cutting or destroying nerves that provide sensation to painful facet joints in the spine.

ously, they provide only short-term relief because, when the anesthetic wears off, the pain impulses start to flow again.

Morphine and other opiates decrease pain another way: They bind to receptors in the brain that alter our perception of pain. Although technically you still feel the pain, you don't perceive it as so sharp or noxious.

Can surgery alter pain impulses? Yes, of course it can. Some surgical treatments interrupt pain pathways between the pain receptor and the brain. Rhizotomy is a surgical procedure in which the doctor cuts some spinal sensory nerve roots, so we no longer feel pain in the areas formerly supplied by those nerves. Surgeons commonly perform this operation in joints in the base of the spine. Although this operation might seem like a cure-all, it is not. In many cases, the nerves grow back, so pain is felt again.

OUR NATURAL PAIN KILLERS: ENKEPHALINS AND ENDORPHINS

We actually produce a type of natural morphine in our brains, as Hughes and Kosterlitz discovered when, in 1975, they found two chemicals that bind to the same receptors in the brain as morphine. These two substances, named neuropeptides, act almost exactly like morphine.

Neuropeptides are proteins made by nerve cells. Sacs called vesicles transport them to the synapse. There, they act as neurotransmitters, the ferries that help signals to cross the gap between neurons.

Two very important neuropeptides are the enkephalins and the endorphins. They both play crucial roles in pain reduction. You can think of them as the body's natural pain killers. Enkephalins and endorphins are concentrated in various parts of the brain, including the thalamus, hypothalamus, and the limbic system, as well as along spinal cord pathways that relay pain impulses.

Think of the enkephalins and endorphins as our on-board opiate system. They stimulate opiate receptors in the brain and decrease our pain perception, as well as creating a general feeling of euphoria. The very same process occurs when we receive a morphine injection. Isn't it amazing? Our bodies produce chemicals that can almost totally suppress many pain signals entering the brain.

Have you ever wondered why some people become addicted to jogging? It's because jogging (and other repetitive aerobic activity) stimulates endorphins, which decrease pain and produce euphoria, causing the "runner's high." As you might imagine, this can be positively addictive! In fact, we call this a "positive addiction." In addition to the euphoria runners feel, they're also experiencing positive physiological changes. This positive addiction is a definite win-win for our bodies. It is also an excellent reason to pursue athletic activity, aside from its benefit to the cardiovascular system.

If you've ever spoken with friends who've been jogging on a daily basis for years and then sustained an injury, you most likely noticed that they seem depressed. One of the sources of this depression is the drop in endorphin levels they've experienced.

Enkephalin, our other natural pain killer, stops substance P, a neuropeptide in sensory nerves, spinal cord pathways, and parts of the brain that are associated with pain transmission. Neurons release substance P (which we'll discuss in detail in Chapter 3), which transmits pain information from the outlying areas to the brain. Enkephalin suppresses the release of substance P and, therefore, decreases painful input to the brain.

The Movement Toward Alternative, Natural Pain Treatment

As we discussed in Chapter 1, we're in the midst of a great movement toward using natural and alternative medical methods to treat every conceivable malady, including pain.

Studies show that acupuncture alleviates pain. During acupuncture, the practitioner inserts very fine needles into various points in the body and twirls them. We don't know exactly how acupuncture works, but some researchers believe that it lessens pain by stimulating the brain to produce endorphins.

Massage and chiropractic manipulation stimulate the large pain fibers that carry sensations of pressure and warmth. These sensations can limit the number of pain messages transmitted along the smaller pain fibers. Techniques like massage produce muscle relaxation and decrease the pain impulses generated by prolonged muscle spasm. This is why hands-on physical therapy is much more effective than passive treatments like hot packs. It also explains why rubbing your toe after you stub it can decrease the pain.

Starting a program of positive thinking in the midst of continual, chronic pain is very difficult. Fortunately, the natural anti-inflammatories (foods, herbs, and supplements) described in *Nature's Pain Killers* may be just what you need to turn the tide against your pain and toward better health. That you are investigating natural treatments indicates that you have already started to think positively in this regard. A direct result of positive thinking is relaxation, and a direct result of relaxation is a *decrease* in muscle spasm and, therefore, pain.

Decreasing muscle spasm results in a better quality of life because you have less pain on a daily basis. While reaching for a pain killer may seem to be the solution at first, if you are a chronic pain patient, then you know this is not the answer. It is, in fact, counterproductive in the long run. Your pain and stress inevitably reemerge shortly after the pill wears off. In addition, you find that the pills don't work as well when taken on a regular basis. The true solution, in addition to finding natural substances that lessen your pain, lies in realizing that your emotional and mental outlook has a tremendous effect on the way you cope with pain.

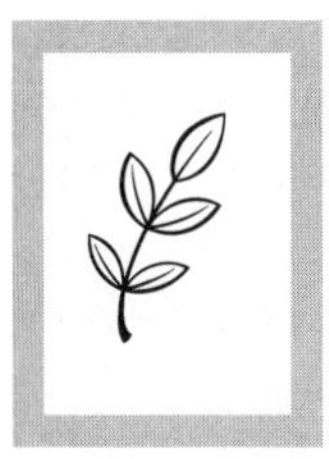

Chapter 3 THE PAIN-IMMUNE SYSTEM CONNECTION

Pain perception is hard-wired in our nervous systems. We've learned that and a great deal more about pain over the last few decades. We have isolated and identified the agents of pain, which include neurotransmitters and other chemicals. We have traced pain's pathways, and even created an anatomical road map for pain. If we understand pain so well, then why can't we treat it more effectively?

We now know that pain is even more complex—and fascinating—than we previously thought. For instance, scientists recently discovered that, contrary to a long-held belief, the nervous system does not govern pain by itself. Even pain researchers were surprised to learn that the immune system is a vitally important player in this biological drama. In fact, we now realize that the nervous and immune systems are equal partners in producing pain.

Injury to any region of our bodies—our bones, skin, internal organs, or any tissue—sets off an alarm that's instantly interpreted by the brain as pain. This alarm uses specific chemicals to carry the pain signal through our tissues until it reaches its target destination: the brain. Any interruption in this biological alarm system can have devastating consequences: Imagine the danger you'd be in if you couldn't feel the pain of a cut, burn, or worse.

Have you ever wondered why diabetics sometimes have toes, or even part of a leg, amputated? It begins when the disease causes numbness in their extremities. Because of such numbness diabetics can't feel cuts or burns on their feet—they don't feel pain (or anything else) there. In rare instances, this numbness allows neglected cuts or burns to develop very serious infections, so serious that they can't be treated with antibiotics or with anything else for that matter. Should the infection spread, it could be fatal. So, the only way to save the patient's life is to amputate part or all of the infected leg.

Thus, as we've noted, *acute* pain truly protects us. *Chronic* pain, however, is very problematic. When pain becomes chronic, pain is our enemy instead of our ally.

Chronic Pain's "Open" Circuit

An interaction between the brain and immune system causes pain signals to remain permanently turned "on" in chronic pain conditions. In fact, chronic pain signals are amplified by a biological circuit without a working breaker. This continuously "open" circuit results in a cycle of pain, inflammation, and more pain.

Interaction between the brain and the immune system plays a vital role in chronic pain conditions like rheumatoid arthritis and fibromyalgia (among many others), in which pain signals stay permanently turned "on." With chronic pain, the nervous and immune systems form a biological circuit without a working breaker. This continuously "open" circuit results in a cycle of pain, inflammation, and more pain.

Because understanding this cycle provides clues about how to treat pain more effectively, it's important that we discuss what fuels it.

THE IMMUNE SYSTEM'S CONTRIBUTIONS TO PAIN

When we injure ourselves or suffer inflammation for another reason, like arthritis, the immune system makes a variety of chemicals that transmit pain signals to the brain. These chemicals include the prostaglandins; cytokines (which are the immune system's hormones), such as the interleukins, including interleukin-1 (IL-1), IL-6, IL-8, and IL-12; peptides like substance P; a neurotransmitter, glutamate; and the gas nitric oxide, which acts as a chemical messenger in the nervous and immune systems and interferes with healing (see Table 3-1). In this chapter, you'll become intimately familiar with all of these agents of pain.

The Chemicals That Produce Pain

- prostaglandins
- cytokines such as the interleukins, including IL-1, IL-6, IL-8, and IL-12
- peptides like substance P
- the neurotransmitter glutamate
- nitric oxide, a gas that acts as a chemical messenger in both the nervous and immune systems, and interferes with healing

Prostaglandins are notorious agents of pain. Enzymes called cyclooxygenases, or Cox enzymes, make prostaglandins. As we discussed in Chapter 1, there are two Cox enzymes, Cox-1 and Cox-2. In many diseases, the Cox-2 enzyme makes the prostaglandins that induce inflammation.

The Cox-2 enzyme is crucial in generating the inflammation that causes pain—neither the inflammation nor the pain would exist without the Cox-2 enzyme. Many new drugs that stop this enzyme, called Cox-2 inhibitors because they prevent Cox-2 from making "bad" prostaglandins, are now being developed, and several are already on the market. You may know someone who's already taking one of these "super aspirins" for rheumatoid arthritis or another pain syndrome.

In addition to prostaglandins, the immune system produces cytokines named interleukins. Cytokines are hormones that jump-start specific immune pathways. They are messengers, carrying signals from the immune and nervous systems to our body's other systems (and back again, of course). They also control the white blood cell traffic in and out of various tissues. We make numerous interleukins; some of them are proinflammatory, and others are not.

We recently learned that IL-1 is linked to numerous inflammatory diseases, including all of the arthritic conditions. Medical studies find high concentrations of IL-1 in painful joints, suggesting it contributes to pain as well as inflammation. Immune cells called macrophages make IL-1. During any inflammation, IL-1 produces both *direct* and *indirect* effects.

Table 3-1
THE CHEMICAL AGENTS OF PAIN

The Chemical	What It Is
Prostaglandins	These hormonelike substances are important agents of pain.
The interleukins: IL-1, IL-6, IL-8, and IL-12	Cytokines that induce inflammation and pain.
Substance P	A peptide that binds to receptors in the brain and spinal cord and stimulates pain.
Glutamate	An excitatory amino acid that is often the principle neurotransmitter for pain.
Nitric oxide	A gas that acts as both a neurotransmitter and a cytokine; it is released by macrophages when we experience inflammation or infection.

IL-1's direct actions break down collagen and other connective tissue, increase prostaglandin production, and dilate blood vessels surrounding the injured area. All of these actions create pain. IL-1's indirect effects include influencing our sleep, inducing fever, and causing behavioral and hormonal changes.

Although IL-1 is an immune system chemical, the brain also responds to increased levels of it, providing a classic example of the brain-immune connection in pain. In fact, when the brain discovers that injured tissue is producing increased amounts of IL-1, it starts making increased amounts of this cytokine, too. If you have more IL-1, you have more inflammation and, therefore, more pain. IL-1's rather surprising ability to induce pain provides us with compelling evidence that immune system chemicals make major contributions to pain. This is further evidence of the equal partnership between the brain and immune system.

Other interleukins that contribute to inflammation are IL-6, IL-8, and IL-12. These pro-inflammatory cytokines contribute to the symptoms we experience in diseases like osteoporosis, rheumatoid arthritis, and other autoimmune diseases. IL-6 is a powerful pro-inflammatory chemical, and IL-12 has been associated with numerous types of autoimmune diseases. Substances that interfere with these interleukins' activity decrease inflammation and, therefore, have the potential to limit pain.

Nitric oxide is not, strictly speaking, either a cytokine or a neurotransmitter, but this gas acts like both. When we suffer from inflammation or infection, our macrophages—the same immune-system cells that produce IL-1—release nitric oxide. At high levels, it appears to interfere with healing by stimulating osteoclasts to destroy bone—which is not exactly helpful if you're trying to heal an inflamed and/or fractured bone.

Chronic Pain's Feedback Loop

We have learned that the nervous and immune systems work together as equal partners to produce pain. Following an injury, a pain signal makes the immune system release chemicals that produce inflammation. These immune system chemicals affect the nervous system, making it release its own chemicals. Some of the nervous system chemicals act on the spinal cord and brain, causing pain.

When the brain detects these new pain signals, it again instructs the immune system to make inflammatory chemicals, and the whole cycle begins again, worsening both pain and inflammation. These immune and nervous system chemicals work together like this:

- Immune system cells release inflammatory chemicals, including prostaglandins.
- Prostaglandins stimulate the release of the inflammatory cytokine IL-1.
- IL-1 causes substance P to be released in the spinal cord.
- Substance P then directly stimulates the brain to perceive pain, which also provokes the release of prostaglandins, beginning the cycle all over.

A pain–inflammation–more pain cycle is thus created between the brain and immune system. This continuous feedback loop causes chronic inflammation and pain.

Substance P exists predominantly in the spinal cord. It binds to receptors in the brain and spinal cord, *directly* producing pain. Substance P may also act *indirectly* on the immune system, however, to increase inflammation. Researchers have now shown that it stimulates the production of prostaglandins and IL-1 which, as you know, both cause pain.

The final players in this orchestra are neurotransmitters called "excitatory" amino acids, with glutamate the most prominent. Like substance P, glutamate binds to specific receptors called NMDA receptors. Drug companies are actively seeking agents that block NMDA (N–Methyl–D–Aspartate) receptors to develop into pain killers. In fact, many drugs that block the interaction between glutamate and the NMDA receptors, and that are used to treat other conditions, also inhibit pain. These include Gabapentin (also sold as Neurontin), which appears to be very effective in treating some pain states, including diabetic neuropathy (pain in the arms and legs).

How The NMDA Blockers Work

- Glutamate, a neurotransmitter, binds to NMDA receptors, which causes pain.
- The neurotransmitter Gaba balances glutamate's effects in the brain. Enhancing Gaba's actions may reduce glutamate's ability to bind to NMDA receptors and create pain.
- An artificial drug named Gabapentin enhances the effects of Gaba, stopping glutamate and the pain it causes when it binds to the NMDA receptors.
- The "branched-chain" amino acids—isoleucine, leucine, and valine also mimic Gaba, as does taurine, another amino acid. These amino acids have potential as natural NMDA receptor blockers and, therefore, as natural pain killers.

Gabapentin works like this: The neurotransmitter glutamate causes pain by binding to the NMDA receptors. Another neurotransmitter, Gaba, blocks glutamate and stops it from causing pain. The drug Gabapentin enhances Gaba's effects, preventing glutamate from binding to the NMDA receptors and stopping it from causing pain.

For their part, the "branched-chain" amino acids—isoleucine, leucine, and valine—work like Gabapentin, enhancing Gaba's actions. (Taurine, while not a branched-chain amino acid, also possesses this ability.) These three amino acids, as well as taurine, have potential as natural blockers of this pain pathway.

An odd fact was uncovered by research into the glutamate-NMDA connection: Drugs that stop glutamate from binding to NMDA receptors also stop us from developing tolerance to opiate drugs like morphine. This is a very important finding, especially for people who have cancer pain. Cancer patients often require higher and higher doses of morphine or other narcotics to relieve their pain. Wouldn't it be exciting to discover natural, nontoxic, nonaddictive treatments that stop cancer pain?

As you now see, an extremely complex array of chemicals works together to create pain. Immune system cells release inflammatory chemicals, including prostaglandins, which play an important role in producing pain. Prostaglandins, besides their inflammatory effects, stimulate the release of pro-inflammatory cytokines like IL-1 (and the other pro-inflammatory interleukins, IL-6, IL-8, and IL-12). IL-1, in turn, stimulates the release of substance P in the spinal cord. Substance P then directly instructs our brains to perceive pain. It also stimulates the release of even more prostaglandins, creating a cycle of pain, inflammation, and pain. Unless we interrupt it, this continuous feedback loop between the nervous and immune systems repeatedly generates inflammation and pain. This is how we end up suffering from chronic pain.

How can we interrupt this vicious circle? In addition to opiate drugs like morphine (with all their side effects), numerous natural substances stop these pain-inducing chemicals. Let's explore these gifts from nature.

NATURAL COMPOUNDS THAT DECREASE INFLAMMATION AND PAIN

Substances That Block Prostaglandins

We can use our knowledge about how the immune system contributes to pain to discover new—hopefully natural—pain killers (see Table 3-2). In fact, many pain medications already on the market rely on this knowledge. For example, nonsteroidal anti-inflammatory drugs (NSAIDs) like Motrin and Advil inhibit prostaglandin production, and

Table 3-2
NATURAL COMPOUNDS THAT DECREASE INFLAMMATION AND PAIN

Compound	How It Works
Polyunsaturated fatty acids (i.e., fish oil containing gammalinolenic acid, or GLA)	These essential fatty acids inhibit pro-inflammatory prostaglandin production.
Turmeric	This Indian spice contains curcuminoids, which inhibit the breakdown of arachidonic acid, a potent pro-inflammatory fat. It also decreases the activity of IL-1 and IL-8.
Boswellia	This gum resin from the boswellia tree inhibits the Cox enzyme pathway and so reduces the pro-inflammatory prostaglandins.
N-acetylcysteine	This sulfur-based amino acid and dietary supplement inhibits IL-1.
Magnesium	This mineral inhibits IL-1.
Extracts from Philippine sponge: Manoalide, scalardial, and hymenialdisine	These natural marine products appear to inhibit the effects of IL-1 and the production of pro-inflammatory prostaglandins.
Ginseng	Ginsenosides, the active component in ginseng, inhibit substance P.
Serotonin's precursor, 5-hydroxytryptophan (5-HTP)	This precursor of the neurotransmitter serotonin "inhibits" substance P.
Amino acids: isoleucine, leucine, valine, and taurine	These amino acids stop the pain-inducing activity of glutamate.
Vitamin D	The only vitamin that acts like a hormone, vitamin D inhibits the pro-inflammatory cytokines IL-1 and IL-12.

Table 3-2 **NATURAL COMPOUNDS THAT DECREASE INFLAMMATION AND PAIN *(cont.)***	
Vitamin E	IL-6 activity is higher when vitamin E levels are low, but appears to decrease when vitamin E levels are adequate.
Quercetin	A powerful antioxidant, quercetin also inhibits the pro-inflammatory cytokine IL-8.
Pycnogenol®	This extract of pine bark controls nitric oxide metabolism and limits the amount of autoimmunity it induces.
Ipriflavone	Derived from natural estrogens called isoflavones that are found in soy foods, the new supplement ipriflavone decreases activity of IL-1 and IL-6, as well as nitric oxide.

so reduce inflammation. The problem with NSAIDs, however, is their many side effects, including gastrointestinal bleeding and kidney damage.

Aware of the potential risks of NASIDs, researchers have sought alternative ways to reduce prostaglandin production and inflammation. One promising natural anti-inflammatory is fish oil. In a recent study, Harvard Medical School researchers tested natural treatments for rheumatoid arthritis, a painful joint condition that affects millions of people. Among the natural treatments they tested was fish oil, which acts as an anti-inflammatory agent by inhibiting leukotrienes. As we discussed in Chapter 2, immune system cells release leukotrienes, which induce inflammation. When the rheumatoid arthritis patients involved in the study took fish oils, which contain the essential fatty acid gamma-linolenic acid (GLA) and other polyunsaturated fatty acids, their symptoms improved significantly. The Harvard researchers also showed that these patients' leukotriene activity levels were reduced, proving that tender joints and morning stiffness can be improved by stopping leukotrienes. Isn't that amazing? This study revealed that doing something as simple as adding fish oil (or fish oil supplements) to your diet can actually decrease pain by shutting down the leukotrienes. These beneficial, polyunsaturated fatty acids also reduce levels of the pro-inflammatory interleukins IL-1 and IL-6, other chemicals that cause inflammation and pain.

The Harvard study was so compelling that researchers in England decided to test whether or not essential fatty acid supplements could replace NSAIDs, the mainstay of rheumatoid arthritis treatment. After twelve months, rheumatoid arthritis patients who took supplemental fish oil had significantly less pain, and were able to use NSAIDs far less often.

Prostaglandin Blockers

- essential fatty acids like those in fish oil
- curcumin from the spice turmeric
- boswellic extracts
- manoalide, scalardial, and hymenialdisine, three drugs extracted from Philippine marine sponges

A variety of other natural substances can inhibit pain-inducing prostaglandins, including the Indian spice turmeric and boswellic extracts. Turmeric contains compounds called curcuminoids, which, in laboratory experiments, possess anti-inflammatory agents. Curcumin acts like aspirin, because it inhibits both the Cox-2 enzyme pathway (as aspirin does) and the breakdown of arachidonic acid, which produces prostaglandins. However, curcumin *selectively* inhibits prostaglandin synthesis—and remember, not all prostaglandins are bad. Certain prostaglandins help our blood clot and, without them, we can develop bleeding problems. Both aspirin and the new "super aspirin" Cox-2 inhibitor drugs inhibit these "good" prostaglandins; curcumin does not. It's possible that the usefulness of the currently approved Cox-2 inhibitors will be limited because they interfere with normal blood clotting.

Boswellia, gum resin from the boswellia tree, also has potent anti-inflammatory properties. It, too, inhibits the Cox-2 enzyme pathway and, therefore, reduces "bad" prostaglandin production. Perhaps because of this action, which researchers have discovered in animal studies, boswellic acids reduce inflammation.

Natural Substances That Inhibit the Interleukins

Interleukin production is the second step in the cascade of inflammatory pain. We now know that a number of natural substances inhibit the interleukins.

IL-1 is a very important, pro-inflammatory cytokine that increases pain and calls the nervous system into action. Vitamin D, the only vitamin that acts like a hormone, inhibits IL-1's action. N-acetylcysteine, a sulfur-based amino acid and dietary supplement, is currently being investigated as an antiarthritic agent because it inhibits IL-1.

Researchers have also investigated the mineral magnesium as an IL-1 blocker. Magnesium deficiency *increases* levels of IL-1, which increases the pain-inflammatory response. It seems reasonable to speculate that getting enough magnesium—by taking supplements, if necessary—may help our bodies block IL-1, and so decrease pain and inflammation.

There is a new supplement named ipriflavone that is derived from the natural estrogens found in soy products (called isoflavones). More and more women are using natural estrogens (isoflavones or ipriflavone) to prevent osteoporosis after menopause instead of taking estrogen replacement therapy, which may cause breast and uterine cancer. As a result of this increased use of ipriflavone, we have learned that besides protecting our bones by acting like a natural estrogen, it reduces IL-1 and IL-6 activity.

Omega-3 essential fatty acids, like those found in fish oil and fish oil supplements, stop both IL-1 and IL-6. We have also learned that the pro-inflammatory activity of IL-6 *increases* when we suffer from vitamin E deficiency. Quercetin, a very strong antioxidant, inhibits the damaging activity of IL-8.

Interleukin Blockers

- N-acetylcysteine, a sulfur-based amino acid, inhibits IL-1.
- The mineral magnesium blocks IL-1.
- Three Philippine sponge–derived drugs (manoalide, scalardial, and hymenialdisine) inhibit IL-1.
- Vitamin D is a strong anti-inflammatory substance that inhibits the activity of IL-1 and IL-12.
- Omega-3 fatty acids block both IL-1 and IL-6.
- Vitamin E apparently inhibits IL-6 activity; vitamin E deficiency *increases* IL-6 activity.
- The antioxidant quercetin inhibits IL-8.

Other natural treatments that address the brain-immune connection in pain include gifts from the sea: marine sponges that can literally wipe away pain. Three potent anti-inflammatory compounds derived from sponges found in the oceans of Indonesia and the Philippines—manoalide, scalardial, and hymenialdisine—appear to inhibit both IL-1 and the pro-inflammatory prostaglandins. Drug companies are currently investigating their potential.

Using Nature to Block Substance P

Many natural compounds appear to reduce substance P, including ginsenosides, the main pharmaco-active molecules of ginseng. Of course, traditional practitioners of Chinese medicine have known about ginsenosides' antipain properties for hundreds of years, but scientists have only recently elucidated their pain-fighting mechanism, when Korean researchers discovered that ginsenosides specifically inhibit substance P.

Substance P Blockers

- the serotonin precursor 5-hydroxytryptophan
- ginsenosides (from ginseng)

Other natural compounds inhibit substance P, including 5-hydroxytryptophan (5-HTP), the precursor of the neurotransmitter serotonin. In a fascinating experiment, Japanese scientists stimulated the brains of animals to release 5-HTP and then measured the amount of substance P found in inflamed tissue. They discovered that, when 5-HTP was present in high enough concentrations, it completely inhibited substance P activity.

Neutralizing Nitric Oxide

Nitric oxide, a gas, carries signals for both the nervous and immune systems, acting as both a neurotransmitter and a cytokine. Immune system cells called macrophages—the same ones that make IL-1—release more nitric oxide when we develop an infection or inflammation. Unfortunately, this extra nitric oxide doesn't help us heal; instead, it breaks down bone and *slows* healing. Pycnogenol, however, a pine bark extract and a powerful antioxidant, stops nitric oxide production. The new supplement ipriflavone, which, as we just discussed, comes from the natural estrogens found in soy foods, also decreases nitric oxide's noxious actions.

Antagonizing Glutamate

A final approach to inhibiting pain uses our current knowledge of glutamate, the amino acid that stimulates pain pathways. Other amino acids antagonize (or stop) the effects of glutamate. These include the branched-chain amino acids isoleucine, leucine, and valine, as well as a fourth amino acid, taurine. Finnish researchers in the Department of Anesthesiology at Turku University Hospital investigated branched-chain amino acids as a way to raise the pain threshold. When used in combination with morphine, they found that branched-chain amino acids markedly decreased pain sensation.

Isn't it astonishing how the brain and immune system work together to protect us, even if it's painful? Now that you understand this complex, pain-producing interaction, it's time to look at the other system that causes us lots of pain: the musculoskeletal system.

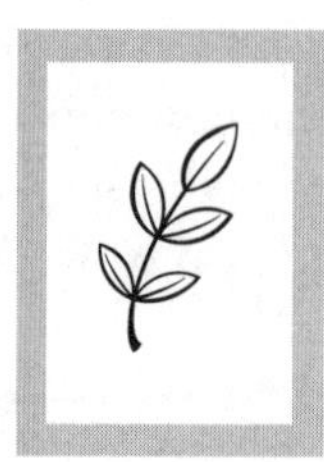

CHAPTER 4

SEARCHING FOR THE CAUSE OF YOUR BACK PAIN

Many different health-care professionals treat back pain. If you are having back pain, you will probably consult your family physician first. He or she will then refer you to an orthopedic surgeon, a neurosurgeon, or a specialist in physical medicine and rehabilitation. Many people choose to see chiropractors or acupuncturists because some of their techniques are quite successful in alleviating back pain. No matter which medical professional you choose, the process should start in the same way, with a thorough medical history and a complete physical examination (see Table 4-1).

The purpose of the history and physical is to diagnose the exact cause of your back pain. Trust us: The best way to determine the cause of your pain is to follow tried-and-true methods.

Unfortunately, a definitive diagnosis can sometimes be elusive, even when your doctors employ reliable methods. In many cases, it is more important to determine what is *not* the cause of your pain if its origin is unclear. For example, cancer and infection are two conditions your doctor should rule out early.

THE MEDICAL HISTORY

A complete medical history has many separate parts: the *chief complaint* (what is really bothering you the most), *history of the present illness, past medical history, family history, review of systems,* and *social history* (see Table 4-1). Each of these parts of the history is equally important, and the doctor should ask you about each and every one of them. This may sound dogmatic, but it is essential to be thorough in gathering your history so the physician doesn't miss any hints about a correct diagnosis.

You are undoubtedly all too familiar with your pain, so be sure to describe it in detail. If you have back pain, it's important to know whether it's just in your back, or if it goes down your leg as well. If it travels down your leg, is it sharply painful, or is it a dull sensation? Does walking make it better or worse? Does it wake you up? Are you more comfortable if you are standing, sitting, or lying down? Does coughing or sneezing make the pain worse? What can you do to make it better? What makes it worse? Does the pain go into your testicular or vaginal area? Does having a bowel movement affect your pain in any way? While the doctor should elicit this information from you, if he or she doesn't ask, bring it up. Think about the answers to these questions before you visit the doctor. You might even jot down a few notes so that you remember the details. For example, if your back pain started the day after you played softball with the neighborhood kids and has been getting worse ever since, the doctor needs to know.

In order to solve your back pain problem, it is crucial for you and your physician to form a partnership. If you feel that your doctor (or other health-care professional) doesn't particularly seem interested in your problems, doesn't relate to you, or treats you like an inanimate object rather than an individual, it is time to move on to someone else. It is critically important for you to have a physician you can talk to, and who is truly interested in you and your back pain.

You also need to tell the doctor how you have treated your back pain so far. Have you been taking strong pain killers, anti-inflammatory medication, or muscle relaxants? Have you consulted a physical therapist, a chiropractor or an acupuncturist? If the answer is yes, did you get an exercise program to strengthen and stretch your back muscles? Your doctor needs to know.

How is your health in general? Give the doctor specific answers about your physical health, as well as your psychological state. As we've discussed, stress can generate pain, so it's very important for the doctor to know whether your life at work or at home is stressful. Stress can create muscle spasm, which directly causes serious back pain. If you aren't crazy about your job, the doctor should know whether you have a happy, balanced home life, or if your wife or husband or kids are also driving you 'round the bend.

The doctor may ask questions that offend you. It is crucial for you to answer them, however, because you can provide important clues about the cause of your pain. While you may not recognize that these bits of information are meaningful clues, your doctor may identify a distinct pattern that explains why you're in pain.

Your family history is nearly as important as your personal history. Many back problems have a genetic factor, so your physician needs to know whether other people in your family have had back pain as adults or even as children. Speaking of childhood, did you ever hurt your back as a child?

Last but not least is your social history. How much coffee and alcohol do you drink? Both of these substances are directly associated with osteoporosis (thin bones). Additionally, smoking has a definite association with poor recovery after back surgery.

We've discussed how important it is for you and your physician to form a partnership when trying try to solve your back pain problem. Remember: It is critically important for you to have a physician you can trust, you can talk to, and who is truly interested in you and your back pain.

Even if you've had dozens of negative experiences with the medical profession, don't despair. Many doctors care, and are willing to talk to you like a friend and colleague. They'll give you the sense of trust and security you need to form a partnership. Truly dedicated practitioners want such a partnership as much as you do.

THE PHYSICAL EXAM

After the doctor has taken your history, he or she should give you a thorough physical examination. If your pain has lasted a long time, either your family doctor or a specialist must do a complete physical to evaluate you properly.

Now, so that you can appreciate what the doctor is looking at during the physical exam (and on X rays and MRIs), and why back pain can be so difficult to diagnose, let's take a closer look at the spine.

The Spine

The thirty-three bones that make up the spine are the vertebrae. We divide the spinal column into five basic regions, named (from top to bottom) cervical, dorsal, lumbar, sacral, and coccygeal (pronounced serv-a-cal, door-sul, lum-bar, say-cral, and cock-sidg-e-ul). The vertebrae are numbered within each region. Therefore, the first cervical vertebra, the one at the very top of the spine, is C1; C2 lies below it, C3 below C2, and so on down the spine.

Cervical Region

The cervical (Latin for "neck") region is the uppermost part of the spine, located directly under the skull. Within the cervical region, there are seven vertebrae. They are the smallest of the entire spine.

Dorsal Region

This region has twelve vertebrae that are bigger than those in the cervical region, but smaller than the lumbar vertebrae. The dorsal vertebrae are also distinguished from others by the presence of additional facets, "demi facets" on the sides of the vertebrae, to which the ribs attach. Conveniently enough, twelve ribs attach to the twelve dorsal vertebrae.

Lumbar Region

The lumbar region consists of the five largest vertebrae; they sit at the base of the spine.

Sacral and Coccygeal Regions

These regions contain nine bones during our earlier years. As we age, they naturally fuse together to form two bones, the sacrum and the coccyx. The sacrum is triangular and the entire spinal column rests on it. The coccyx is more commonly known as the tailbone. The adult spine has twenty-four vertebrae plus the fused sacrum and coccyx.

The Vertebrae

A vertebra possesses two major portions: the vertebral body and the vertebral arch. The "facet joints," in the center of the vertebrae, attach them to each other. The vertebral body is in front (i.e., next to the body cavity containing our internal organs), and is the largest part of each vertebra. It is somewhat cylindrically shaped (see Figure 4-1).

The outermost portion, the vertebral arch, looks like a horseshoe. There is a "spinous process" in the middle of each arch; they form the "bumps" you can see on the back of a lean person.

Each vertebra fits snugly into the bone above and below it by using the articular facets. These "facets" are simply surfaces surrounded by a capsule; they contain cartilage (see Figure 4-2).

The spine is very complicated, but we can picture it simply. Despite all of the structures in the spine, when you think about it, think doughnuts. Imagine twenty-four doughnuts stacked on top of each other (i.e., twenty-four doughnuts instead of twenty-four vertebrae—or twenty-four tires, whatever works for you). What goes in the hollowed-out section? The spinal cord runs through the center of the vertebrae. The vertebral bodies are in front, the vertebral arches are in back, and the spinal cord is in the open space in the center of the doughnuts.

To understand how the spine functions, let's examine the vertebrae in the cervical spine (neck). The C5 vertebra attaches to the C4 above it and C6 below it. We can make simple movements like nodding our heads because the muscles and spinal joints act together. In other words, muscles and spinal joints help us run, walk, bend, and twist. When the joints of the spine function normally, life's movements seem effortless and, additionally, you probably feel pretty good.

However, various physical stresses we encounter in life, such as falling, lifting heavy objects, repetitive stress, poor posture, old traumas, car accidents, or sleeping on an unsupportive bed, cause spinal joints to malfunction. If a spine joint is stuck and not moving as well as it should, we call it "hypomobile." A joint that moves more than it should is "hypermobile."

Why do we need a biomechanically sound spine? Each of our spine's

Table 4-1 **THE HISTORY AND PHYSICAL EXAM**	
The History	
Chief Complaint	What is the main thing that is bothering you?
History of present illness	What kind of pain are you having? What makes it better or worse? Does it "travel" to another area of the body, like your leg? Does coughing, sneezing, or having a bowel movement make the pain worse? Are you taking pain killers, anti-inflammatories, or muscle relaxants? Have you seen a chiropractor? Are you doing exercises to strengthen or loosen your back? Have you had this type of pain before? Did you ever hurt your back as a child?
Review of systems	You will be asked a series of questions to help determine if there is a problem with any other organ system.
Past medical history	What serious illnesses have you had in the past? What medications are you currently taking?
Family history	Are there any hereditary illnesses in your family? Do any other family members have back problems?
Social history	How much do you smoke or drink? Are you having any problems at work or with your family?

Table 4-1 THE HISTORY AND PHYSICAL EXAM *(cont.)*	
Physical Exam	
General posture	How do you stand and walk? Are you swaybacked? Are you round-shouldered? Do you have a curved spine?
Range of motion test	How far can you bend to the front, side, and back? Does bending in any direction cause pain?
Soft tissue exam	Are any of your muscles in spasm? Do you have "trigger points" that hurt when touched?
Neurological exam	Are your reflexes normal? Do you have any areas of numbness? Do you have any muscle weakness?
Vaginal and/or rectal exam	Some back problems can cause troubles in these areas.

functional units—composed of two adjacent vertebrae, the disk that separates them, and all the soft tissue connecting them, like ligaments—must protect the spinal cord and its nerves. Unfortunately, this protection must occur in a very hostile environment. We continually place weight on the spine at the same time as it must bend, as well as cope with shearing, tensile, and compressive stresses, all of which affect the spine's functional units.

In addition to serving as a modified shock absorber, the disk also provides some degree of stability to the spine. The disk separates the two adjacent vertebrae from each other. With age, the disk loses its water content and we develop degenerative arthritis, which is also known as osteoarthritis or degenerative disk disease.

Numerous spinal ligaments acts as stabilizing structures, attaching the vertebrae to each other and holding the front and back of the vertebrae together. It is these very strong and thick ligaments of the spine that provide stability between the vertebral segments (see Figure 4-2).

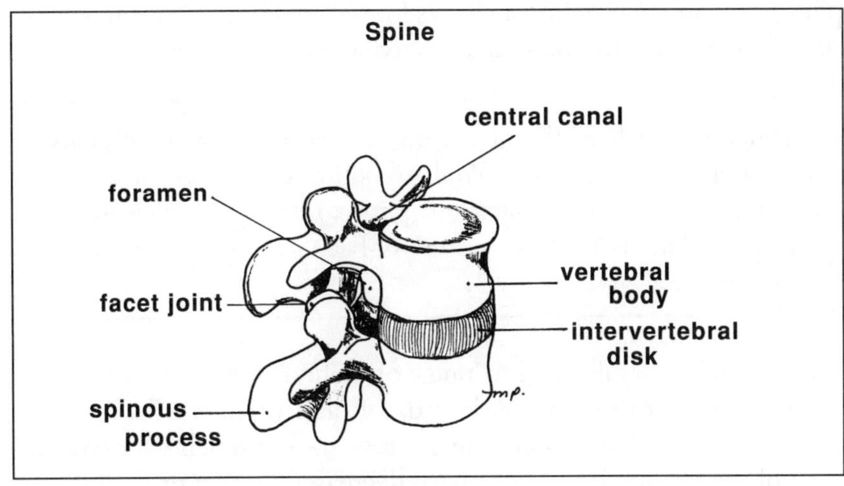

Figure 4-1

EXAMINING THE LOW BACK

The low back exam itself has several basic parts. You must undress down to your underwear for the doctor to do the exam properly. If the doctor examined you fully clothed, then it is time to find another doctor. An appropriate exam requires looking at and touching your body, not your clothes.

The doctor will examine your general posture first. Are you round-shouldered or swaybacked? Is there any evidence of curvature of the

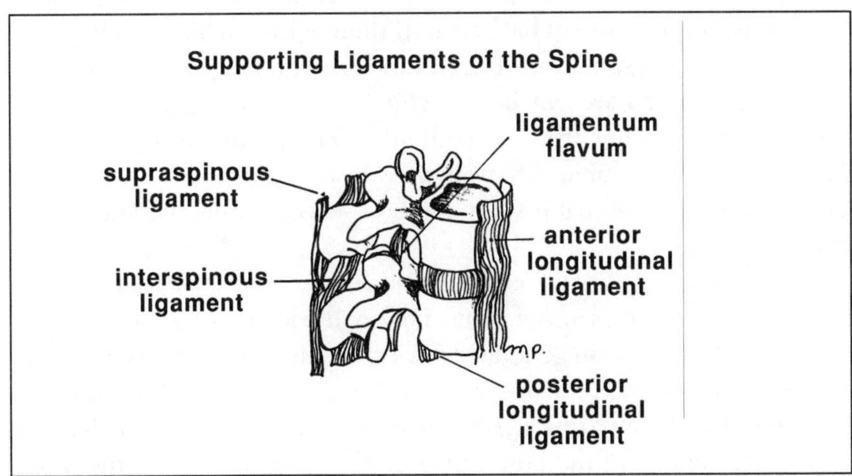

Figure 4-2

spine, or scoliosis? The doctor checks for scoliosis by having you bend in half (90 degrees) at the waist and observing how you do so.

> Did you ever hear the old saying "When you hear hoof beats, think horses, not zebras"? Well, sometimes the hoof beats *are* made by zebras, and a similar exception to the rule applies to low back pain: The most obvious cause of back pain is not necessarily its *true* cause.

The doctor generally does a "range of motion" exam next. During it, you will bend forward and backward, left and right; you'll rotate this way and that, and put either your neck or back through whatever full range of motion you can. If you have decreased motion or flexibility, it could be due to a multitude of causes, including arthritis, congenital problems, inflammatory conditions, and many others.

While you bend, the doctor will also determine whether any particular movement evokes pain. This is important because, if you have a herniated disk, you'll probably experience pain when you bend to the side. If you have spinal stenosis, in which nerves in the spinal canal are crowded by abnormal bone, you will usually feel more comfortable when you bend forward and experience more pain when you bend backward.

Next, the physician will watch you walk. Do you walk with a limp? Is there any evidence that one leg is longer than the other? This is a surprisingly common cause of back pain. If there is even a hint of this problem, the physician should measure both legs with a tape measure. Can you walk on your toes *and* heels? This tests the strength of your leg muscles, which comes from nerve impulses that pass through the low back area. If you are unable to walk on your toes or your heels, you may have a pinched nerve that is stopping those muscles from working properly.

A thorough "soft tissue" examination is next. The physician should palpate all the muscles around your neck and back looking for spasm or tightness. Muscle spasm generates powerful pain impulses, and can also be a clue that there is a pain-producing area underneath the muscles. The body has an amazing ability to protect itself, and if you have a painful area in one of the bones in your spine, it's normal for the muscles overlying that area to go into spasm. The only way to detect spasm is for the doctor to feel your muscles with his or her hands. If you had a back exam that omitted this, then you didn't have a complete exam.

The doctor should also identify trigger points. These little, knotted-up areas in the muscle are very tender to touch. When you press on them, a pain may shoot down an arm or leg, depending on their position. Trigger points are quite common in large segments of the population. When trigger points occur in the muscles that overlie the neck or cervical spine, they perpetuate spasm in those muscles, which can also cause headaches. How do they do so? When the muscles that attach at the base of the skull go into spasm, they pull on the area and cause an occipital headache. This kind of headache generally starts in the back of your skull and spreads toward the front or around the sides of your head.

> Testing muscle strength is an important part of the neurological examination. If you have muscle weakness, it may indicate that there is pressure on the nerve going to that muscle.

People who use computers for many hours a day have a notoriously higher-than-normal number of trigger points and muscle spasms in their necks, because they hold their heads in the same position all day long. While we once thought that these headaches were related to radiation from the computer screen, we've learned that most of them are caused by constant muscle spasm in the neck and the presence of many little knots (trigger points).

Later in this chapter, we'll discuss two conditions in which muscle spasm, pain, and tender trigger points are very important: myofascial pain syndrome and fibromyalgia.

The neurological portion of the back exam is one of the most important. The reflexes at your knees, ankles, elbows, and wrists are checked, and the doctor runs a small pin up and down your arms and legs to see if you feel touch normally. If you have numb areas on your skin, you may have a pinched nerve in your spine. Believe it or not, an area of numbness can identify precisely which nerve in your spine is pinched, because each spinal nerve supplies feeling to very specific areas of skin. Therefore, if you are numb in one particular area of skin, it's a tip-off about where the problem in your back probably is.

Testing muscle strength is an important part of the neurological examination. You've already walked on your toes and heels, but now all of your muscles must be tested for weakness. If you have muscle weakness, it may indicate that there is pressure on the nerve going to that muscle.

The combination of all these tests helps the doctor make a diagnosis. If you have decreased reflexes, numbness in a part of your leg, weakness of certain muscles, and possibly a shrunken thigh or calf muscle, you most likely have pressure on a nerve root. In most cases, either a herniated disk or pressure from surrounding bones is the problem. In this instance at least, you may need to have other tests, such as an MRI, to determine whether the initial diagnosis is correct.

Did you ever hear the old saying "When you hear hoof beats, think horses, not zebras"? Well, sometimes hoof beats *are* made by zebras, and a similar exception to the rule applies to low back pain: The most obvious cause of back pain is not necessarily its *true* cause.

It's quite common, for example, for circulatory problems to produce leg numbness that mimics a herniated disk. For this reason, it's important for the doctor to check the pulses in both of your legs to see if there is good blood flow.

The straight leg-raising test is another important part of the back exam. While you are lying down, the physician lifts your leg from a horizontal position to see whether the motion creates any pain or numbness in that leg. Lifting the leg stretches the sciatic nerve that runs down it. If you feel pain when the doctor lifts your leg off the table, it's an indication that you might have pressure on the nerve roots in your back. A reasonably flexible person without any significant back problems or extremely tight hamstring muscles should be able to have his or her leg lifted to approximately 90 degrees.

Did you know that it's not unusual for a patient with significant hip problems to have back pain? That's because arthritis of the hips (and other hip joint disease) can lead to decreased motion, which we frequently feel as low back pain. Therefore, the doctor will put your hips through a full range of motion to see whether they move normally.

The doctor will also carefully feel the little bumps, called spinous processes, running down the middle of your neck, mid-back, and low back. Tenderness right over a bone can indicate a tumor. To determine if you have a tumor—a *very* rare situation—requires other tests, like a bone scan.

> Laboratory tests must be used along with the history and physical examination; nothing can replace a careful history and physical. The new laboratory tests are so sensitive that they detect even the smallest physical changes, which often just show normal wear and tear—they don't mean anything. Only by combining these sophisticated lab tests with a complete history and physical can we get the entire picture and determine whether a test result is significant.

Last but not least, you should have a rectal or vaginal exam. Back pain can be caused by problems in these areas of your body. Most commonly, your gynecologist or internist will do your pelvic and rectal exam. You *must* have these exams to have a complete evaluation.

In the best of all possible worlds, the doctor would always know the cause of your back problem after the history and physical examination. He or she will have obtained answers to questions about prior surgery, preexisting back injury, the possibility of a tumor or significant arthritic problem, the potential for pressure on nerve roots, and some indication about whether or not psychological factors play a part in causing your back pain. It's entirely possible that you will walk away from the history and physical with a definite diagnosis such as muscle strain, a facet problem, a herniated disk, or degenerative arthritis. Unfortunately, we are not always able to make an absolute diagnosis after the history and physical. In fact, when this happens—and it does fairly frequently—it's necessary to employ additional laboratory testing.

DIAGNOSTIC TESTING

Researchers have made tremendous advances in medical technology during the past decade, which give us a new diagnostic edge. Many of the medical tests available today didn't even exist in science fiction movies twenty-five years ago.

Laboratory tests *must* accompany the history and physical examination; they cannot replace a careful history and physical. The new laboratory tests are so sensitive that they detect even tiny changes that often

Table 4-2
DIAGNOSTIC TESTS

Test	Condition(s) It Diagnosis	How It's Done	Potential Adverse Effects
Plain X rays	Fractures, arthritic changes, significant mal-alignments of the vertebrae. May show cancer. (Can't image soft tissue structures clearly).	An X ray machine emits radiation which catches the image of the bones and bony structures on X-ray film.	Exposure to radiation if overutilized.
MRI	All of the above in addition to many conditions affecting soft tissue structures.	Patient is placed into a magnetic field and a computer is used to generate cross-sectional images of the body.	Claustrophobia from being in a closed MRI unit (which can be avoided by using an open MRI machine); allergic reaction to contrast dyes, if used (very rare).
CT or CAT scan	Extremely accurate for bony lesions and somewhat helpful for soft tissue.	X ray and computers create cross-sectional images of the spine and other parts of the body at various levels.	Exposure to radiation
Myelogram and CT/myelogram	Pressure on the nerves and spinal cord with extreme accuracy.	Dye is injected into the sac surrounding the spinal cord. X rays and then a CT scan are done.	Headache; allergy to the dye (very rare)
Diskogram	Used to determine the cause of leg and/or back pain when other tests have been negative. May reveal internal disk disruption.	First saline and then dye are injected into the disk followed by CT scan of the disk.	Allergy to injected dye; pain
Bone scan	Areas of increased metabolic activity such as fractures, tumors, and infection that may not show up on plain X rays.	Radioactive isotope is injected into the blood and followed by scanning.	Allergy—extremely rare
Electrodiagnostic studies: EMG and nerve conduction	Pinched or entrapped nerves.	Fine needles are inserted into the muscles to measure electrical activity.	Pain from needle insertions
Blood tests	Diseases of various organ systems, infection, arthritic disorders.	Blood sample is analyzed.	None

just show normal wear and tear, and which shouldn't concern you. Only by combining these sophisticated tests with a complete history and physical can we get the entire picture and determine whether a test result is really significant.

Even with all these new, sophisticated tests, when you first see your doctor for back pain, he or she will probably start out with the traditional X ray. There is a growing trend in the United States not to do initial X rays, but to wait and see if the patient just gets better. Unfortunately, we could miss a cancer this way and, in the world of managed care that tries to cut down on laboratory testing, physicians shouldn't forget this possibility.

Traditional X rays typically show fractures, arthritic changes, and significant misalignments of the vertebrae. In other words, they show us the bony structures. However, X rays can't give us information about the soft tissues, such as ligaments and muscles. For that, we need a more sophisticated type of imaging test, like an MRI (see Table 4-2).

Magnetic Resonance Imaging (MRI)

Magnetic resonance imaging (MRI) is a state-of-the-art test. During the MRI, a patient is placed into a strong magnetic field and, with the assistance of computers, we get an extremely clear picture of almost all of the structures in and surrounding the spine. You aren't exposed to X rays during an MRI, which is an added advantage.

The MRI shows us the nerves, ligaments, and even muscles. As you know, a lot of pain involves these soft tissues. MRI lets us actually see into a person's body and visualize more than just bones (which is all we can see on X rays).

People used to have no choice but to slide into a narrow, closed tube to have an MRI test. As you can imagine, this was a real problem for people with claustrophobia. Recently, however, researchers developed units called open MRI machines that have eliminated this problem.

If you choose to go into the MRI tube, many facilities now provide headphones so you can listen to your favorite music while you have the test done. The headphones also help to drown out the thumping sounds the MRI machine makes. Although the open MRIs are a definite option for patients with claustrophobia, some physicians feel the closed machines usually produce better images. Therefore, many physicians prefer the test done in closed machines, if possible. If this really bothers you, however, speak up! Your doctor should be willing to work with you.

When should you have an MRI? If you undergo treatment for your back pain, consisting of conservative therapy and medication, for four to six weeks and do not improve, then you should have an MRI. If your physical exam suggests that a herniated disk is putting pressure on a nerve, you should have an MRI to confirm or to rule out that diagnosis. Additionally, MRIs clearly reveal infections and tumors of the spine which, although rare, do occur.

MRI exams frequently show aberrations that are not at all significant, and this is their biggest disadvantage. Studies reveal that, when people forty to sixty years old have MRIs, 30 to 50 percent of them show evidence of a herniated disk, even though they have no back pain whatsoever. We've learned that a herniated disk can be "normal" in aging individuals. Just because something shows up on an MRI doesn't mean that it's important.

If we see an abnormality on an MRI exam, *it's only significant if the physical examination concurs with it*. For example, if your history and physical exam show that you have low back pain with sciatica (pain) down your left leg, the MRI result is important if it shows a herniated disk at a particular point on your left side. If it shows a herniated disk at the *right* side but your pain is in your *left* leg, then that MRI finding means nothing. Therefore, it's very important to give MRIs only the importance they deserve.

The vast majority of us have normal wear and tear degenerative changes in our spines. Again, this is normal. If you are over forty, you're an oddity if your MRI doesn't show normal aging changes, so you shouldn't worry about them. If your MRI shows the moderately advanced changes of normal wear-and-tear arthritis and they match your physical exam, then they *might* be important. As you can see, we always return to a thorough history and physical exam, the backbone of the entire diagnostic process.

Computed Tomography (CT) Scan

Before MRIs were readily available and affordable, we used computed tomography (CT) scans (also called CAT scans) instead. A CT scan is an X ray picture of the spine; computers assist in making the final images. "Tomography" means that we take pictures in slices down the spine; in other words, the CT looks at a cross section of the injured area—but without slicing you open! Unfortunately, CT scans emit a fair amount of X rays, but the exposure never exceeds the safe range.

CT scans show bones very accurately, which is their greatest advantage. It shows disks and nerves, too, but not nearly as distinctly as an MRI can. Since so many back problems involve tissues other than bone, MRI is now the test of choice, although your doctor may order a CT scan if he or she feels it will give a better picture of the bones.

Myelograms and CT-Myelograms

The word "myelogram" invokes fear in the hearts of many patients, because they know it's an invasive procedure. During this test, the doctor inserts a needle into your back to do a spinal tap. He uses the needle to inject dye into the dural sac, the sac of fluid that surrounds the spinal cord.

You will then lie on an X ray table that tilts back and forth, and the technician takes X rays. The dye shows up white on the X ray. If there are any problems, the doctor can see indentations on the sac of dye that shouldn't be there. Years ago, we only had oil-based dyes and, at the end of the procedure, we had to remove them. Now we have water-soluble dyes, which the body absorbs. Water-soluble dyes cause fewer side effects, so myelograms are much safer than they used to be.

> If we see an abnormality on an MRI, it is only significant if the physical examination matches it. For example, if you have low back pain with sciatica down your left leg, the MRI result is important if it shows a herniated disk at a particular point on your left side. If it shows a herniated disk on the *right* side but your pain is in your *left* leg, then that MRI finding means nothing. Therefore, it's very important not to rely too heavily on MRIs.

A myelogram is an exceptionally useful procedure. After we inject the dye, we put the patient in a CT scanner and get extremely accurate cross-sectional views. This is a CT-myelogram. It is so accurate because the dye totally outlines many structures that we normally can't see so clearly on a plain CT scan.

Many spine surgeons think the CT-myelogram most accurately determines what is happening in the spine. For this reason, a surgeon may use a CT-myelogram if an MRI scan doesn't explain the patient's back and leg pain. In fact, a CT-myelogram can show a tiny defect pressing on a nerve that an MRI doesn't show.

The most common side effect of a myelogram is a headache, which can develop if spinal fluid leaks out of the hole through which the doctor injected the dye. Headaches are rare, however, and they're even less likely if you stay in bed for several hours after the myelogram and drink plenty of fluids.

Diskogram

If you have a herniated disk, it may be difficult for your physician to diagnose, even with all the sophisticated tests available today. If you have pain in your back running down one leg, your doctor will definitely suspect a herniated disk, and your history and physical will provide important clues. An MRI is the next diagnostic step to take, but you (like many people with herniated disks) may have a negative MRI. You may even have a negative CT-myelogram. If your test results come back in this pattern, you may have an "internal disk disruption."

In this situation, the disk is abnormal or cracked, but it is not pinching a nerve. Even so, the abnormal disk creates significant back pain and, sometimes, leg pain. A CT diskogram is necessary to diagnose this type of abnormal disk.

> In these days of managed care, it is sometimes difficult for a physician to order all the tests he or she believes are necessary in order to make an accurate diagnosis. In the best of all possible worlds, we would be able to do every test we feel might be helpful. The course of action outlined here is obviously an ideal one. Of course, every patient, doctor, and situation is unique. If your physician doesn't think you need certain tests described here, that decision reflects your very individual situation.

The CT diskogram is an X-ray procedure. A physician inserts a needle into the disk and watches its placement with X-ray guidance. First saline, or salt water, and then dye are injected into the disk. A normal disk only absorbs a few drops of saline because it is intact. If the disk is abnormal, it is easier to inject much more fluid. After the dye is injected, you lie in a CT scanner, and the technician takes cross-sectional X rays. From them, the doctor can see if the dye leaks out of the disk. If the disk is normal, it shouldn't leak. If it does leak, then the doctor can be fairly certain that the disk itself is the site of your problem.

Bone Scans

A bone scan test measures the metabolic activity of bone cells—how fast they absorb nutrients, expel waste products, and grow. Certain rare conditions, like tumors or infections, create areas of increased activity. As uncommon as they are, it is always important to rule them out. Physicians often perform bone scans on patients over forty years old who have continual, unrelenting, and unexplained back pain, just to make sure a tumor or infection is not the cause of the pain.

During a bone scan, the physician injects radioactive isotope into a vein in your arm. Then—here's a shocker—you wait for several hours. Normal bone cells only absorb a small portion of the isotope injected. Abnormally active cells, however, collect a much larger amount of isotope. Two hours after the injection, we use a Geiger counter to measure and record the radioactivity over several areas of the bone. In an abnormal bone scan, there are darkened areas in the bone. We call them "hot spots."

As you might imagine, if a bone has been broken and is still in the healing stages, it will show up as a hot spot on a bone scan. This is because as a fracture heals, it's naturally more active in the areas that are healing; the bone scan *should* look abnormal. So this test can also tell us whether a fracture is new or old.

Osteoporosis, or fragile bones, affects a large segment of the population, and one of its cardinal findings is "compression" fractures of the spine. If an elderly woman has back pain, and traditional X rays show a compression fracture, we sometimes perform a bone scan to determine if the fracture is old or new. If it is new, the bone scan is positive (that is, abnormal), and she must wear a back brace until the fracture heals. If, on the other hand, the fracture is old, the bone scan is normal (no matter what the X ray looks like). In this situation, it is not necessary to wear a brace.

Blood Tests

As we know, with managed care it is sometimes difficult for a physician to order all the tests he or she believes are necessary in order to make an accurate diagnosis. Needless to say, we still believe that we should leave no stone unturned in our search; we should do every possible test to discover the source of a patient's pain. For example, we generally use traditional X rays to see if there is an easily identifiable source of pain. At the same time, there are certain blood tests that we occasionally require just to assure us that we've made every attempt to find the source of the pain.

The vast majority of back pain is due to muscle strain, ligament strain, a herniated disk, or arthritis. Sometimes, however, an infection or unusual form of arthritis is the source of the problem. In these cases, it is necessary to do some blood tests to find out exactly what went wrong in the first place.

One blood test, an erythrocyte sedimentation rate (ESR or sed-rate), although it is not all that specific a test, is very sensitive. For example, a sed-rate test will detect the presence of almost any inflammation in the body. If you have cancer or an infection that is causing significant inflammation, your sed-rate will be elevated. This is a good indication that we should look further, and possibly perform a bone scan to reach an accurate diagnosis.

Multitudes of blood tests exist for specific arthritis disorders. The RA Latex test is for rheumatoid arthritis and the HLA-B27 test is for a disease called ankylosing spondylitis, a form of rheumatoid arthritis that causes inflammation and stiffening of the spine. A patient who has had back pain for a long time should have at least a routine blood count and a blood chemistry profile to check for abnormalities in other parts of the body that could cause the back pain.

Electrodiagnostic Studies

Nerves and muscles play very significant roles in many types of back pain. We use two tests, electromyography (EMG) and nerve conduction studies (NCS), to measure the electrical activity and the function of nerves and muscles. With these tests, we can determine if a disruption exists in the normal electrical activity in nerves.

During an EMG test, a small wire is inserted into a muscle, and then attached to the machine that records the electrical activity of the muscle. The machine's report looks like a graph. The EMG shows whether or not the muscle is getting enough stimulation from the nerves. It can even determine if there is overstimulation, as when a muscle is in a chronic state of spasm.

Nerve conduction tests measure how fast the nerve impulse travels down the nerve toward the muscle. In fact, it's like having a speedometer attached to your nerves. We know that the impulses should go at a certain rate; if they go slower than they should or are blocked, that helps determine exactly what the problem is.

Nonetheless, electrodiagnostic studies are not the most pleasant experience for patients. To perform such studies, physicians or other medical staff must stick you with many different, small needles. Fortunately, electrodiagnostic studies are extemely helpful and can aid physicians in identifying exactly where a problem exists. For back pain sufferers, that's good news! The studies are especially useful in finding pinched nerves.

Now that you know how we determine the cause of back pain, let's take a look at what some of those causes are.

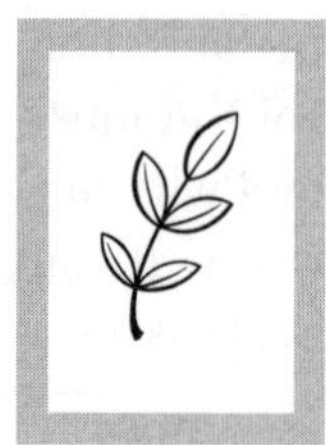

Chapter 5 COMMON CAUSES OF BACK AND MUSCULOSKELETAL PAIN

If you have back pain, you're probably frustrated by the unanswerable question, "Where is my back pain coming from?" (see Table 5-1). You may have been told by your doctor that your back pain is "idiopathic"—a big word doctors use when they don't know what causes a condition or disease. In this chapter, we're going to delve into the common causes of back pain to help you understand what makes your back hurt, and how Western physicians generally classify and deal with it. Of course, you understand by now that both medications and surgery have serious drawbacks. While you may need traditional medical care (even surgery) if you are severely injured, the best way to conquer pain is to take responsibility for your own care. In later chapters, we'll tell you about herbs, supplements, exercises, and psychological techniques you can use to control your pain safely, without the risks and side effects of surgery or medication.

You may have wondered why so many people have low back pain. Well, here's the answer: The low back, the lumbar area, is under more stress than any other section of the spine. Just standing puts quite a bit of pressure on the spine, and you'll probably be surprised to learn that sitting *increases* the pressure by an additional 50 percent. All of this nonstop stress puts a constant strain on the structures of the low back, which eventually malfunction just as any machine would. The area under the greatest stress is at vertebrae L4-5 and L5-S1 (refer back to Chapter 4 to review comments and images on the structure of the spine), which is why the majority of problems occur there.

What Contributes to Low Back Pain?

- Being overweight
- Poor posture
- A sedentary lifestyle
- Weak abdominal and back muscles
- Continual heavy physical work
- Work that requires twisting and bending
- Work in machinery that vibrates (like trucks and other heavy machinery)

You're more likely to have back pain if you have weak muscles in the abdomen and back. Remember, the muscles in the abdomen and those overlying the spinal column support the body. They also provide increased resistance to injury. If you have poor muscle tone from lack of exercise or a sedentary lifestyle, you are at greater risk for back pain.

Certain types of work are problematic for people prone to back pain. Continual heavy physical work that involves lifting accelerates normal wear-and-tear arthritis in the back, and can lead to disk problems. Work done without changing positions or its opposite, work that involves frequent bending and twisting, can cause back problems. Constant vibration is associated with many back problems and, not surprisingly, many truck drivers have serious back problems.

If you are overweight and need a good reason to start a diet, now you have it: losing weight can only help alleviate your back pain. A large, protruding abdomen shifts your center of gravity forward and makes the muscles in your back work harder to hold you upright. This puts increased stress on your lumbar spine, particularly the facet joints (they connect the vertebrae and the disks that separate them). If you are overweight, the first thing you can do to help yourself is to start a diet and an exercise program (after checking with your physician, of course) that is appropriate for you.

You should also try to improve your posture, because bad posture is associated with back pain. You'll find, however, that your posture will improve automatically when you've lost even a few pounds and start ex-

Table 5-1
COMMON CAUSES OF LOW BACK PAIN

Cause of Pain	**What It Is**
Ankylosing spondylitis	An inflammation and stiffening of the spine. A form of arthritis that may affect other joints and organs. Occurs mostly in young men.
Arachnoiditis	Scarring of the membranes which cover the spinal nerves. Typically a result of multiple surgeries. May result in incapacitating back and leg pain.
Coccyx pain	Known as coccygodynia. Results from a fall on the "tail bone."
Degenerative arthritis	Normal "wear and tear" arthritis of the spine. A degenerative disease which is a normal process of aging.
Degenerative disk disease	A manifestation of degenerative arthritis in which the disks lose water. Shows up on X ray as narrowing of the disk space with bone spurs.
Diskitis	Bacterial or viral infection of a disk space. It causes pain, fever, and malaise.
Fibromyalgia	Chronic muscle spasm associated with sleep disturbance and localized "tender points." Depression and/or anxiety frequently accompany this disorder.
Herniated lumbar disk	When the soft central portion of the disk, called the nucleus pulposus, herniates through the outer fibers of the disk and pinches a nerve to the leg causing sciatica. May be associated with neurological deficits such as numbness and weakness.

Table 5-1
COMMON CAUSES OF LOW BACK PAIN *(cont.)*

Cause of Pain	What It Is
Lumbar strain	When a muscle, tendon, or ligament is stretched beyond its normal limit. The most common back injury. Typically back pain without leg pain.
Myofascial pain syndrome	Chronic muscle spasm associated with "trigger points." Pressure on the trigger point may cause a "twitch response."
Osteomyelitis	Infection of the bone itself. There is a gradual onset of fever, with pain, severe spasm, and tenderness.
Rheumatoid arthritis	A crippling form of arthritis. The presence of "rheumatoid factor" in the blood can help make the diagnosis.
Spinal stenosis	A narrowing of the spinal canal through which the spinal cord and nerve roots traverse. Caused by degenerative disk disease and degenerative arthritis of the facet joints. Typically causes back pain and leg pain which is worse with walking.
Spondylolysis and spondylolisthesis	Spondylolysis is a defect in a part of the vertebrae called "pars interarticularis." May result in spondylolisthesis when one vertebra slips forward over another one.

ercising. Losing weight and exercising won't just help your back—it'll make you healthier and look better, so you'll feel better about your body and your life.

COMMON CAUSES OF LOW BACK PAIN

Lumbar Strain

Lumbar strain is the most common kind of low back pain. A "strain" is limited to the back; its pain doesn't radiate down the legs. If you have a strain, you have probably suffered some type of mechanical stress in that area, like a lifting injury or a sports-related accident that causes a muscle, ligament, or tendon to be stretched beyond its normal limit. The injury causes bleeding and inflammation. If a strain is slight, your muscles will spasm, either because they are injured, or to decrease motion in an injured segment of the spine right underneath them.

Lumbar strains come in two forms other than slight: the acute and the chronic form. "Chronic" means that the painful condition lasts longer than the typical healing period, which for lumbar strains is approximately six weeks. Poor posture or repetitive heavy-duty lifting can also cause chronic lumbar strains. Repetitive twisting and rotational motions can aggravate them. The inflammation that results from a chronic strain may be more widespread and so more difficult to treat than an acute strain.

When you have a lumbar strain, there is usually tenderness over the injured area. Range of motion testing (which we discussed in Chapter 4) increases the pain. In this instance though, a neurological exam will usually turn out normal, because there is no pressure on the nerve roots for the exam to spot.

Fortunately, studies in Sweden and elsewhere show that *the vast majority of lumbar strains heal without any problems whatsoever under normal circumstances*. When due to the strain, bleeding in the injured structure starts the normal inflammatory process, and there is usually great improvement within seven days. Complete healing with scar tissue replacing the injured or torn area, of course, takes longer, even up to several months. Complete healing, however, does not mean that the damaged muscle or ligament will function completely normally, because scar tissue is inelastic—it doesn't stretch, as muscle and ligaments do. For this reason, people who have had a lumbar strain are more prone to injure themselves in the future. Exercise is important here as well. Exercise can increase the strength of the abdominal and back muscles to overcome the scar tissue's potential weakness. All of this is in the normal process of things. Most people recover fully enough to resume their usual activities.

In the past, treatment for a lumbar strain involved prolonged bed rest. Thankfully, we know better now. In fact, if you stay in bed for a long period, your muscles progressively weaken, making you more likely to suffer *another* lumbar strain. Therefore, bed rest should be either nonexistent or limited to no more than forty-eight hours. Increase your activity in duration and intensity as soon as the pain allows you to.

Yes, physical therapy or chiropractic care can decrease muscle spasm and increase mobility here, but the most important aspect of the treatment is a good exercise program. Exercise is essential to strengthen the abdominal muscles in the front of the spine and the muscles behind the spine. Combine your exercise program with stretching, which alleviates the pain from chronic muscle spasm. Passive physical therapy—application of heat, ultrasound, massage, and traction—can certainly make you feel better, but none of these is as important as an exercise program.

Treatment for Lumbar Strain

- Most lumbar strains get better all by themselves in less than twelve weeks.
- After a *short* period of rest, return to normal activity as soon as possible.
- Exercise to increase abdominal and back muscle strength.
- Physical therapy (heat, ultrasound, massage, traction).
- Chiropractic care.
- Anti-inflammatory medication.
- Stress management.
- Prolonged bed rest is *not* recommended. In fact, bed rest can further weaken muscles, leading to repeated lumbar strains.

What about anti-inflammatory medication? Anti-inflammatories help to decrease pain as well as muscle spasm. Some physicians prescribe muscle relaxants like flexeril, and/or narcotic analgesics. Whatever physicians prescribe in this regard, know that many of these drugs are addictive and you should avoid them, except in very unusual cases. Prolonged use of strong muscle relaxants and narcotics can create a host of problems that are much more difficult to deal with than lumbar strain, which usually heals itself.

Psychological factors are also important. Stress and anxiety can definitely contribute to increased spasm and, if not dealt with appropriately, can cause significant depression. This creates a vicious cycle: Stress causes additional pain and spasm, which in turn cause an increase in the already present stress, tension, and pain. This vicious circle can turn a simple strain into chronic back pain that just won't disappear. You cannot always rely on your physician or chiropractor to address this issue. We'll discuss it a great deal more in Chapter 10.

Fibromyalgia and Myofascial Pain Syndrome

Just as a lumbar strain is a soft tissue injury, fibromyalgia is a soft tissue *syndrome*, a collection of symptoms. We also call it "fibrositis." Patients with fibromyalgia have discrete tender-point areas as well as a profound sleep disturbance. It occurs quite commonly in people who are somewhat obsessive-compulsive.

Only now do physicians recognize fibromyalgia as a distinct disease that affects a tremendous number of people. Some studies estimate that more than 10 million Americans have fibromyalgia. We find it most commonly in Caucasian women. The average age of these patients is thirty. It closely resembles (but is distinct from) myofascial pain syndrome, which we'll discuss separately.

The major symptoms of fibromyalgia are generalized aches and pains that seemingly have no explanation. Additionally, there are numerous tender points at set locations over the body, sleep disturbance, generalized fatigue, chronic headaches, and neck pain with a sensation of swelling in the neck or back.

We can identify distinct, tender areas around joints (elbow and knee) and over various ligaments, tendons, muscles, or bony bumps. Stiffness ranges from lasting a few minutes to all day long. While there's nothing objective to explain the patient's pain, we know that cold and humidity aggravate fibromyalgia, whereas warmth and dry weather improve it.

Some investigators think fibromyalgia is a psychological disorder. Many physicians, in fact, doubt that fibromyalgia is a distinct disease at all, primarily because researchers found no inflammation when they studied muscle tissue from fibromyalgia patients. Others feel that fibromyalgia patients become depressed because they live with chronic pain for so long. Rest assured, however, that the person who suffers with fibromyalgia has a genuine problem that the medical establishment must—and can—deal with appropriately.

There are no specific physical or laboratory findings that help diagnose fibromyalgia. It's significant to find twelve or more tender points in typical body areas. Other diseases sometimes occur along with fibromyalgia, including rheumatoid arthritis, osteoarthritis, connective tissue diseases, thyroid and parathyroid disease, chronic infection, and

HIV infection. If you have fibromyalgia, don't be frightened by this list—you do not have to be a statistic.

Treatment of Fibromyalgia

- Anti-inflammatory medication, like NSAIDs.
- Exercise and physical therapy.
- Psychological support at home and work.
- Injecting tender points with Novocain, or Novocain and a long-acting steroid, to stop pain and inflammation.
- Antidepressant medication that boosts serotonin levels.

We need to attack fibromyalgia from many different directions. It's important to continue to work and be productive as you learn exercises and receive physical therapy, because work provides the psychological support that we all need to heal ourselves with. We usually treat fibromyalgia with anti-inflammatory medication, like NSAIDs. We can inject the tender points of fibromyalgia with either Novocain (a local anesthetic) or a combination of Novocain and a long-acting steroid (a strong anti-inflammatory) (see Figure 5-1). As with lumbar strain, narcotics have no place in fibromyalgia treatment.

Antidepressant medication, on the other hand, can be extremely helpful in treating fibromyalgia. Tricyclic antidepressants and selective serotonin re-uptake inhibitors (SSRIs) are effective because fibromyal-

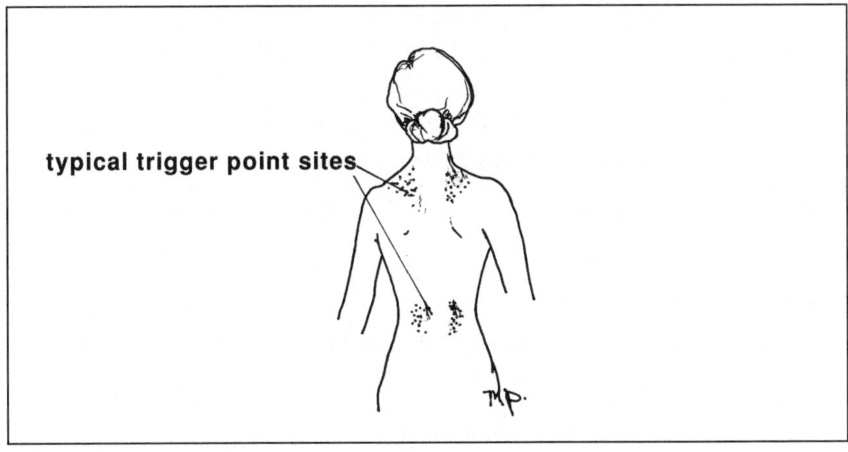

Figure 5-1

gia patients have decreased levels of the neurotransmittor serotonin, which these drugs have the potential to boost.

If you have fibromyalgia, it's important for you to learn as much about it as possible. Studies show that fibromyalgia patients who are not educated about their disease become even more depressed and less responsive to treatment with time. Be assured though, that we can treat fibromyalgia symptoms in many cases. If your pain and movement limitations are depressing you, please get whatever help you need.

Myofascial pain syndrome, which is somewhat different from fibromyalgia, was brought to public attention by Dr. Janet Travell, then President John Kennedy's personal physician.

In myofascial pain syndrome, you can actually feel the trigger points in the muscle, unlike the tender points in fibromyalgia. When the trigger point is pressed, there is a specific area of pain (which can be referred pain—it's not necessarily at the trigger point itself). Muscles are extremely tender to the touch, and trigger points cause a painful "twitch response" (a flickering of the muscle fibers) when pressed. Low back pain and neck pain is frequently associated with myofascial pain syndrome.

Myofascial pain syndrome involves a localized painful area, whereas fibromyalgia is a diffuse pain syndrome. Unlike fibromyalgia, myofascial pain syndrome is a definite, distinct disease that we can treat more successfully.

The goal of treatment is to get rid of the trigger points and muscle spasms caused by them. A local injection of Novocain, dry needling, or what we call "ischemic compression" can relieve symptoms. Ischemic compression is best performed by a physical therapist skilled in the technique.

Treatment of Myofascial Pain Syndrome

- Injecting trigger points with Novocain, or Novocain and a steroid.
- Spray and Stretch Technique—muscles are sprayed with a cooling spray and stretched out to length by a skilled physical therapist.
- Dry needling.
- Ischemic compression, which pinches off the blood supply to the trigger point. This must be done by a trained physical therapist.
- Exercise and a stretching program.
- Consideration of antidepressant medication.

In the first treatment, we inject the trigger points with Novocain, spray the muscles with a superficial cooling spray, and stretch them. This is the Spray and Stretch Technique®.

Some practitioners have reported excellent results by using dry needling of the trigger points as well. Utilizing this technique, a needle alone is passed through the trigger point several times without injecting any substance. In many cases, this causes the trigger point to go away and subsequently the muscle spasm decreases.

In ischemic compression, a skillful physical therapist can actually pinch off the blood supply to the trigger point. Once the trigger point is gone, the muscles relax and the symptoms dissipate. Ischemic compression must be combined with a twice-a-day exercise and stretching program.

Be that as it may, a significant number of orthopedic patients are still dismissed by physicians as having psychiatric disorders simply because neither they nor a colleague bothered to do a thorough soft tissue exam and to look for trigger points. Many of these long-term pain patients simply have myofascial pain syndrome, which is curable, not a mental problem. Without appropriate trigger-point injections and physical therapy, however, many of these people suffer needlessly for years and years. The lesson here is simple: If you feel you suffer from myofascial pain syndrome, make sure your physician does a soft tissue exam and looks for trigger points.

Herniated Lumbar Disk

The disks act as shock absorbers or cushions between the vertebrae. A great deal can go wrong with a disk, but all disk problems begin the same way—with the normal degeneration of aging.

When we hit thirty or forty, our disks have already started to degenerate. Over time, the cartilage-like disk gradually loses water, becomes less elastic and, therefore, less functional as a shock absorber. In an extreme stage, a disk can even become totally stiffened (calcified).

X rays, of course, can identify disk degeneration. Here the spaces between the vertebrae clearly narrow. On the X ray itself, it's not the disk that appears (because it's made of cartilage instead of bone), but the space where we know the disk is. Again, as this space narrows naturally with age, we can also see small bone spurs called osteophytes bridging the space if, in fact, they're there.

It's quite normal for a simple bulging disk, or even a number of bulging disks, to appear on an MRI. Many studies have revealed that up to 50 percent of MRI scans done on patients who have no back pain whatsoever reveal severely degenerated and in many cases herniated disks. A herniated disk may therefore certainly be a normal part of aging. As a disk loses water and degenerates, it has an increased propensity to herniate. It does not always cause pain, however.

Most lumbar disk problems occur at the bottom of the lumbar spine, the area under the greatest amount of stress and so the most susceptible to injury. Disk problems can start when the material inside, which is gelatinous, starts to push out beyond the retaining wall of the disk. It can eventually rupture, and put pressure on the spinal nerve that runs right next to it.

Studies reveal that herniations occur most commonly between ages thirty-five and fifty-five. Heavy lifting and athletic accidents can cause herniations, or they can just occur by themselves as a disk degenerates.

Symptoms and Diagnosis of Herniated Disks

A simple bulging disk is serious only if it begins to cause symptoms. Ninety percent of all herniations occur at L4-5 or L5-S1 and cause back pain with pain in the buttock, back of the thigh and calf, and occasionally down to the heel and foot. A herniation causes limitation of motion and muscle spasm just as a strain does. The leg pain, however, is much more severe. Herniated disks usually cause some degree of numbness, weakness, and reflex changes, depending on the extent to which they are pinching the nerve root running nearby. If the herniation is significant enough to put pressure on the nerve root, it will most likely cause leg pain (when the pressure occurs in the lumbar area), or neck and arm pain (when the herniation occurs in the cervical spine or neck area; see Figure 5-2). The situation becomes even more serious if the disk herniates and puts pressure on the nerve root, causing sciatica (which we discussed in Chapter 4; see Figure 5- 2).

A severely pinched nerve at the L4-5 interspace can result in a foot drop, a condition in which people walk with an abnormal gait because their leg muscles don't have the ability to lift their toes. If you have foot drop, you can't walk on your heels during a physical exam (as we described in Chapter 4).

Please understand that disk herniations typically occur in *well-*

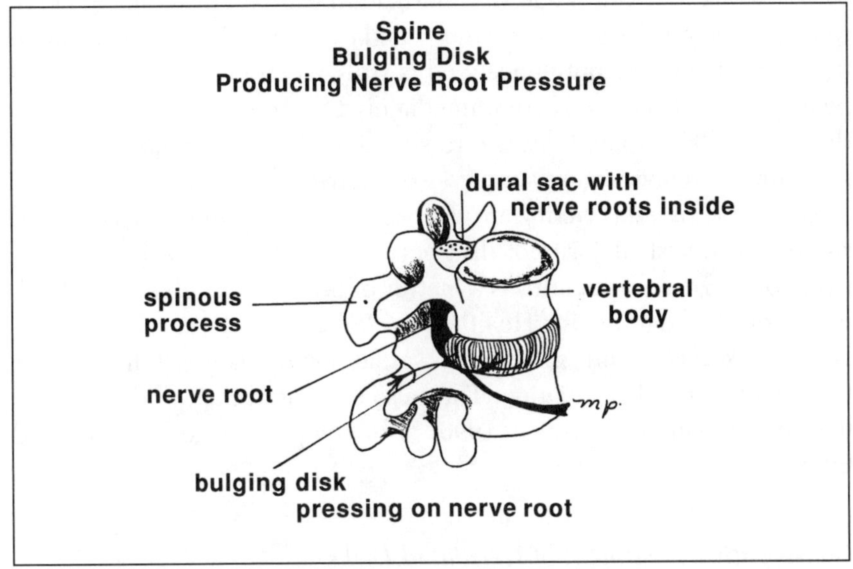

Figure 5-2

established places: In the lumbar spine, they occur at L4-5 and L5-S1 and in the cervical spine, they usually occur at C5-6 and C6-7. If a doctor tells you that you have a disk herniation at a different location and that you need surgery, it is wise to get a second—and maybe a third—opinion before you go under the knife.

The MRI, which physicians now usually ask for to help in diagnosing disk problems, has pretty much replaced both myelograms and CT scans. If you appear to have a pinched nerve with numbness, muscle weakness, and reflex changes, your doctor should order an MRI to confirm or to rule out a disk herniation.

Symptoms of Herniated Disks

- Back pain
- Sciatica—pain in the buttock, running down the back of the thigh and into the calf, sometimes into the heel and foot
- Numbness
- Weakness
- Reflex changes
- Muscle spasm
- Limitation of motion

Occasionally, a very large disk herniation can compress many nerve roots in the region known as the "cauda equina." This can result in bowel or bladder incontinence, and is truly an emergency. If this happens, you must have surgery immediately to remove the disk and free the nerves. It is, thankfully, a rare situation. The vast majority of disk herniations do not require surgery; we can treat them conservatively.

Don't become a victim in the epidemic of unnecessary spinal surgery. The vast majority of disk herniations improve with conservative, nonsurgical treatment. As a matter of fact, the Panel on Low Back Pain from the Agency for Health Care Policy and Research endorsed aspirin, exercise, and short-term spinal manipulation (chiropractic treatment) for disk herniation. They also estimated that, of the $20 billion spent on medical costs in 1990, $7 billion paid for services that did little good.

Conservative Treatment of Herniated Disks

Bed rest is an effective treatment for a herniated disk (as opposed to a lumbar strain, for which we do *not* recommend bed rest). Actually, this is probably the *only* common spinal disease that we treat this way. You should lie on your back with a pillow placed underneath the knees to decrease stretch on the irritated nerve root in the low back area.

Even so, prolonged bed rest—over one week—is not advisable. The body loses muscle strength rapidly, so you should begin physical therapy right away. You should also learn muscle strengthening and stretching exercises so you don't lose the muscle strength you have.

Epidural steroid blocks give immense relief to the pain of herniated lumbar and cervical disks. In this procedure, we inject an anesthetic and cortisone solution into the area surrounding the herniated disk, bathing the disk and nerve root. This decreases the amount of substance P and prostaglandins produced in response to inflammation and, therefore, the pain they cause.

Conservative Treatment of Herniated Disks

- Bed rest, up to a week
- Muscle strengthening and stretching exercises
- Epidural steroid blocks (injection of cortisone and anesthetic)

Did you know that we can do epidural blocks as outpatient procedures? It's true. Depending on how you respond, the doctor will do between one and three of them, but if you don't respond at all to the first one, there's no sense in doing any more. Epidural blocks work especially well in the cervical spine where the normal stresses of the lumbar spine are not present.

It's amazing though how well people with disk herniations recover without surgery. Let us share with you the story of a flight attendant who had a herniated disk at L4-5 with a complete foot drop. Not only was she in severe pain, she had a partially paralyzed leg. She absolutely refused to have surgery because she didn't want a scar on her back. After several weeks of bed rest and exercises, her foot drop totally disappeared, and she went back to her normal life.

The lesson here is never rush into surgery for a herniated disk unless there is a severe neurological deficit like bowel or bladder incontinence, which is truly a surgical emergency. The other definite indications for surgery are incapacitating pain which has not responded to conservative treatment measures or significant muscle weakness.

Surgical Treatment of Herniated Disks

In this procedure, the surgeon removes the herniated disk which he or she is able to get to after a part of the bony architecture of the vertebra called the lamina is removed. This is why it is called a laminectomy and diskectomy. Unfortunately, a high proportion of the people who have this operation don't do well, despite the fact that the operation appears to have gone without a hitch. It probably did. Unfortunately, the nature of the beast is such that many people who have had lumbar laminectomy and diskectomies either continue to have pain or have a short period of pain relief followed by recurring pain despite the fact that the operation went as planned. The MRI scan may even show that the herniated disk is gone. So why do some people continue to have pain?

There are many different structures, particularly nerves, in the lumbar spine area that surgery can easily damage. Even a tiny amount of scar tissue around these nerves (which lumbar disk surgery can create) results in incapacitating pain that doesn't go away—a condition called arachnoiditis. Since the results are so dismal, you should have this procedure only as a last resort.

Surgery's Success Rate

According to some sources, most back surgery's success rate is only about 60 to 70 percent—and that's for the first surgery. The success rate for a second surgery, if the first fails, is 30 percent, for a third surgery, 25 percent, and only 5 percent for a fourth surgery. Sadly, many people whose back surgery is not initially successful have many more back surgeries, leaving them with intractable pain.

Unfortunately, as we've noted, many feel that the success rate for most back surgery is not that encouraging. Because of a rather relatively high failure rate, we strongly advise that you make every effort to avoid surgery altogether and treat your problem more naturally and with appropriate exercise and other modalities discussed in this book. Nor do the statistics just mentioned reflect another troubling aspect of surgery—the many people who have increased pain and disability *because of* repeat surgery.

As the statistics show, the most dismal cases involve people who have had multiple back surgeries, which is all too common. The truth of the matter is that if the first back surgery didn't work, the second back surgery probably won't work either. According to Dr. A.A. White, a well-known spine surgeon and researcher on back surgery, the chances of success diminish with each successive surgery: only 30 percent for a second surgery, 25 percent for a third, and 5 percent for a fourth. With each operation as well, the nerves and muscles endure additional trauma, and the growth of inflexible scar tissue increases. I'm sure by now that you can guess the result: increased pain and disability, and an ongoing nightmare for patient and physician alike. It's only necessary to have repeated surgeries if a second condition develops.

Timing is also an important aspect when considering surgery and how you wish your surgery to turn out. Most physicians now advocate waiting at least six weeks to see if your pain improves before having any surgery. In this regard, Dr. White suggests that herniated disk patients who wait less than sixty days have a better surgical prognosis than those patients who wait longer. Thus, if you elect to have this surgery, the ideal time is forty to fifty days after your leg pain began. Other patients who wait longer, undergoing disk removal after eighteen months, for example, get only half as much pain relief as those patients who have surgery earlier. In addition, if a foot drop goes on too long—more than three to six months—there is a good chance that it may never disappear, even after surgery.

Why do people do poorly if they wait too long to have surgery? One theory holds that constant compression and inflammation can irreparably scar the nerve roots. This is one reason why using anti-inflammatory substances is critical in treating a herniated disk.

Degenerative Arthritis, Degenerative Disk Disease, and Spinal Stenosis

We'll discuss these three topics together because the same process causes all three: normal wear-and-tear arthritis of the lumbar spine, also known as osteoarthritis. "Arthritis" is a general term that means joint inflammation. It can develop in any joint in the body, and at more than one site. Other names for osteoarthritis are degenerative arthritis or spondylosis. Remember that "-itis" means inflammation and, as you know, inflammation and pain go hand in hand.

Two common sites for osteoarthritis are where our vertebrae join each other at the intervertebral space (where the disk is), and at the facet joints (refer back to Chapter 4 if you've forgotten what these structures are).

There are many, less common forms of arthritis, such as rheumatoid arthritis and ankylosing spondylitis, but they all produce inflammation and pain.

Symptoms of Facet Syndrome

- Back pain, with pain going down to the knee, but *not* below (if you have pain that extends below the knee, you probably have a herniated disk).
- The back pain is made worse by bending backwards.
- Tenderness over the inflamed facet joints, just to the side of the midline of the back.

Osteoarthritis generally involves inflammation of the facet joints, which is why it's called "facet syndrome." The smooth cartilage that covers the ends of these joints starts to degenerate over time, as they lose water. Then they become inflamed, which causes pain. As inflammation increases, it affects the surrounding structures.

Inflammation of one or more of the facet joints produces back pain, along with referred pain that goes down to the knee, but not below it. That is the doctor's tip-off that you have facet syndrome instead of a herniated disk (sciatic pain from a herniated disk usually goes below the knee and may extend to the ankle and foot). If you have facet syndrome, you'll also have back pain that's made worse by bending backwards.

We can treat pain from facet syndrome very effectively with anti-inflammatory medication, either oral or injected right into the facet joint. A facet block, is a procedure in which a combination of an anesthetic and cortisone is injected right into or just around the joint.

Degenerative disk disease is a form of arthritis of the spine in which the soft central portion of the disk loses its water content. This process begins at about twenty years of age and continues throughout life. Most degenerative disk diseases cause no symptoms. Sometimes, however, people develop "mechanical low back pain," which is caused by increased activity. X rays show narrowing of the disk spaces, as well as small bony spikes (osteophytes). If degenerative disk disease advances, there can be a complete bridging of disk spaces by these bony growths.

When degenerative disk disease produces symptoms, we can treat them most effectively with anti-inflammatory medication and a good exercise program to increase muscle strength and spine flexibility. Degenerative disk disease usually doesn't require surgery.

Spinal stenosis is a narrowing of the spinal canal that runs through the vertebrae. It squeezes the spinal cord or, sometimes, just the nerve roots in the low back area. When osteoarthritis involves the facet joints, they enlarge, and this can narrow the canal and cause stenosis. Stenosis can occur in one spot, or it can run up and down the spine. It occurs in both the central canal and the space where the nerve roots exit on their paths to the arms and legs.

Symptoms of Spinal Stenosis

- Low back pain with thigh pain
- Leg cramping that is worse with walking
- Weakness
- Numbness
- Changed reflexes
- Pulses in the legs are normal, which differentiates stenosis from vascular claudication, in which there is inadequate blood supply to the legs.

Some people have a congenital (inborn) narrowing of the spinal canal. People with this condition are more prone to develop spinal stenosis from arthritis as they age.

Spinal stenosis usually occurs in people who are sixty years of age or older. Initially the symptoms are quite vague: low back pain, followed by thigh pain, as well as leg cramping that gets much worse with walking. Sitting down or just resting relieves the pain. There may also be weakness, numbness, and reflex changes. Straight leg-raising tests are usually normal (as opposed to a herniated disk, in which they are abnormal). It's important to distinguish this condition from vascular claudication, in which the blood supply to the legs is simply not sufficient, and so walking causes leg pain. For this reason, it's important that your examining physician check your pulses.

Spinal stenosis treatment involves a back exercise program and anti-inflammatory medication. If you are overweight, you should slim down, and it's usually necessary to curtail strenuous activities. We can use epidural cortisone injections, but they don't give long-lasting pain relief.

If conservative measures don't work, you may need to have a surgical procedure called a "decompressive laminectomy." With this procedure, the surgeon removes bone from the back of the spinal canal to widen it. This gives the nerves more room and relieves the pressure from the stenosis. Unlike other forms of surgery, the decompressive laminectomy works very well and has a high cure rate. Spinal stenosis shows up easily on an MRI or CT scan, and if you don't respond to conservative treatment, you can be happy about the fact that the surgical results are usually quite good.

Rheumatoid Arthritis and Ankylosing Spondylitis

When you hear the phrase rheumatoid arthritis, you probably picture a person with deformed hands and replacements for their knees, hips, and other joints. Unfortunately, rheumatoid arthritis also occurs in the spine, although it is infrequent. Routine X rays and specific blood tests that detect "rheumatoid factor" are helpful diagnostic aids here.

Ankylosing spondylitis is a form of rheumatoid arthritis that can involve the joints of the spine. It occurs predominantly in young men. Appropriate lab tests as well as X rays can diagnose it.

Both of these conditions can result in significant disability. Their

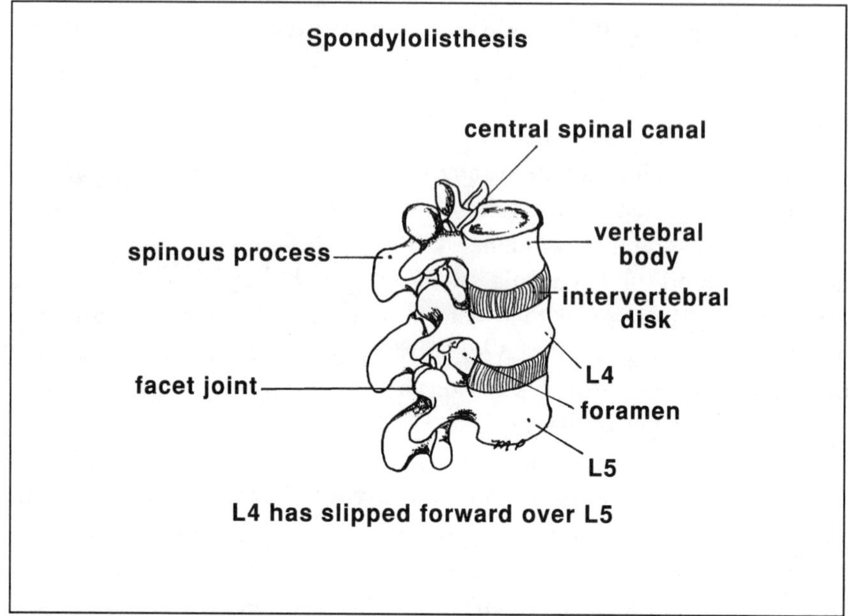

Figure 5-3

treatment involves a combination of anti-inflammatory medications and exercises. Newer medications have recently been developed for these conditions.

Spondylolisthesis and Spondylolysis

In spondylolisthesis, one vertebra slips forward over another one (see Figure 5-3). A normal spine, when viewed from the side, shows the vertebrae perfectly lined up. In spondylolisthesis, L5 has usually slipped a little bit forward onto S1, or L4 has slipped a little bit forward on L5. This is usually due to a stress fracture in a part of the vertebra called the pars interarticularis. Most people feel it occurs in childhood and doesn't heal. It has the ability to later allow the vertebra to move forward. The crack itself is called a spondylolysis, and the actual slipping is called spondylolisthesis.

As you might imagine, this condition is frequent in childhood athletes who participate in contact sports like football. We also find this condition in ballerinas and gymnasts, who stretch their backs and legs repeatedly, probably resulting in stress fractures.

Sometimes it is very hard to find the fracture on a plain X ray and we must resort to a bone scan, which will show a fracture as a small area of increased activity or a "hot spot." If a child or teenager complains of unrelenting back pain, the doctor should order a bone scan to see if spondylolysis is the culprit.

If the scan is positive, or additional X rays (or a CT scan) show a defect in the bone, the child should wear a brace for four months. Obviously, activities are also limited during this time. If the defect does not heal and allows the vertebra to slip forward later in life, it can cause a mechanical back pain that frequently requires a spinal fusion. The results of this surgery are also usually quite good.

Arachnoiditis

Earlier in this chapter, we contemplated the dismal results of most back surgery. When surgical procedures inflame and scar the tissues around the nerve roots, it causes a painful condition called arachnoiditis. (The arachnoid is one of the membranes that surrounds the nerves.)

Patients with arachnoiditis have unrelenting pain, as well as numbness and weakness from the back into the lower extremities. Unfortunately, arachnoiditis does not typically respond well to traditional therapy.

Arachnoiditis treatment involves physical therapy and exercise, as well as epidural steroid injections and oral anti-inflammatory medication. In severe cases, after all other measures fail, a device called a spinal cord stimulator, made up of electrodes and wires, may be implanted in the back. These stimulators theoretically work by blocking out painful nerve impulses. Unfortunately, they don't work very well, and we frequently have to remove them.

Remember that surgery may *cause* arachnoiditis, and the easiest way to make it worse is to have *more* surgery. Unless a new, identifiable lesion shows up that requires additional surgery, the best course is to stick *entirely* to conservative treatments.

Diskitis and Osteomyelitis

You know by now that "-itis" means inflammation. Diskitis, therefore, means inflammation of the disk. When the cause of back pain is difficult to identify, the doctor should order a bone scan. Diskitis shows up as a "hot spot."

A bacterial or viral infection between the vertebrae usually causes diskitis. Fever, malaise, and pain accompany the infection and inflammation.

Diskitis is unusual in the general population. We find it, however, with increasing frequency in injection drug addicts, as well as diabetics and individuals with immune deficiency. The appropriate treatment is high-dose antibiotics after cultures determine which bacteria is the culprit. Since the advent of antibiotics, infections of the spine have not been very common, and we have been successful in avoiding their sometimes serious complications.

The medical name for bone infection is osteomyelitis. It usually causes a gradually increasing fever, with pain over the involved area of the back, as well as severe muscle spasm and tenderness. Blood tests reveal an increase in the body's infection fighters, white blood cells—called leukocytosis—and the sed-rate is elevated. Initially, while X rays are normal, a bone scan can be more helpful. After three to four weeks of onset, however, the infection will show up on the plain X ray as a clear area, which indicates that it has destroyed bone.

Treatment involves hospitalization to culture the infection, which we treat with intravenous antibiotics. Wearing a brace to immobilize the area is also helpful. While this treatment sometimes solves the problem, if the infection is difficult to control, surgery to remove the infected tissue may be a final necessity.

Osteoporosis

Osteoporosis is a disease in which we develop thin bones because we've lost bone mass. It has become a major health problem, affecting 25 million Americans and causing approximately 1.5 million fractures per year. Fifty percent of women and 20 percent of men over the age of sixty-five eventually sustain a fracture from osteoporosis. These "compression fractures" often involve the vertebrae, but they may also involve the wrist, hip, or other areas. Hip fractures are especially dangerous for elderly people. Because of the fact that patients who have sustained hip fractures are so less mobile, up to 30 percent of them die within the first year following the fracture. This typically occurs from medical problems like pneumonia.

Women start to lose bone mass at age thirty-five, and the process speeds up rapidly when they reach menopause, usually around the age of fifty. This is because of a drop in estrogen levels, which causes an increase in bone resorption. Calcium intake, which should be about 1200 milligrams a day for nonpregnant adults, is usually closer to 450 milligrams in the typical American diet. Additional risk factors are smoking and excessive alcohol consumption.

It's possible to tell whether you have osteoporosis by taking a test called a dexa scan, which measures your bone density. The dexa scan is quite safe and perfectly painless. Afterward, when your test results are in, you can decide with your physician whether additional supplements or medications are appropriate for you. In any case, do try to prevent yourself from getting osteoporosis. A good exercise program and an appropriate diet, including food sources high in calcium and vitamin D, are an excellent way to start—if you haven't already.

Coccyx Pain

A hard fall on your tailbone can result in an extremely painful condition called coccygodynia. The coccyx is that bony structure at the very tip of the spine. It is also possible to get pain around the coccyx just from sitting for prolonged periods on a hard chair if you don't have a lot of padding on your derriere.

The correct treatment is to sit on a rubber tube for a few weeks. This will free the coccyx from touching anything and reduce local pressure around it. Anti-inflammatory medication and a local injection of an anesthetic and cortisone are frequently required. Coccygodynia can be an extremely problematic and long-lasting "pain in the butt" for many patients. Nonetheless, it does not require surgery. In fact, many people who have had their coccyx removed are frequently worse off afterward than they were before the surgery.

Cancer

When it comes to back pain, being thorough means looking for every possible cause, even when nothing readily shows up on diagnostic tests. Unfortunately, certain cancers can start in the back, and others can spread there. You sometimes have to look hard to find them.

It's possible to have a benign tumor in a vertebra—that is, a tumor that's not cancerous, but which causes pain and inflammation. Displacement of normal bony tissue can make it worse. Benign tumors are usually not much to worry about, and we can remove them easily.

Malignant tumors, however, can either start in the bone itself or spread (metastasize) to the bone from another area. Tumors that spread to bone in the spine are usually from the breast, kidney, lung, prostate, or thyroid gland.

Back pain caused by a tumor is usually worse when lying down or when trying to sleep. Generally, the bone is tender to touch. When patients state that they are awakened during their sleep by back pain, that's a clue that cancer may be present. The doctor should order a bone scan to find out. If cancer is present, it will show up as one or more "hot spots," and a biopsy will show where the cancer started. MRI, CT, and plain X rays can also show cancer. It's then possible to biopsy the vertebra using specialized needles to extract a specimen that can be looked at under a microscope. The type of treatment will depend upon the tumor, and where it came from.

If you've had back pain for a prolonged period and your physician has not ordered a bone scan, you might want to ask him or her about it. It's extremely unlikely that cancer is the cause of your problem. A bone scan will reassure you and your physician, however, that you don't have a life-threatening disease.

A sed-rate, although a very nonspecific blood test, is also a good indicator of whether or not any increased metabolic process like cancer is going on in your body. A sed-rate, therefore, is a good screening test for somebody who has back pain without an obvious cause. If the sed-rate is elevated for no apparent reason, that is a good enough reason to order a bone scan and any other studies necessary to determine why.

MISCELLANEOUS MUSCULOSKELETAL CONDITIONS

Tennis Elbow and Olecranon Bursitis

The elbow joint consists of two bony connections, or articulations. One is between the bone of the upper arm (the humerus) and one of the bones of the forearm (the ulna); the other is between the humerus and the other bone of the forearm (the radius). The elbow has inherent

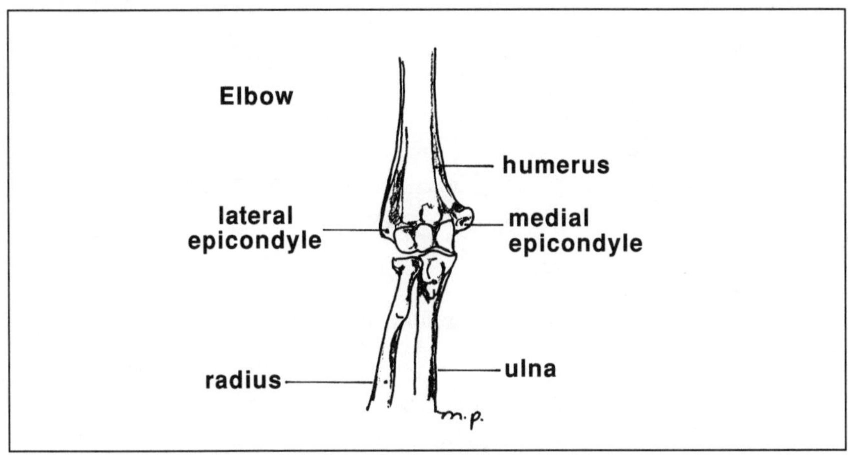

Figure 5-4

stability because of the "hinge" articulation between the humerus and the ulna. The tip of the elbow is the olecranon; the triceps muscle attaches to it (see Figure 5-4). Overuse can easily cause inflammation and pain in this area.

Tennis elbow, or lateral epicondylitis, develops when repeated strain causes inflammation in the region of the bump on the *outside* of the elbow.

Repetitive strain to the outside of the elbow can occur from a variety of activities, but we call it "tennis elbow" because physicians see it commonly in tennis players, who develop it because of repeated stress from swinging the racket, especially the backhand stroke. Tennis elbow is also common in golfers, carpenters, and people in a multitude of other occupations involving this motion.

Medial epicondylitis is an inflammation of the *inside* of the bump on the elbow, caused by overuse and by performing activities that involve repetitive wrist flexion or forearm rotation. This subsequently leads to micro-tears in the tendon; inflammation and pain follow.

Medial epicondylitis occurs when the inflammation develops at the tendon on the inside of the elbow. Though it is not as common as lateral epicondylitis, it has the potential to cause irritation and inflammation of the ulnar nerve, which is in the same area. This can cause numbness along the inside of the forearm, and the ring and little fingers. If it goes on long enough, it can cause muscle weakness and loss of fine motor coordination in the hand.

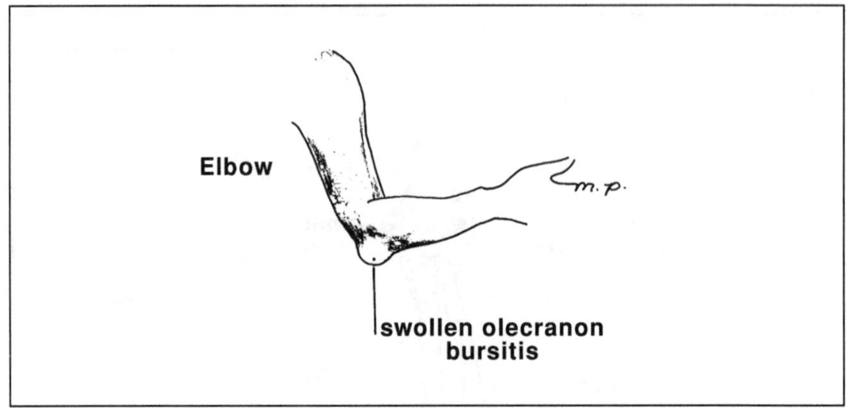

Figure 5-5

Both medial and lateral epicondylitis cause exquisite tenderness. Bending the wrist *backward* causes pain in lateral epicondylitis, and bending it *forward* causes pain in medial epicondylitis.

If the ulnar nerve is involved, there will be a positive "tingle sign": A slight tapping over the ulnar nerve produces an electrical sensation that shoots down the forearm into the hand. It also causes a "tingling" in the elbow and fingers as though you've hit your "funny bone." Nerve conduction studies are useful to confirm ulnar nerve inflammation and entrapment.

Olecranon bursitis develops in the olecranon bursa, a sac of fluid that can develop between the skin of the elbow and the tip of the elbow bone itself (see Figure 5-5).

As you can see by feeling your elbow, there is not much soft tissue coverage at its tip, and it is easily irritated and inflamed. When that happens, the bursa is injured, and we develop olecranon bursitis. The bursa fills with fluid. The inflammation causes pain and, in some cases, the bursa itself can develop a bacterial infection, so pus fills it, instead of clear fluid.

Treatment of Tennis Elbow and Bursitis

We should try to treat both of these conditions conservatively. Anti-inflammatory medication and ice massage are helpful. To compress the muscles and decrease their force on the elbow, place a strap around the upper forearm. This is a "tennis elbow brace." If the anti-inflammatory medication and brace does not work, a steroid injection into the area is usually helpful.

Physical therapy, using massage and ultrasound, is also quite helpful. Naturally, you must avoid the repetitive motions that caused the condition and you should begin an exercise program to strengthen the involved muscles, which usually reduces the chance of recurrence.

Conservative treatment almost always works on tennis elbow. In occasional cases, surgery is necessary to release the tendons. The surgery releases them so they can slide down and, therefore, exert less force.

Modifying activities and taking anti-inflammatory drugs also treats medial epicondylitis. If the ulnar nerve is involved, surgery must free it around the elbow and move it to a position in front of the elbow, where it is under less stress. This is "ulnar nerve transposition," and it's very effective.

To treat olecranon bursitis, we use a needle to remove the fluid from the enlarged and inflamed olecranon bursa. If there is an infection, which is unusual, we treat it with antibiotics and possibly surgical drainage. The best treatment is oral anti-inflammatory medications; if they don't work, we inject cortisone into the bursa, which usually works quite well. Nonetheless, if the olecranon bursa sac remains thickened and painful, we must remove it surgically. This simple operation is also usually very effective.

The Shoulder

The ability to swing a golf club or to throw a baseball is testimony to the excellent range of motion our shoulders have. Unfortunately, the shoulder can only achieve this kind of motion by sacrificing some inherent stability, which makes it extremely susceptible to injury.

Our shoulder consists of many separate, smaller joints (see Figure 5-6). The rotator cuff, which is best visualized as a large flat band of tendons that goes over the top of the upper-arm bone, stabilizes the shoulder joint. The biggest muscle in the shoulder, the deltoid, moves the arm out to the side of the shoulder. A person with a completely torn rotator cuff has difficulty in making this movement.

It's easy to injure the rotator cuff, especially by repetitive overhead lifting. One of the most common conditions we develop is "rotator cuff

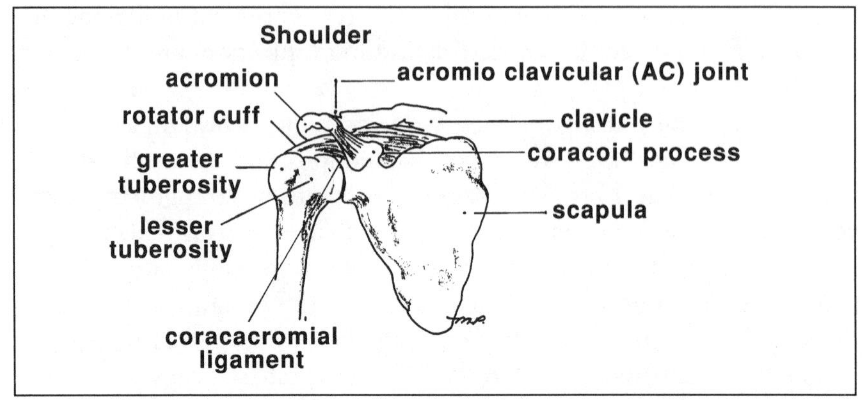

Figure 5-6

tendinitis." Inflammation often occurs during overhead lifting, when the bones squeeze the rotator cuff structures, causing "impingement syndrome."

The pain of rotator cuff tendinitis or impingement syndrome is usually in the front of the shoulder joint, but it can also radiate down the arm to the elbow. It generally occurs at night and wakes people up when they roll onto their sore shoulder.

The first line of attack in treating impingement syndrome or rotator cuff tendinitis is anti-inflammatory medications and cortisone injections to decrease inflammation. It's very important to stretch as well as strengthen the muscles that form the rotator cuff. The strengthening phase usually has to wait until the inflammation is finished because it is too painful before that. Ultrasound and massage may help to reduce inflammation.

If a rotator cuff tendinitis persists indefinitely, it is possible for the cuff itself to give way and actually tear. Continual inflammation eventually causes thinning and scarring of the rotator cuff itself, and older people are especially susceptible.

The primary tendon in the rotator cuff does not have many blood vessels supplying it. Its healing potential, therefore, is not very good, and another reason it's very susceptible to trauma. A torn rotator cuff has all the inflammatory symptoms we described earlier, but there can also be weakness when you lift or rotate the arm. If there's a large tear, you may actually have a very difficult time just holding your arm out to the side. An MRI is best for diagnosing a rotator cuff tear.

We don't always have to repair rotator cuff tears surgically. Older people, for example, function quite well with partial tears of the rotator cuff, and sometimes even with significant tears.

An impingement syndrome that doesn't respond to conservative therapy—anti-inflammatory medications, cortisone injections, and a good physical therapy program—benefits from an arthroscopic procedure called an acromioplasty. We insert instruments through small holes to widen the space between the humeral head and the acromion by grinding away some bone and thus widening the area. This relieves the pressure on the pinched rotator cuff and decreases inflammation.

Some surgeons still prefer to do this surgery openly as opposed to arthroscopically using larger incisions. Even so, the recovery period is much faster when we do it arthroscopically.

Biceps Tendinitis

The biceps muscle is the one you commonly see on the front of your arm when you "make a muscle." It has two tendons that attach it to the bone. Bicipital tendinitis involves irritation of the long head of the biceps tendon. It often occurs in people who have rotator cuff tendinitis.

Biceps tendinitis causes pain in the front of the shoulder that's aggravated by overhead lifting. There is also exquisite tenderness to touch right over the tendon itself. If this tendinitis continues too long without appropriate treatment, it is possible for the tendon to rupture, which can deform the arm.

Symptoms of Biceps Tendinitis

- Pain in the front of the shoulder that's aggravated by overhead lifting
- Tenderness to touch over the tendon
- A ruptured biceps can deform cosmetic appearance of the arm and require surgery

Treatment for biceps tendinitis involves physical therapy, anti-inflammatory medication, and local cortisone injections. Biceps tendinitis usually responds quite well to this regimen. If the tendon ever does rupture, most patients have it surgically repaired, which restores full function of the biceps muscle.

Hip Joint and Thigh

The hip is a classic ball-and-socket joint. As opposed to the shoulder, the hip is a very stable joint. Both the basic ball-and-socket configuration and the soft tissues contribute to the stability of the hip. Very thick, ligamentlike structures make up the "capsule" of the hip that surrounds the bones.

Trochanteric Bursitis

Trochanteric bursitis is an inflammation of the lubricating sac located between the bump on the outside of the hipbone called the greater trochanter and the tendons of some of the muscles around the hip joint. Flexing the hip repetitively and direct pressure over the bone aggravate this condition. Pain is usually on the outside or lateral aspect of the hip.

A disturbance in gait causes 95 percent of cases of trochanteric bursitis. There are many reasons why someone may have an abnormal gait. It could be due to lumbar disk disease, leg length inequality, or disorders of the sacroiliac joint, or it could be idiopathic. Any abnormal pattern of walking or standing has the potential to increase friction or to cause uneven contractions of the hip muscles. Both of these situations lead to an irritation of the bursa. The hip develops bursitis just like other parts of the body.

Trochanteric bursitis causes pain over the outer thigh and difficulty walking. It's not unusual to see a person with trochanteric bursitis rubbing the outside of the thigh in the region of the hip, as if to help relieve pain. It is also common to have pain when lying on the side on a hard surface, or even when rolling over in bed onto the affected hip. Standing for prolonged periods can be problematic because this causes muscle contraction, which increases tension and inflammation at the site of the bursitis.

This condition is easy to diagnose: Pressure over the greater trochanter causes the patient to jump. Obviously, as with any type of joint pain, the physician should do a full examination, even if you have this very identifiable response to pressure.

Table 5-2
MISCELLANEOUS MUSCULOSKELETAL CONDITIONS

Condition	What It Is
Tennis elbow	Also known as lateral epicondylitis. Inflammation of the tendons attaching to the lateral epicondyle. Results from repetitive extension of the wrist
Biceps tendinitis	Inflammation of the tendon that attaches the large biceps muscle in the upper part of the arm to the shoulder. Produces shoulder pain
Trochanteric bursitis	Pain on the outside of the hip caused by inflammation of a lubricating sac between the tendons and the bone
Costochondritis	Chest pain caused by inflammation of the joints where the ribs attach to the sternum
Chondromalacia	Softening of the cartilage on the back of the kneecap (patella). Most common in adolescents. Causes pain in the front of the knee.
Prepatellar bursitis and patellar tendinitis	Inflammation of the patellar tendon (tendinitis) or of the bursal sac (prepatellar bursitis) in front of the kneecap
Pes anserine bursitis	Pain on the inside of the knee caused by an inflammation of tendons and bursa in this area
Ankle sprain	A stretching or tearing of the supporting ligaments of the ankle joint
Heel spur and plantar fascitis	Inflammation that develops where the plantar fascia attaches to the heel bone (calcaneous). If it continues long enough a heel spur forms in that location.
Achilles tendinitis	An inflammation of the Achilles tendon where it attaches to the calcaneous or where the calf muscle attaches to the tendon.

Even with such joint pain, X rays are usually normal. In long-standing cases, however, some flecks of calcification are sometimes visible near the outer aspect of the hip.

The goal of treatment is to reduce inflammation in the area of the bursa, as well as to correct any underlying abnormalities. For example, if a leg-length discrepancy is the cause of an abnormal gait, you should get an appropriate shoe lift. As with other inflammatory conditions, you should treat it with anti-inflammatory medications and physical therapy, including exercises to stretch the muscle and to decrease the tension.

Costochondritis

Many people complain of chest pain, but it comes from the heart in only a minority of cases. One of the most common causes of chest pain is inflammation of the chest wall cartilage.

The cartilage, which attaches all of the ribs to the breastbone (sternum), is an extremely common site of inflammation. This can be extremely painful, not to mention scary, because the patient frequently fears that he or she is having a heart attack.

It's easy to distinguish this condition from cardiac pain because there is direct pain when you touch the ribs where they attach to the breastbone. In severe cases, there can also be swelling, or Tietze's syndrome. Your doctor should perform an electrocardiogram (EKG) and other tests if there is any doubt as to whether or not the pain is coming from your heart.

The treatment of costochondritis involves anti-inflammatory medication and, if necessary, local steroid injections over the tender areas. Phonophoresis, a procedure in which a gel containing hydrocortisone is massaged into the affected area using an ultrasound machine, can be quite helpful in this condition.

While frightening because of the location and intensity of the pain, the vast majority of cases of costochondritis improve by themselves within four to six weeks. Most often, even injections are not necessary. If you have this condition, don't worry; it may hurt but it's not serious.

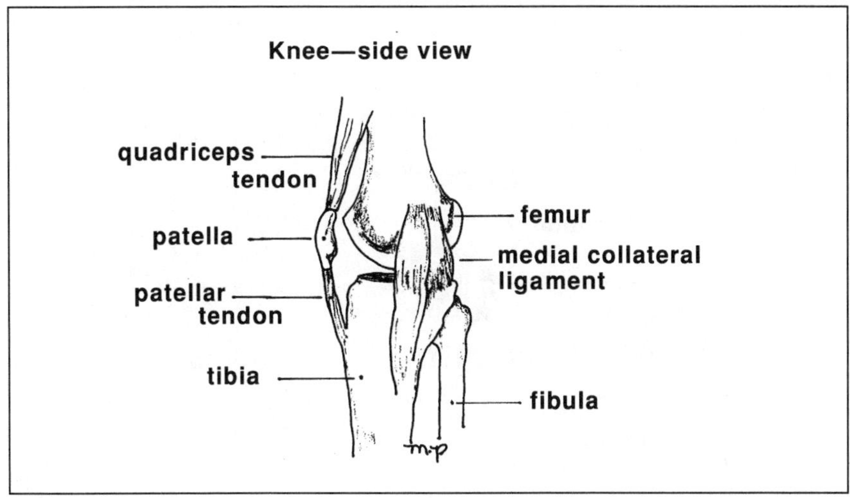

Figure 5-7

Inflammatory Conditions of the Knee

The knee joint is a complex hinge joint that needs both stability and mobility. A gliding and rotational motion accompanies the knee's hinge-type motion. Both are necessary for the many athletic endeavors we engage in.

The joint itself is composed of the femur above and the tibia below (see Figure 5-7).

A smooth, gliding type of cartilage, hyaline cartilage, covers the ends of these bones. Like all joints, the knee has a synovial membrane, which secretes fluid to lubricate the joint. The knee can develop degenerative arthritis as well as many other forms of arthritis.

Because the knee joint relies on ligaments for stability, these ligaments are stressed and frequently injured.

Patella Problems

The patella is the kneecap. It lies in a groove on the front of the femur and, in the best of all possible worlds, tracks smoothly when you bend and extend the knee (see Figure 5-8).

Since all of us are a little bit knock-kneed (this is normal), the patella is often pulled toward the outside of the leg as the knee bends. If you

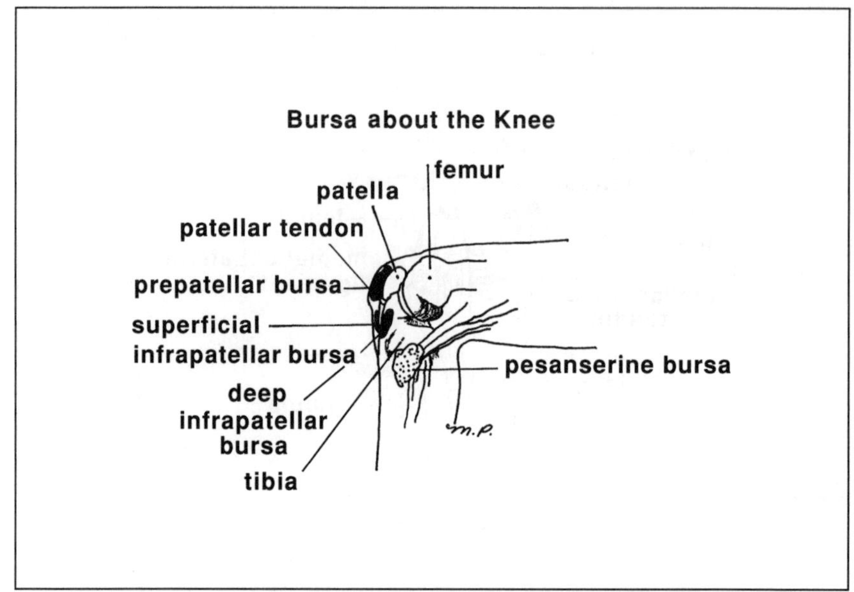

Figure 5-8

are more knock-kneed than typical, there is a good chance that you will be subject to a patella femoral disorder. The most common complaints are generalized front-knee pain, giving way of the knee, and pain when going up or down stairs. Abnormal moving of the patella over the front of the femur causes irritation, inflammation, cartilage breakdown, and pain.

Chondromalacia patellae is a condition that involves degeneration of the back of the patella, where it rides along the front of the femur. An increased knock-kneed deformity or misalignment of the patella causes this condition to develop faster because of increased forces on the kneecap. However, it can also occur in individuals with no tracking problems at all.

You can develop chondromalacia from direct trauma to the knee, like hitting your kneecap on the dashboard of your car. However, it is more commonly the result of repetitive irritation from abnormal tracking. Runners know this quite well, as it is the most common cause of knee pain they suffer. For that reason, we call it "runner's knee." If you are a jogger and develop knee pain, statistically, you most likely have chondromalacia.

The doctor diagnoses chondromalacia by having you lie on your back and pushing your kneecap toward the outside of the leg, pressing on the back of it. It will be quite tender and painful if chondromalacia is the problem. In advanced cases, bending and extending the knee reveals a grinding sensation underneath the patella itself, as if there were sand in the joint.

Treating Chondromalacia Patellae

- Anti-inflammatory medication
- Strengthening exercises for the quadriceps muscle
- Arthroscopy to shave down uneven cartilage on the back of the patella that's causing the inflammation

As with other inflammatory conditions and arthritis disorders, our first line of defense is anti-inflammatory medication. Exercises that strengthen the quadriceps muscle on the front of the thigh are essential. When this muscle gets stronger, it stabilizes the patella and the pain usually decreases.

If conservative treatments are unsuccessful, you will probably need arthroscopy, which has good results. When your physician looks into the knee with an arthroscope, he or she will see what appears to look like crab meat hanging down from the back of the patella. This "crab meat" is actually broken up cartilage. It it's there, we'll remove it surgically with what is known as the patella shaver. This is used to smooth down the cartilage on the back of the kneecap. With this type of surgery and a good exercise program, you shouldn't have too much to worry about. The success rate here rises to nearly 80 percent.

In advanced cases in older people with severe degenerative arthritis of the back of the kneecap (patellar femoral arthritis), sometimes it is even necessary to remove the patella itself. Although this sounds drastic, it is totally possible to live without a patella and function quite normally. It produdes a cosmetic defect and perhaps a bit of weakness. Be that as it may, most people function quite normally after surgery.

Patellar Tendinitis and Prepatellar Bursitis

The patella tendon is a band of connective tissue that goes from the patella itself to the front of the shinbone (the tibia). As with other tendons subjected to repetitive motion, this one can develop an inflammatory condition, patellar tendinitis, where the patellar tendon attaches to the bones. Its treatment is similar to that of other cases of tendinitis we have discussed.

Prepatellar bursitis is a painful thickening of the sac overlying the patella, under the skin. Trauma, like bumping your knee, or a penetrating wound that causes an infection in the bursa itself, can cause it. This can happen if you kneel down on a foreign object, like a piece of metal or glass and, a few days later, you might notice that your knee has grown hot and swollen.

The doctor diagnoses what type of bursitis you have by withdrawing some fluid from the bursa and looking at it under a microscope. If he or she sees bacteria and an extremely high number of white blood cells, the diagnosis is infection. If the fluid simply shows a moderate number of white cells and no bacteria, then irritation is the culprit. We must treat infections aggressively with antibiotics and, frequently, surgical drainage. If it is simply an inflammation, you can treat it as we have already described.

Pes Anserine Bursitis

Since so many baby boomers started jogging, a whole new range of inflammations in the knee has become more frequent. Pes anserine bursitis is an inflammation of the bursal sac, which is located on the inside of the knee under a group of tendons called the pes anserinis.

This condition produces pain on the inside of the knee, just below the joint. It is extremely tender to touch. The most common cause is an abnormal gait. Although normal activity like walking doesn't stress the mechanical relationships between the knee, hip, and pelvis, joggers are frequently subject to multiple problems because they stretch many structures beyond the normal limits of a sedentary life.

Treatment includes anti-inflammatory medication and, if necessary, a steroid injection to the painful site. Combined with an anesthetic, this treatment confirms the diagnosis because the injection takes all the pain

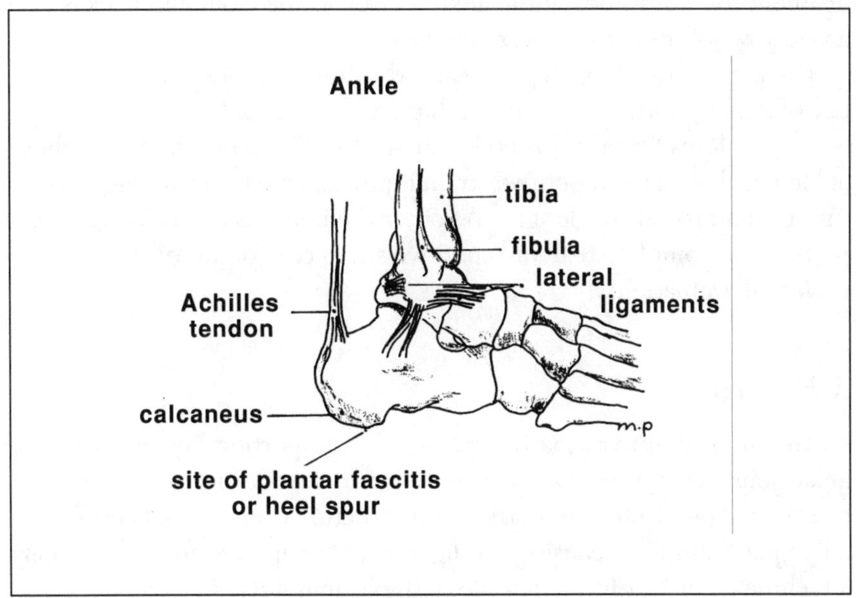

Figure 5-9

away. Applying ice is helpful in alleviating acute symptoms. You shouldn't squat, kneel, or bend your knee repeatedly, because these motions all aggravate this problem. As with other inflammatory conditions, physical therapy is helpful.

Ankle and Foot

The design of the ankle is better than that of any other joint in the body. We're lucky that it is, because the ankle bears up to five times our body weight with just normal walking. It is a complex hinge joint. The bony configuration of the ankle provides its stability, along with a complex structure of ligaments that further reinforce the joint (see Figure 5-9).

It's important that the two bones of the lower leg, the tibia and fibula, don't separate during athletic activities, or we'd develop tremendous instability. The ankle ligaments also maintain the correct distance between the tibia and fibula.

A single strong ligament reinforces the inside of the ankle, and a vast complex of ligaments stabilizes the outside. Along with this multitude of ligaments on both sides of the ankle as well as the front and back is also a vast array of tendons, nerves, and blood vessels.

The popularity of jogging has caused a dramatic increase in the number of ankle disorders, as it has in hip and knee problems. It may cause acute problems like a ruptured ligament. In many cases, however, these ankle problems are "repetitive strain injuries," due to stretching a structure beyond its normal length. Whether the injury is a microscopic tear, partial tear, complete tear, or repetitive strain type of injury, it always involves inflammation.

Ankle Sprain

An ankle sprain is a partial tear of the supporting ligaments of the ankle joint. Inversion (when your foot turns underneath you) usually causes it. You stretch and stress the structures on the outside of the ankle joint and foot, causing the ligaments to separate from their bony attachments or tear in the middle of the ligament itself.

Many "weekend warriors" make the big mistake of treating an ankle sprain as a minor injury. An ankle sprain can be a very serious injury because, if ligaments don't heal back into their taut position, the result is chronic instability. This may require surgery later to reinforce and replace ligaments that could have healed properly the first time if they had been treated appropriately.

> Why is ankle instability so serious? First of all, it is very difficult to walk on an ankle joint in which the bones are not tightly attached. Second, the abnormal motion between the bones in an unstable joint will eventually lead to advanced arthritis of that same joint.

There are three grades of ankle sprains. Grade One involves a stretch in the ligaments but no actual tear. Upon testing, the ankle has no instability. A Grade Two sprain involves some tearing of ligaments but still no ankle instability. Grade Three injuries involve not only a complete tearing of the ligaments but also gross instability of the ankle.

An ankle sprain produces pain, swelling, bruising, and "giving way" of the ankle. In some cases, we take stress X rays to compare the injured side to the normal side. In a bad sprain with instability, an abnormal space is present between the bones. Your doctor will most likely check to make sure that there hasn't been any separation between the tibia and the fibula at the ankle joint, because this can create serious instability.

Why is instability such a problem? First, it's very difficult to walk on an ankle joint that has loose bones. Second, the abnormal motion between the bones in an unstable joint will eventually lead to advanced arthritis in that joint.

In treating an ankle sprain, your goal is clear: having the ligaments of the ankle reattach to their normal bony sites. Elevating your ankle and placing ice compresses on it for the first few days will help to decrease swelling and pain.

Treating an Ankle Sprain

- All sprains: Elevation, ice, anti-inflammatory drugs, staying off the ankle, using a brace, Ace bandage, and crutches, if necessary.
- Grade One and Two: Anti-inflammatory drugs, a brace to immobilize the joint, crutches (if necessary), and an exercise program.
- Grade Three: A short leg cast for six weeks, along with all the treatments used in Grade One and Two, as appropriate and as the ankle heals.

Grade One and Two sprains may be treated with a brace that provides some degree of stability while allowing minimal upward and downward motion at the ankle joint, immobilizing the joint so it can't be reinjured. We also prescribe anti-inflammatory drugs. As swelling decreases, your doctor should also give you a range-of-motion exercise program along with a muscle-strengthening program.

You will soon be able to gradually resume your athletic activities but don't be impatient. It takes about six weeks for connective tissue to heal. In many cases, it takes several months for the swelling to disappear completely and, therefore, it's hard to predict how long it will be until the weekend warrior can resume his or her weekend activities at full tilt.

Grade Three injuries, which are associated with instability of the ankle, require complete immobilization, like a short leg cast, for six weeks. Usually, you'll be able to bear weight on the cast after approximately two weeks, since the cast immobilizes the ankle and the ligaments will not move. They will hopefully heal in their normal position and restore the stability to the ankle.

Some people have recurrent ankle sprains. A careful physical examination, possibly with the use of stress X rays, confirms a diagnosis of chronic instability. Immobilization in a cast will not help a chronically unstable ankle to heal. Surgery is necessary, in which a tendon is used to make new ligaments that attach to the bones through drill holes. It is impossible to sew together torn ends of a chronically torn ligament. Although the results of ankle reconstructive surgery are quite good, extensive physical therapy is still necessary to achieve the best possible result.

Heel Spurs (Plantar Fascitis)

Heel pain is a common affliction of mankind. It is also quite difficult to treat.

The problem is an inflammation of the ligament that runs along the sole of the foot and creates the arch. That ligament starts on the heel bone (calcaneus). Poorly fitting shoes, walking on concrete, prolonged standing, and obesity are all factors that contribute to the development of heel spurs.

How does it happen? A chronic inflammatory process develops where the ligament attaches to the heel bone. If the inflammation continues long enough, a heel spur forms in that location. The heel spur itself is not really the cause of the discomfort, but is more or less a sign that there is a chronic inflammation.

The Causes of Heel Spurs

- Poorly fitting shoes
- Obesity
- Walking on concrete
- Prolonged standing

Heel pain is exceptionally disabling in the morning. One of the most painful moments you can have is getting out of bed and putting the first pressure on the heel. The pain gradually improves during the day, but any increased activity can exacerbate tenderness on the bottom of the heel. If you are thin enough, you can actually feel the heel spur.

If you have heel spurs, be conservative in your treatment, using anti-inflammatory medications and a heel cup. The heel cup is a rigid plastic structure that fits inside the shoe and squeezes the soft tissue on either side of the heel, increasing the thickness of the padding under the heel spur itself. Heel cups are quite wonderful mechanisms and are actually more effective than expensive orthotics in most cases.

It generally takes steroid injections to cure this condition. As you might imagine, these injections are very painful, because skin on the heel is quite thick and can be difficult to penetrate. More than one injection is frequently necessary, and for that reason, find a doctor you trust to treat you gently.

Heel spurs occasionally require surgery. But be aware that this surgery can sometimes be difficult, with more pain occurring afterward than before. Newer surgical techniques using arthroscopy are showing increased promise, but avoid surgery whenever you can.

Achilles Tendinitis

The Achilles tendon attaches the muscle mass in the back of the calf to the heel bone. Contracting the major calf muscle allows us to flex our foot and stand up on our toes. This tendon can be the site of many problems though, particularly in athletes like basketball players (even weekend amateurs).

In fact, it's quite common to sustain a total rupture of the Achilles tendon. This usually occurs as your foot is forced upward while you are contracting the muscles that push it downward. These antagonistic forces pull the Achilles tendon apart. The usual site of rupture is one to three inches from where the tendon attaches into the heel bone. For a total rupture, surgical repair is the only way to go.

Achilles tendinitis, on the other hand, has a slow, rather than an abrupt, onset. This is an inflammation of the junction where the muscle attaches to the tendon or where the tendon attaches to the heel. It is due to repetitive irritation and persistent inflammation that may lead to micro-tears. It's common in runners who don't stretch properly before running. The most immediate symptom is pain behind the ankle that is worsened by walking, running, or even prolonged standing.

What type of running shoes you wear are very important here. If the heel on your running shoe is lower than the heel on your everyday shoe, this places increased stress on the tendon. When runners compete in races, some runners may also use heels that are lower than their usual training shoes. This is one reason Achilles tendinitis often follows participation in a race that wouldn't have caused a problem if the runner had simply been using his or her normal running shoes, with a higher heel.

Treatment should decrease inflammation as well as increase flexibility in the calf muscles. Your doctor will most certainly prescribe anti-inflammatory drugs. A heel lift can be quite helpful by decreasing stretch on the Achilles tendon and, therefore, aid in the healing process. Using heel lifts on a regular basis helps some patients with chronic Achilles tendinitis.

Ice massage and phonophoresis (described above) are also helpful. Although Achilles tendinitis can drag on for months, it will gradually improve with time. It's important to get it under control because tendinitis that persists for prolonged periods can eventually cause the tendon to rupture.

Although steroid injections are helpful for many tendon conditions, you should avoid injections for Achilles tendinitis, because they can cause this tendon to rupture.

There are many standard medical treatments for these and other conditions; let's explore them now, before we enter the exciting world of alternative therapies. See Table 5-2 for a summary of the conditions discussed in this section.

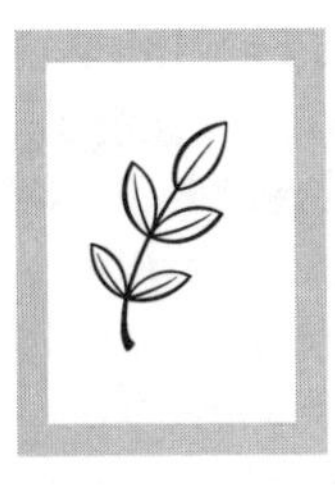

CHAPTER 6

TRADITIONAL MEDICAL TREATMENT OF COMMON BACK PROBLEMS

Most of us think that there is *always* a definitive, objective link between injury and pain. In reality, however, the amount of pain we experience is not always proportionate to the severity of the injury and, in fact, pain doesn't always result from physical damage. This is why we've adopted the Gate Control Theory of Pain, as we discussed in Chapter 2.

In some joint problems, the link between the amount of physical damage and the severity of symptoms is obvious, as we discussed in Chapter 5. We know, for example, that throwing a baseball over and over again for days on end will probably give you pain in the elbow or shoulder. In this case, the link between injury and pain is easy to see.

We've learned from chronic pain conditions like fibromyalgia, however, that there *isn't* always a definite relationship between injury and pain. In the majority of fibromyalgia patients, the injury occurred so long ago that we can't even relate it to the pain we need to treat now.

Research shows that numerous factors influence the amount and type of pain we experience, including our previous experiences with pain, our remembrances of them, and our ability to understand the cause of our pain. Education plays a vital role in this latter factor.

Although *Nature's Pain Killers* describes both natural and traditional anti-inflammatory and antipain substances, we have one goal in using all these substances—to diminish pain. As you now know, a direct link exists between inflammation and pain. While the pain experience is different for every individual, its root organic cause is usually inflammation.

Acute pain syndromes are easier to treat than chronic ones are. They generally have a definable cause, and we know from experience that, if we attack them aggressively without wasting any time, the results are quite good. We can cure the pain you feel and help you avoid developing a chronic pain syndrome.

Unfortunately, many people have chronic pain syndromes, and they require every tool we possess, both traditional and alternative, to treat their pain. Combining traditional and alternative medicine can provide the best of both worlds to both patient and physician. Many refer to this as "integrative medicine," since it integrates the two methods.

As caregivers, whether we're using traditional or alternative means, quality care, patient rights, caring, and making ethical decisions are uppermost in our minds. Each has an important role in determining the effectiveness of a pain management program. Caring, particularly, is integral to quality health care and it's a fundamental patient right, as well. As caregivers, we must educate ourselves about every traditional, alternative, and new form of treatment that might possibly help. We need to communicate to our patients that his or her wellness is our most important concern.

> Time is perhaps the most important part of the patient-doctor interaction. Doctors must spend time studying all the different methods available to help a patient, and then spend a lot of time talking with the patient about every aspect of the current problem, as well as about his or her life in general.

This kind of care stands in direct opposition to the experiences of so many patients whose office visits end without them having had a chance to speak up, or being given an opportunity to become a member of a "treatment team" with their physicians.

It all goes back to the basic patient-doctor interaction. It may not make much scientific sense, but anyone who has been in practice long enough will tell you that patients who have a true affinity with their physicians improve much faster than those who feel virtually abandoned by their doctors. It is almost as if the patient wants to get better to please the doctor, because the patient knows that the doctor cares about him or her and his or her family.

Time is perhaps the most important part of the doctor-patient interaction. Doctors (and other health-care providers) must spend time studying all the different methods available to help a patient, and then spend time talking with the patient about every aspect of the current problem, as well as about his or her life in general.

A hands-on approach is the second-most-important element to the doctor-patient interaction. It's simply impossible to determine what's wrong with an individual by sitting across the room and taking a quick history. It's necessary to palpate the muscles and take the time to look for trigger points and muscle spasm. An accurate diagnosis cannot be made by X rays alone either. Nor will the most sophisticated MRI unit replace the value of a thorough doctor-patient rapport.

Unfortunately, health-care professionals who are sensitive to these issues haven't risen up in a large group to challenge the way many doctors treat patients. Only a very human connection between physician and patient will allow for an accurate diagnosis to proceed smoothly to a successful treatment regimen.

> The only truly effective way to overcome pain is to do something about it yourself. Your plight will generally improve when you exercise regularly, make an effort to change your outlook, and attempt to place pain low on the scale of significant aspects of your life. In other words, you must change your attitude by changing how you respond to pain.

In the last two decades, we've made major breakthroughs in health care. Believe it or not, much of our current knowledge about pain-management techniques dates only to the mid-1970s.

As we've discussed, traditional methods often are not effective in treating chronic pain (see Table 6-1). We've been thoroughly conditioned to believe that there's a pill for every symptom we suffer, but that is not always true for chronic pain (although, of course, some medications are necessary, as we discussed in Chapter 1). Nevertheless, this belief leads to a large segment of the population becoming overly dependent on doctors and drugs.

Mental attitude contributes significantly to chronic pain. The only truly effective way to overcome pain is to do something about it yourself. Your plight will generally improve when you exercise regularly, make an effort to change your outlook, and attempt to place pain low on the scale of significant aspects of your life. In other words, you must change your attitude.

It's not wise to stop any kind of treatment you've been undergoing for a long period unless your doctor approves stopping it. Nevertheless, total reliance on any drug is unwise when, as you now know, our bodies make natural chemicals that fight pain effectively. Some drugs actually inhibit the body's ability to heal itself and, naturally, we should avoid them.

Despite the fact that we spend increasing amounts on health care every year, the statistics quite clearly reveal that people are turning to alternative or integrative medicine in record-breaking numbers. As a matter of fact, some therapies once thought to be on the fringe of established medicine are now so accepted that it would really be improper to consider them "alternative." For example, a significant percentage of the medical profession has viewed the fields of chiropractic and osteopathy with disdain in the past. Today, both are completely acceptable to most M.D.s. The same is true of relaxation therapy, acupuncture, and many other alternative treatments. We owe much of this new attitude to the practitioners who are beginning to recognize that our physical problems frequently have emotional, mental, and spiritual underpinnings that treatment must address. We should think of ourselves as being made up of these four parts—physical, emotional, mental, and spiritual—in an environment composed of home and family, work, hobbies, and social activities.

In this chapter, we'll examine traditional medical treatment of common back conditions, before we plunge into the world of integrative medicine.

ANTI-INFLAMMATORY MEDICATIONS

As their name implies, anti-inflammatory medications reduce inflammation. In Chapter 1, we described the inflammatory process, how it causes pain, and how anti-inflammatory medicines interrupt pain signals. If you've forgotten the details, please refer back to Chapter 1 for a complete description of the inflammatory process, and how NSAIDs and steroids work.

MUSCLE RELAXANTS

Many musculoskeletal system disorders, as we've discussed, produce muscle spasm, which is not only painful but can also be disabling. Repetitive stress injury, traumas that result in inflammation, and chronic back pain all involve muscle spasm.

> Practitioners generally agree that when muscle relaxants work, the patient may appear to be a little bit woozy. He or she is not really drunk, of course, but is responding to the drugs' sedative effects. Many strong muscle relaxants cause not only lassitude but, over time may cause depression. Mental functioning slows, so patients taking muscle relaxants should not drive or use heavy machinery. Naturally, you should *never* mix muscle relaxants with alcohol.

Many researchers think that muscle spasm is a natural, protective mechanism that the body uses to help heal itself. Unfortunately, the spasm does produce pain. Anti-inflammatory medications ease much of this pain by taking care of the inflammation. The spasm usually dissipates as the underlying condition heals. It's only when muscle spasm is *the prominent feature* of a problem that we need to use muscle relaxants.

In general, we should use muscle relaxants sparingly because they have a host of unwanted side effects. Another drawback to muscle relaxants is that many act on the brain. Causing relaxation in the central nervous system, for instance, makes the muscles in outlying areas relax. Other types of muscle relaxants act in the muscles themselves. However, even these drugs cause changes in the central nervous system. Practitioners generally agree that when muscle relaxants work, the patient appears to be a little bit drunk. He or she is not really drunk, of course, but is responding to the drugs' sedative effects. You should also note that muscle relaxants cause not only lassitude but, over time, may cause depression. Mental functioning slows, so patients taking muscle relaxants should not drive or use heavy machinery. Naturally, mixing muscle relaxants with alcohol is a "no-no."

It's best to use muscle relaxants in the evening, if you need to use them, for insomnia caused by muscle spasm pain. Muscle spasm can interrupt rapid eye movement (REM) sleep, the deep sleep we need to feel refreshed in the morning. If you are unable to rest at night, then a short course (seven to ten days) of a muscle relaxant before bedtime can be helpful.

In the past, some practitioners used antianxiety agents like Valium to reduce muscle spasm. If these medications work, it's a good clue that your pain may be stress-related, and you should pay attention to that. In addition, antianxiety medications can be addictive, and they also may cause depression in the long run.

Quite simply, muscle relaxants (or antianxiety drugs) are not necessary to treat back pain. Anti-inflammatory medications remain our first line of defense, and if chronic spasm is an important factor in pain, other avenues like biofeedback and relaxation training are better choices than mind-altering medications.

ANALGESICS (PAIN MEDICATIONS)

As health-care providers and people who genuinely try to care for our patients' well-being, one of the most frustrating problems we face is caring for people who have been prescribed tremendous amounts of narcotics for a condition (like a simple lumbar strain) that didn't need them. Narcotics are among the most widely used medications for back pain. Unfortunately, these drugs often hurt more than they help. Narcotic analgesics *are* necessary in some circumstances; treating cancer pain is an example of when we require narcotics. In the vast majority of musculoskeletal conditions, however, they should be used only infrequently and for a short time. In fact, pain relievers are rarely necessary for more than two or three days.

Pain medications range from over-the-counter drugs like Tylenol to narcotics like morphine and the synthetic morphine derivatives. Most of them are unnecessary, since anti-inflammatory medication will alleviate pain. Narcotics like Hydrocodone, codeine, and Percodan, for example, are almost never necessary to treat back pain. If your pain is severe and incapacitating, they may be useful for two to three days only. They also keep postoperative pain in check. However, they should never be used alone, but always in conjunction with other treatments.

> Many chronic back pain patients' primary problem is addiction to narcotics. Some practitioners find it easier to prescribe narcotics than to listen to their patients' problems. The body rapidly accommodates to the medication's effects, and larger doses are needed over time to gain the same pain relief. This is called tolerance.

Pain killers produce many side effects, including nausea, lethargy, constipation, depression, sedation, and the potential for addiction and/or tolerance. Even Tylenol, the most widely used over-the-counter analgesic, can cause deadly liver damage with excessive use.

Many chronic back pain patients' primary problem is addiction to narcotics. In fact, there are some practitioners who find it easier to prescribe narcotics than to listen to their patients' problems and attempt to deal with them. So, as the body rapidly accommodates to the medication's effects, larger doses are needed over time to gain the same pain relief, and the patient's tolerance level rises.

The symptoms of dependence frequently follow those of tolerance. When you stop taking the narcotic, you may develop sleep disturbance, cramps, and agitation as a result of your withdrawal from the narcotic.

The entire medical community does not share the views we have expressed here. Many physicians are strong believers in pain medication and feel that most pain is not adequately treated and, occasionally, they are correct.

For example, a person who has an acute herniated lumbar disk may develop severe low back pain with unrelenting pain down the leg. Because this pain may not be relieved by NSAIDs alone, narcotics will be necessary, along with bed rest and physical therapy. The chance of becoming addicted to narcotics during a *short course* of therapy is quite small. It is thus safe to take sufficient doses of narcotics for short periods when absolutely necessary.

In more serious cases, like those of bone cancer, we do need to use long-term narcotic therapy. Cancer in the spine often causes compression fractures and constant, incapacitating back pain. In response we use several narcotics, like Oxycontin, for long-term treatment.

Chronic low back pain in the absence of a serious injury, however, does not require narcotics. Chronic pain patients who take narcotics experience all the toxicities and side effects of these medications, but none of their benefits. Before other, more natural therapies like stress reduction can work, however, the person must rid his or her system of the narcotics he or she has been taking. The physical and mental problems that accompany prolonged narcotic use can easily hinder the capacity of other treatments to help patients with chronic low back pain.

ANTIDEPRESSANTS

Unlike narcotics, antidepressants are useful in treating chronic pain, which can severely affect a person's social, emotional, and financial condition. People who suffer from chronic pain also frequently fall prey to clinical depression. And why shouldn't they? They seem to face an unbeatable, ever-present foe. Adding clinical depression to chronic pain, however, can make for a very serious set of conditions that affects both bodily and mental health.

Depressed people commonly develop anxiety and feel "jittery" a good deal of the time. Some may have out-and-out panic attacks with feelings of vertigo, rapid breathing, and fears of asphyxiation. More commonly, chronic pain patients feel sad, irritable, and worried. Anxiety, however, will cause additional muscle spasm, which creates more pain, resulting in a vicious cycle that must be taken seriously and dealt with appropriately.

> Antidepressant medications have many side affects, including constipation, fatigue, and bladder emptying problems. Newer antidepressants, the selective serotonin reuptake inhibitors (SSRIs) like Prozac, have fewer side effects. The sedative effect of many antidepressants which is a drawback during the day, can be overcome by taking the medication in one dose just before bedtime.

For people with chronic pain, antidepressants work like analgesics. They relieve pain by affecting two neurotransmitters, norephinephrine and serotonin. As you may recall, our neurotransmitters act like ferries at nerve synapses, the place where one nerve cell meets another. The neurotransmitters carry messages from cell to cell, including those that make for pain or pleasure.

Many antidepressants act like sedatives as well. When taken at night they allow patients with chronic pain to rest and to sleep more comfortably. Indeed, getting more restful sleep not only improves our coping abilities upon waking, but our capacities to heal as well. Nonetheless, antidepressant medications have many side effects that you may not enjoy, including constipation, fatigue, and problems with bladder emptying. The newer antidepressants, the selective serotonin reuptake inhibitors (SSRIs) like Paxil and Zoloft do have fewer side effects, although reliance on them and addiction to them can be difficult to distinguish. Their sedative effect of some, which is definitely a drawback during the day, can be overcome by taking the medication in one dose just before bedtime.

If other, more natural methods of pain relief haven't worked, trying antidepressant therapy may be an option. Still, trying something and having it work can be different things. However reasonable it may seem, there is no absolute guarantee that this kind of drug therapy will work for *you* or *your* particular kind of pain.

EPIDURAL INJECTIONS

The dura is a sac that surrounds the nerve roots in the lower spine. One very effective method of treating mild nerve root compression produced by a herniated disk or spinal stenosis is having your physician inject steroids and an anesthetic agent into the epidural space just outside the dura. Medication injected into this space has a direct anti-inflammatory effect on the nerve roots, as well as on other connective tissues in the area.

Physicians used epidural injections for years to anesthetize the pelvic area and the legs, especially during childbirth. Epidural injection is similar to spinal anesthetic, except that the anesthetic agent is placed outside the membrane ("epi" means "outside"), rather than inside. It's not necessary to make a hole in the dura and, therefore, side effects like

Table 6-1
TRADITIONAL TREATMENTS FOR LOW BACK PAIN

Treatment	Used to Treat	Advantages	Disadvantages
Muscle relaxants	Condition in which muscle spasm is the primary cause of the problem	Stop muscle spasm Aid in sleep deprivation	Many act on the central nervous system and cause lethargy. Long-term use may cause lassitude and depression
Anti-anxiety drugs like Valium.	Used to treat some types of chronic pain and anxiety related disorders	Produce muscle relaxation and reduce anxiety. If effective it's a sign that the problem may be stress related	These medications can cause lassitude, depression and may be addictive
Narcotics	Used for acute pain from surgery or severe sciatica or cancer	Used for short periods of time they can be very helpful	Many side effects including nausea, constipation, lethargy, tolerance, and addiction.
Antidepressants	Chronic pain and the depression that frequently accompanies it	Can be very effective when used for chronic pain by affecting neurotransmitter levels	Side effects of lassitude, constipation, fatigue and so forth
Epidural injections	Lumbar spine conditions like herniated disks, arachnoiditis, and spinal stenosis	May be an alternative to surgery when effective	Long-term effectiveness not guaranteed
Facet joint injections	Used to treat facet syndrome	May relieve mechanical back pain from facet syndrome	Long-term effectiveness not guaranteed
Laminectomy and diskectomy	Herniated disk pressing on a nerve root	Very effective for definite herniated disk with significant neurological deficit	Possibility of a bad result—could be worse after surgery
Traction	Muscle spasm	Noninvasive	Most studies show it's not effective
Collars, corsets, and braces	Immobilize the painful area and therefore relieves muscle spasm	Noninvasive	May produce muscle weakness if overused
Trigger point injections	Myofascial pain syndrome and fibromyalgia	Very effective when used in conjunction with other modalities	Pain from needles. Usually needs to be repeated
Chymopapain injections (chemonucleolysis)	Herniated disk pressing on nerve root	No incision	High rate of complications

headaches or nausea don't occur very often. Injecting a combination of a steroid and anesthetic bathes the nerve roots and directly relieves irritation and inflammation. It is an extremely effective method for treating lumbar spine conditions, and it's a good alternative to surgery in many cases.

The medical literature is filled with studies of epidural blocks, both pro and con. Some report only a transient decrease in pain, leaving the long-term situation unchanged. Other reports, however, describe significant beneficial effects. The best results are found in people with uncomplicated low back and leg pain that may be due to a mildly herniated disk. People who have had sciatica and/or neurological problems for a long time, on the other hand, can respond poorly. As described in this book, some people with significant disk herniations have also been able to avoid surgery by using eipdural blocks.

> Trying up to three epidural blocks before resorting to surgery for a herniated disk without severe neurological problems is reasonable. If the first epidural block is not successful at all, it's senseless to proceed with additional ones.

Just as you choose the best lawyer or accountant, you want this procedure done by the person who is both skillful at and who does many such procedures on a consistent basis. It's just like having your car fixed—you wouldn't want your transmission replaced by someone who'd only done one other transmission replacement in his career! This is especially true when you're considering having nerve blocks done in your back. Experience is the best teacher, and there is a direct relationship between skill and experience of the person doing the injections and your end result.

Absolutely critical is the correct placement of the needle. Many physicians do epidural blocks "blindly," instead of using an X ray to see exactly where the medication is injected. Using an X ray along with a small amount of harmless dye reveals the exact placement of the needle before injecting the steroid and anesthetic, which definitely leads to more consistently good results.

Trying up to three epidural blocks before resorting to surgery (for a herniated disk without severe neurological problems) is reasonable. If the first epidural block is helpful in relieving the pain, you might consider doing two more. The next two blocks can be done one week apart. If the first epidural block is not successful, there's simply no reason at all to proceed with additional ones.

If your doctor tells you the only solution to your pain is surgery on your spine, we strongly recommend that you get a second opinion. This doesn't mean that your doctor is wrong, but surgery on the spine is a big undertaking with no guarantee of good results. If surgery is not an emergency and you have a herniated disk or spinal stenosis, inquire about epidural blocks. The worst that will happen is that you'll have the block and not get a good result. If that happens, you'll have the surgery that you were going to have anyway. If you're lucky, you will get a good result from the block, and you may not require surgery.

FACET JOINT INJECTIONS

We've known since the 1930s that facet joints, where one vertebra attaches to another, are sources of back pain. Like the knee, it's lined with smooth hyaline cartilage and has a membrane that secretes synovial fluid to lubricate the joint.

Degenerative arthritis often shows up in the facet joint. As arthritis overtakes the facet joints, the cartilage cracks, and the synovial fluid increases as a response to irritation. The joint enlarges, and can pinch the spinal nerves that run right next to it. Pressure on a nearby nerve, arthritis of the joint itself, or pinching of the synovial membrane inside the joint all cause facet joint pain.

This "facet syndrome" usually causes mechanical-type low back pain that's made worse by bending backwards. The pain usually radiates down the center of the back to the thigh to the knee, but not below. There can also be tenderness over the joint itself. Muscle weakness is rare.

> Overall, most studies of facet joint injections have not shown good, long-lasting results. The short-term success rate, however, is 50 percent or greater. If nothing else, facet blocks provide a period of pain relief that allows normal motion to resume. With normal motion restored, you can proceed to an appropriate exercise program.

The facet block, which is similar to an epidural block, is an effective treatment for facet joint arthritis. In this procedure, you lie on a fluoroscopy table, and the area around the joint is totally anesthetized. While watching on an X ray, the doctor injects a combination of steroid and anesthetic into the joint.

It's not unusual for the pain to get worse before it gets better, because there's usually some irritation from the injection. This fades within twenty-four to forty-eight hours, the beneficial effects of the steroid take over, and your symptoms start to disappear.

Overall, most studies of facet joint injections have not shown excellent results in the long run. The short-term success rate, on the other hand, is much more optimistic at 50 percent or greater. If nothing else, facet blocks can provide a period of pain relief that allows normal motion to resume so that you can begin with an appropriate exercise program.

Facet blocks, like epidural blocks, are invasive procedures. Each should be done *only* after trying noninvasive, conservative measures like oral anti-inflammatory medication, physical therapy or chiropractic, and a good exercise and stretching program.

LUMBAR LAMINECTOMY AND DISKECTOMY

A laminectomy is a surgical procedure that removes a part of the vertebra called the "lamina," allowing the surgeon to remove a herniated disk from between two vertebrae. "Diskectomy" is removal of the disk. Theoretically, it removes pressure from the nerve root, so that your leg pain and back pain will dissipate. While we always hope for this result, many lumbar laminectomies unfortunately produce far from perfect results.

A laminectomy and discectomy should be done *only* after all conservative measures fail, and either the pain is intolerable or the neurologic problems are severe. There are no other emergencies that *absolutely* require back surgery other than incapacitating pain which does not respond to conservative treatment, or severe neurological problems like bowel and bladder incontinence.

Many surgeons will tell you that lumbar laminectomies produce good results 70 to 90 percent of the time. In reality, a high number of people who have lumbar laminectomies either continue to have back pain, or their back pain goes away for a short period of time and then returns. The pain is frequently worse when it returns, and people in this situation may, in desperation, allow themselves to be operated on multiple times. The final result is failed back syndrome, which is caused by scarred nerves in the back. When nerves are scarred by surgery, the condition is called arachnoiditis.

The pain caused by arachnoiditis is far worse than the original pain from the herniated lumbar disk. Arachnoiditis patients commonly become addicted to narcotic medications, and many of them go to pain clinics. Unfortunately, the results of pain clinic programs are generally dismal.

The sequence of events that leads to the "multiply operated back" has destroyed many lives. The vast majority could have been avoided, if only the problem had been approached by using conservative methods of treatment, and operating only as a last resort.

Don't think that back surgery is your only answer, or that the cure will be immediate and permanent. You now know that, after surgery, scar tissue replaces damaged tissue. When that scar tissue involves nerves, it often produces pain, and frequently translates into a lifetime of misery.

PERCUTANEOUS DISKECTOMY

In a percutaneous diskectomy, a large, hollow needle is placed in the disk space, and the disk material is mechanically sucked out. Still it is much less invasive than surgery, and can be done on an outpatient basis. People are awake during this procedure, just as they are during facet blocks, epidural blocks, and chymopapain injections (described below).

We don't yet know how effective this procedure is. Still, it's being advertised heavily by doctors and hospitals, and success rates above 90 percent are reported.

Many risks and pitfalls are associated with percutaneous procedures, however, including infection and injury to nerves or blood vessels. Repeat herniation is common, with some reports showing up to 30 percent recurrence of symptoms within six months. Large pieces of disk are sometimes left behind in the spinal canal, and they can cause problems later.

Additionally, these are not easy procedures to do. The L5-S1 disk space can be very difficult to enter because of the overlapping pelvic bones, and, as you now know, approximately 50 percent of disk herniations occur in this area.

DECOMPRESSION LAMINECTOMY

In spinal stenosis, the spinal canal narrows, placing pressure on the spinal cord and nerve roots. This happens frequently when degenerative arthritis develops in the disk spaces and facet joints. It can also occur when herniated disks project far into the spinal canal.

If you develop spinal stenosis, your back pain is accompanied by leg pain in the buttocks and down the back of the thighs into the calves. Physical activity will aggravate the pain and rest will relieve it.

To stop the pain surgically, we must enlarge the spinal canal to relieve pressure on the nerves. Fortunately, the results of this surgical procedure are excellent.

Spinal stenosis usually occurs at multiple levels, from L1 to the sacrum. It is much more frequent in patients who are sixty years old or older. When the main problem is central canal stenosis, the results of surgically widening the spinal canal are excellent as well. When it's necessary to remove herniated disks, more caution is advisable. There is an increased chance that surgery will scar the nerve roots which can create a less-than-optimal result. Although epidural blocks can provide some relief in cases of spinal stenosis, most cases do require surgery.

SPINAL FUSION

As we've discussed, the vertebrae are attached to each other with many ligaments and muscles. If the ligaments are cut or stretched, or if bony support has been removed by surgery, the motion between vertebrae increases. We need a certain amount of motion in the spine to be able to bend and twist, but too much motion results in instability and pain.

After a disk (the cushion between the vertebrae that provides stability and strength) is removed or degenerates or the facet joints are affected by degenerative arthritis, the movements between vertebrae can become excessive, causing instability. The commonest sites of this are

L4-5 and L5-S1 (refer to Chapter 4 if you've forgotten where these vertebrae are).

Instability is easily diagnosed by what we call flexion and extension. X rays of a side view of the spine. You first bend forward, and then backward. If one vertebra moves more than half a centimeter over the top of the one below it, we diagnose instability.

The same kind of instability can occur in conditions like spondylolysis and spondylolisthesis, which we discussed in Chapter 5. In these conditions, there is either a defect in the bone itself or one vertebra has slipped forward over the one below it.

Spinal fusions have their own problems. A condition called pseudoarthrosis can occur, in which the fusion didn't take. This means that the same painful motion is still present after the failed operation, and it occurs in up to 25 percent of fusions. Newer techniques that employ devices called pedicle screws and spinal fusion cages have made it possible to lower rates of pseudoarthrosis and produce better surgical results.

Instability may follow surgical procedures that remove bone, like laminectomy. When bone is removed, some ligament is also removed. Too much surgery can cause an unstable spine as well, which can be extremely painful. Its solution involves fusing the vertebrae to each other so they don't move. Eliminating the abnormal motion eliminates the pain.

Spinal fusion is done in a limited area, most commonly at L4-5 and L5-S1 (see Chapter 4 to refresh your memory about where these vertebrae are). The loss of normal motion at the fused vertebrae isn't a problem, because other segments of the spine compensate.

Before undergoing a spinal fusion, you'll be fit with a brace to stabilize the lower back and prevent abnormal motion. If the brace relieves your back pain, it's a good indication that spinal fusion will, too. If you don't want to undergo spinal fusion, continuing to wear the brace is another option. Not many people, however, are willing to spend their whole lives wearing a spinal brace.

Spinal fusions present problems unique to the procedure. A condition called pseudoarthrosis can occur, in which the fusion didn't take. This means that the same painful motion is still present after the failed operation, and it occurs in up to 25 percent of fusions. Newer techniques that employ internal fixation such as pedicle screw fixation and spinal fusion cages have produced much better results with lower failed fusion rates.

> A new technique uses "spinal fusion cages." In this case, two one-inch cylindrical cages with mesh on the outside are filled with bone chips and placed in the intervertebral disk space. There are many varieties of these cages, and their use is growing exponentially. Their results have been excellent, and the pseudoarthrosis rate has dropped tremendously. Some studies reveal that the fusion rate is 95 percent or better.

In recent years, spine surgeons have used many different metal devices to aid fusion. One system is "pedicle screw fixation." It's a system of plates and screws that hold the vertebrae together, while a bone graft grows. This system has greatly increased fusion success rates by preventing motion while the fusion occurs.

A newer technique uses "spinal fusion cages." Here, two cylindrical cages, both one-inch long and with mesh on the outside, are filled with bone chips and placed in the intervertebral disk space. Many varieties of these cages now exist, each with their particular benefit, and their use has grown exponentially. Results so far have been excellent. In addition, the postsurgery pseudoarthrosis rate has dropped tremendously. Some studies reveal that the success rate is 95 percent or better.

Unfortunately, the picture is not completely rosy. Spinal fusion cages and pedicle screw fixation can cause many surgical complications. Some studies have shown significant incidence of damage to the dural sac and nerve roots. These same studies have also shown that the incidence of side effects is much less when a specialist in spinal surgery, with expertise in these procedures, does the surgery.

Nevertheless, these "instrumented fusions" that use hardware to stabilize the vertebrae have a place in spine surgery. They are probably best done by fellowship-trained spine surgeons who've spent years perfecting them. As with anything else, they should be undertaken *only* after a thorough trial of conservative treatment has failed.

TRANSCUTANEOUS ELECTRICAL NERVE STIMULATION (TENS) UNITS

Transcutaneous electrical nerve stimulation (TENS) involves applying low levels of electricity to painful areas by placing electrodes on the skin. TENS units produce low intensity, high frequency electrical stimulation.

Melzack and Wall's Gate Control Theory of Pain (which we discussed in Chapter 1) suggests that electricity can help reduce pain. If touch fibers on the skin are stimulated, the resulting messages passing into the spinal cord can jam pain messages and close the pain gates.

To use a TENS unit, we attach black carbon electrodes with "electro jelly" (jelly pads) under them to the skin over the pain. A battery pack generates electrical current. It produces a tingling sensation, which mixes with the pain sensations and, in the best of all possible worlds, is a pleasant substitute for the pain.

TENS units are not always effective therapeutic aids. For this reason, you should rent one first and, if it helps, then purchase it. Remember though that your need for TENS units should not supercede your use of other, more conservative treatments like anti-inflammatory medications, exercise, and massage. In fact, you should use them together.

We also recognize that TENS units can help some individual patients but only to a point, after which the TENS units become ineffective. For such patients, the therapy just doesn't seem powerful enough. There's also a different type of TENS unit available, a dorsal column stimulator, which is an electrode that's surgically implanted in the epidural space very near to the spinal cord.

> Chronic pain patients undergo a battery of psychological testing to determine if they are appropriate candidates for an implanted dorsal column stimulator, but studies have shown that, in many cases, such patients don't obtain significant long-term relief from these stimulators.

Dorsal column stimulators have been used to treat failed back syndrome and a condition called reflex sympathetic dystrophy. Unfortunately, from a practical point of view, very few of the dorsal column stimulators work for long, and many have to be surgically removed.

ULTRASOUND

Ultrasound uses high frequency sound waves that aren't detectable by the human ear. They can penetrate various tissues in the body, causing heat and relieving pain. Ultrasound works best when used in association with manual therapy, like chiropractic or massage and a good exercise program.

TRACTION

There are two basic types of traction: cervical traction for neck problems, and pelvic traction for low back disorders. In traction, the doctor attaches a halter-type apparatus to the neck or pelvis and applies weights. One stated purpose is to pull the vertebrae away from one another, which may reduce pressure in the disk space. In reality, however, it takes a lot of weight to move the vertebrae at all and traction, as routinely used, is not effective here.

Studies show that traction provides some relief of muscle spasm and enforces a couple of days of bed rest. Unfortunately, it's not very effective in relieving the pressure of a herniated disk or creating good posture.

CORSETS, COLLARS, AND BRACES

These supports are widely prescribed for back pain and neck pain.

A cervical collar supports the head, allowing the muscles in the neck to relax if they are in chronic spasm. A cervical collar also restricts neck movement so that injured and inflamed areas can heal more rapidly.

Lumbar corsets restrict motion in the painful part of the spine, as well as providing abdominal support and correcting posture. Although they provide some pain relief, most orthopedists feel that they should be avoided because prolonged use of a lumbar corset leads to muscle weakness. People who lift moderate to heavy weights all the time while working often use them. Scientific studies show that lumbar corsets don't really protect the back against injury by support alone. However, they remind the worker to lift correctly, bending his or her knees.

INJECTION THERAPY TO SOFT TISSUES

Soft tissue injuries like muscle and ligament tears usually heal in six to twelve weeks. If they don't, they're called chronic strains.

People who have continual soft tissue pain without any bony or disk disease probably have either fibromyalgia or myofascial pain syndrome, which we discussed in Chapter 4. Once the physician identifies the tender trigger points of fibromyalgia or myofascial pain syndrome, he or she should inject and eliminate them so they don't perpetuate chronic muscle spasm and soft tissue inflammation.

> Interestingly enough, many trigger-point areas in the spine correspond with acupuncture points, which we'll discuss in Chapter 11.

Active myofascial trigger points cause pain even at rest, and they prevent full lengthening of the muscles. If they last a long time, the muscle can be weakened. Latent, as opposed to active, trigger points are tender only when pressed, and don't produce tenderness at rest.

Interestingly enough, many trigger-point areas in the spine correspond with acupuncture points, which makes for a striking coincidence between Western and Eastern ideas about pain regulation, and which we'll discuss in Chapter 11.

Treatments for fibromyalgia and myofascial pain syndrome are described in detail in Chapter 5, and include anesthetic injections, dry needling, and Spray and Stretch®. Stretching exercises, heat, massage, and even acupuncture should be used to return normal muscle function.

CHYMOPAPAIN INJECTIONS (CHEMONUCLEOLYSIS)

Chemonucleolysis is an invasive procedure in which an enzyme is injected into the disk to dissolve part of it to relieve pressure on a nerve root. Chymopapain injections were approved in the United States in 1982 and immediately became popular. Compared to a large surgical procedure, they seemed to be a quick fix for leg pain associated with a herniated disk. Doctors performed chymopapain injections while watching needle placement via X-ray fluoroscopy.

Unfortunately, chymopapain injections are also associated with a tremendous number of problems. There were many allergic reactions to the enzyme, as well as neurological complications. In fact, some people were paralyzed from their reaction to the enzyme and other people developed diskitis, an infection of the disk space. For all of these reasons, chymopapain injections are, for the most part, no longer used in the United States, although they are still done in other countries.

Now that you know how the Western medical profession generally treats back pain with medication and surgery, let's enter a whole new world and explore complementary, integrative, and nutritional treatments for pain.

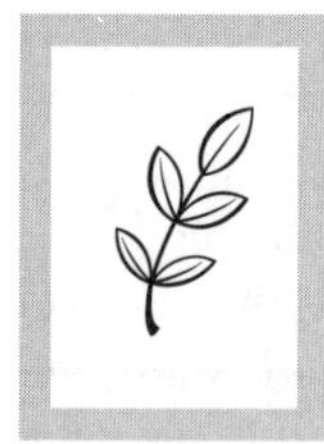

Chapter 7 THE NUTRITION CONNECTION: THE RIGHT DIET

"Fish is brain food."
"An apple a day keeps the doctor away."
"Carrots help you to see in the dark."
"Eating the right foods each day keeps pain and inflammation away???"

It's a wonder that body and mind have survived together for this long. A case in point—eating. The body views eating as an opportunity to replace lost nutrients. When the stomach gurgles and grumbles, it's a sign that the body needs nourishment. Conversely, the mind views eating as satisfying desires—it wants to stop feeling hungry. It also wants eating to be pleasurable. So the mind and body initiate eating for very different reasons. Unfortunately, what the mind wants and the body needs may differ considerably. More often than not, a bag of potato chips suffices for lunch during our busy work days. And there's always room for dessert, even though the salad and vegetables lie on the dinner plate untouched. The body does its best to tolerate what the mind wants—potato chips, chocolate cake, coffee, and pizza. Eventually, however, a lifestyle of satisfying desires leads to a preoccupation with another need: the need to seek medical attention.

Diet plays a pivotal role in health and disease. Cancer, heart disease, and a host of other chronic conditions have their roots in diet and lifestyle. Throughout *Nature's Pain Killers*, we've examined the physiology of pain and inflammation. In this chapter, we'll take the concept of healthy eating into a new realm. We'll examine how diet can ameliorate pain and inflammation, and how your food choices can help you control your pain.

People suffering from the chronic forms of pain described in *Nature's Pain Killers* are most likely to profit from the dietary concepts explored in this chapter. While good nutrition is always important to healing, people with acute forms of pain—like a broken bone, cuts, bumps, or bruises—will find that diet has less impact on their immediate pain.

We won't lie to you—changing your diet is a difficult process that requires commitment and willpower. You may not feel the effects for weeks, but once you integrate the concepts described here into your daily regimen, you'll find that all the hard work was worth it.

After all, we are what we eat. We derive the ingredients for inflammation from our diet. Therefore, the foods we eat and the proportions of nutrients contained in them either *increase* or *decrease* inflammation. It makes sense to alter diet and lifestyle to *decrease* our supply of proinflammatory substances, while *increasing* foods that possess anti-inflammatory and antipain properties.

There are two ways we can attack pain and inflammation with diet: (1) decrease our intake of inflammatory substances and (2) increase our tolerance to pain. Let's begin with decreasing inflammation.

FATTY ACIDS: AFFECTING THE ESSENTIALS OF INFLAMMATION

Dieters regard fat as a formidable enemy which they must face at every meal. Whether we like it or not, dietary fat is as necessary as any other nutrient for optimum health. Fat serves many biological roles other than expanding your waistline.

Triglycerides are the fats we obtain from food. To make triglycerides, three fatty acids attach to a molecule, glycerol, which serves as a backbone. Hence the name triglyceride: "tri" means three, and "glyceride" is another name for glycerol. Think of dietary fat as resembling a comb with three teeth. While fatty acids come in many sizes and shapes, they all fall into two broad categories: essential or nonessential.

We synthesize nonessential fatty acids, the largest category of fatty acids, in the body; therefore, we don't need a dietary source (hence their designation as "nonessential").

Conversely, we obtain essential fatty acids *only* from the diet; we cannot synthesize them internally. Only two—linolenic acid (omega-3) and linoleic acid (omega-6)—fall into this category. They are both polyunsaturated fatty acids. Ironically, the essential fatty acids group, a lightweight compared to the colossal category of nonessential fatty acids, plays the greatest role in the inflammatory process.

We are what we eat. If we took a piece of fatty tissue from a person and examine the fatty acids found in the membranes of those cells, we'd see that the type of fat stored in the body reflects that person's diet. Eat a lot of corn or olive oil, and it invariably shows up in your cells. Different fats influence cellular processes differently. There is no greater example of this than the essential fatty acids. Both linolenic (omega-3) and linoleic (omega-6) acid control inflammation: One promotes inflammation while the other slows the inflammatory process. Therefore, the proportion of these essential fatty acids in the body determines, to a certain extent, the amount of pro-inflammatory and anti-inflammatory products we produce.

As we discussed in Chapter 3, linoleic acid is the major precursor of arachidonic acid, which forms the prostaglandins and leukotrienes. Prostaglandins and leukotrienes, as you'll recall, are major players in inflammation and contribute significantly to causing pain. Most vegetable oils, especially safflower, corn, soybean, and cottonseed oils, are rich sources of linoleic (omega-6) fatty acid. Increased consumption of omega-6 fatty acids provides a pool of raw material for making arachidonic acid, which in turn provides for prostaglandin and leukotriene synthesis in the body (see Table 7-1). All of these substances contribute to inflammation and pain.

Canola oil, walnuts, wheat germ, and hemp oils are rich sources of linolenic (omega-3) fatty acid, which are anti-inflammatory. Another rich source of omega-3 is cold-water fish (see Table 7-2). Unlike humans, these fish are able to convert linolenic acid to eicosapentaenoic acid (EPA) and docosahexaenoic acid (DHA) inside their bodies. Both EPA and DHA are omega-3 fatty acids, and so they are anti-inflammatory fats.

Isn't that remarkable? Fish are not only "brain food," they're also "anti-pain food"!

If we give our cells a choice, they absorb omega-3 fatty acids *instead* of absorbing omega-6 fatty acids and arachidonic acid. In other words, omega-3 fatty acids successfully compete with omega-6 and arachidonic acid for cellular space. If you have enough omega-3 fatty acids in your diet, the amount of pro-inflammatory omega-6, and its availability for prostaglandin and leukotriene synthesis decreases.

Table 7-1
SOURCES OF ESSENTIAL FATTY ACIDS

Linoleic Acid (omega-6):	Linolenic Acid (omega-3):
Safflower oil	Canola oil
Corn oil	Flaxseed oil
Soybean oil	Walnuts
Cottonseed oil	Wheat germ
Most vegetable oils	Hemp oil

If you think back to Chapter 3, you'll recall that not all prostaglandins and leukotrienes are "bad." Some prostaglandins and leukotrienes—those produced from omega-3 fatty acids—actually cool down the inflammatory response.

Think of the cell as resembling a kitchen sink. The hot water represents the omega-6 fatty acids that accumulate from the diet, and the cold water represents the "cooling" omega-3 fatty acids. Open the omega-6 valve more than the omega-3 valve, and you end up with a sink full of scalding water (i.e., lots of inflammation). The more omega-3 you have, the cooler the water.

Decreasing omega-6 while increasing omega-3 fatty acid intake seems to be a practical idea, yet we rarely do it. In fact, the typical Western diet lacks sufficient amounts of omega-3 fatty acids while containing far too much omega-6. It's not surprising to find an omega-6 to omega-3 ratio of 25:1 in the diets of people in industrialized societies, compared to a ratio of less than 2:1 in a pre-industrial society. The result is that people living in a modern society have more omega-6 fatty acids in their cells, creating a greater pool from which to synthesize more arachidonic acid, potentially increasing inflammation and pain.

Consuming a diet rich in omega-3 fatty acids decreases the amount of omega-6 fatty acids your cells absorb. Long-term intake of omega-3 fatty acids may even decrease your long-term need for anti-inflammatory drugs.

What does science have to say about omega-3 fatty acids? The debate over whether increasing dietary intake of omega-3 fatty acid actually decreases inflammation continues. Some studies show that people who eat diets rich in omega-3 fatty acids experience fewer inflammations. Others contend that it's impractical, from a dietary standpoint, to try to consume the high amounts of omega-3 required to elicit a response. Most studies have used supplements of omega-3 (fish-oil supplements) to influence inflammation.

Increasing your intake of dietary omega-3, however, is still practical for several reasons. First, a diet high in omega-3 reduces your dependence on omega-3 supplementation, which should make budget conscious consumers take note. Consuming increased amounts of omega-3 fatty acids decreases the amount of omega-6 fatty acids available to your cells. Finally, long-term intake of omega-3 fatty acids may decrease your need for anti-inflammatory drugs. It seems that you have nothing to lose and everything to gain by altering your diet to include more omega-3 fatty acids and fewer omega-6.

There is no recommended dietary allowance (RDA) for essential fatty acids. The human requirement for omega-6 is approximately 2 to 7 grams daily (about 1 to 3 percent of total energy intake). The optimal intake of omega-3 fatty acids is about 1.1 to 1.5 grams daily. For people suffering from inflammation, the *amount* of essential fatty acids in the diet may not be as important as the *ratio* of the two. The ratio of omega-6 to omega-3 should be around 4:1 to 10:1. In light of the role these two fatty acids play in inflammation, a ratio of 2:1 to 4:1 may be even more beneficial.

Essential fatty acids are highly reactive oils and, because of this, you must protect them. Keep oils containing essential fatty acids (especially omega-3) in the refrigerator. Light can react with essential fatty acids, causing them to turn rancid, so buying them bottled in dark glass is helpful. Additionally, if you plan to cook with oils containing essential fatty acids, minimize their exposure to high temperature, which destroys omega-3. In fact, it's best to use these oils in ways that don't require cooking, such as salad dressing. Alternatively, you can pour a little extra oil on your food after it's cooked.

One study estimated that five to six servings of fish weekly will help elevate omega-3 levels in the body. If you are obtaining this essential fatty acid from a variety of sources, including oils, you can certainly reduce the amount of fish you eat.

Table 7-2 FISH SOURCES OF OMEGA-3	
Atlantic cod	Halibut
Atlantic salmon	Herring
Sockeye salmon	Mackerel
Bluefish	Striped bass
Flounder	Tuna

Arachidonic Acid: Will The Real Culprit Please Stand Up?

Even though omega-6 fatty acids have a tarnished reputation, we need them. Some studies, in fact, disagree about whether omega-6 fatty acids actually contribute to the inflammatory process. In stark contrast to the controversy surrounding both omega-3 and omega-6 fatty acids, however, we know for sure that arachidonic acid is fuel for the flames of inflammation. Thus, eating foods rich in arachidonic acid may be more detrimental than eating a diet rich in omega-6 fatty acids.

Meat is the food that is highest in arachidonic acid; both lean meat and the visible fat that surrounds meat contain high levels of it. Duck contains the highest amount of arachidonic acid in the lean portions, while pork contains the highest concentrations in the visible fat. Beef and lamb are lowest in this pro-inflammatory acid.

If you need a better reason to limit your daily intake of meat and meat products, here's a good one: Consuming large quantities of meat or meat products, which is not uncommon in industrialized societies, can contribute significantly to raising arachidonic acid levels in the body. This may enhance the synthesis of pro-inflammatory chemicals, like leukotrienes.

Several dietary studies support arachidonic acid's role in increasing the synthesis of inflammatory prostaglandins and leukotrienes. For example, one study revealed that some immune system cells require free arachidonic acid to make leukotrienes; this arachidonic acid can either be made internally, or be absorbed from the diet.

So you can now see that altering your dietary intake of omega-6 fatty acids and arachidonic acid can actually alter the inflammatory response.

Now let's examine another astonishing dietary truth: We can use diet to reduce chronic pain.

PAIN AND THE SEROTONIN CONNECTION

First isolated in 1948, serotonin is one of the most actively investigated chemicals in the body (see Figure 7-1). Serotonin is a "jack-of-all-trades," participating in many chemical processes in the body, including smooth muscle contraction, temperature regulation, appetite, behavior, blood pressure, and respiration. Of the many organ functions requiring serotonin, none is better known than its role in the brain. We've investigated the connection between serotonin deficiency and depression extensively, but serotonin's activity in the brain doesn't stop there. Serotonin may also regulate pain.

Ironically, serotonin cannot enter the brain, because it is unable to cross the blood-brain barrier that protects this delicate organ from potentially harmful chemicals and infectious agents. Synthesis of serotonin must begin in the brain itself. This is where tryptophan, an essential amino acid, steps into the picture. It is the raw material for serotonin synthesis, and easily enters the brain. There, enzymes convert it into serotonin.

Hypothetically, increasing tryptophan levels in the brain would increase serotonin levels, which should diminish chronic pain. The only problem with this scenario is that tryptophan supplements are available only by prescription and increasing its levels in the brain by eating more tryptophan-rich foods may not work.

You may ask, "If I eat foods high in tryptophan, won't that enhance tryptophan entry into the brain?" Because tryptophan competes with other amino acids for entry into the brain, the answer to that question is probably "No."

We find tryptophan in high-protein foods like turkey and cheeses (see Table 7-3). The same foods that are high in tryptophan, however, are also high in other amino acids, and there are far more of these amino acids than tryptophan in these foods. Therefore, a high-protein meal, with its large quantity of amino acids competing with tryptophan for entry into the brain, results in tryptophan being "crowded out"—unable to enter the brain and make serotonin. This is analogous to too many people trying to board a crowded elevator, with "Mr. Tryptophan" being at the end of the line.

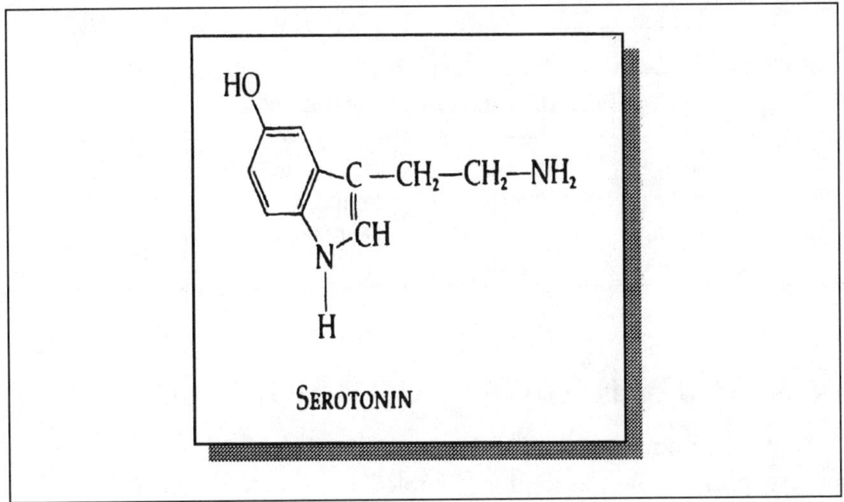

Figure 7-1

Eating a high-protein meal, then, is *not* the answer to increasing serotonin levels. We need to remove the competition so that tryptophan can board the elevator and go straight to the brain. We can do this by eating a carbohydrate-rich diet, which increases tryptophan levels in the brain, leading to a rise in serotonin levels.

Several studies confirm the role of serotonin in pain regulation, suggesting that higher serotonin levels buffer the pain response, while lower levels may exacerbate it. Considering that people afflicted with fibromyalgia appear to have reduced serotonin levels (as we discussed in Chapter 5), these studies may provide a clue about fibromyalgia's cause, which continues to elude researchers.

It seems, therefore, that limiting your protein intake and focusing on carbohydrate-rich foods, like vegetables, fruits, and grains, could play a role in lessening your pain.

Because tryptophan is an essential amino acid, we need a dietary source of it (just as we need to obtain essential fatty acids from the diet). We don't recommend totally eliminating high-protein foods from your diet either. Combining these foods, however, with carbohydrates (like pasta or bread) will allow your brain to absorb tryptophan more easily. Your diet should thus be fairly high in carbohydrates, and contain moderate amounts of fat and protein.

Table 7-3 FOODS HIGH IN TRYPTOPHAN	
Turkey Chicken Pineapple Banana	Unripened cheese Yogurt Dairy products

SIMPLE SUGAR, COMPLEX CASE

Another important issue is the role that simple sugars, particularly sucrose, play in pain perception. Simple sugars are another form of carbohydrates; they're found in table sugar, cakes, candy, and most sweetened food products. Some researchers contend that diets high in simple sugars heighten our perception of pain. They reached this conclusion by observing diabetic patients, who often have dramatic swings in blood sugar levels. The only problem with these studies, however, is that diabetes is a complex condition that alters many metabolic systems. Uncontrolled diabetes leads to pain from nerve damage, as well as from a variety of other conditions associated with the disease. Relatively healthy individuals are able to regulate their blood sugar levels and don't endure the problems seen in diabetics. This fact alone may negate any correlation between sugar intake and pain perception in nondiabetic individuals. In fact, studies in animals and human infants, some of which have been placebo controlled and randomized, have shown the opposite—sugar may, in fact, have an analgesic effect.

Whether through its ability to enhance tryptophan's entry into the brain or through some unknown mechanism affecting the opioid system, sugar appears to offer some relief from pain. This doesn't mean you should routinely order an extra serving of dessert, or begin a diet centered on chocolate bars and Gummi bears. Quite the contrary—these snacks are not only high in sugar, they are very high in fat, and not much else. They're nutritional voids that contribute to weight gain, leading to greater stress on weight-bearing joints, which further aggravates pain and inflammation. Besides, eating too many sugary snacks may be more of an ache than a pain . . . that is, a toothache. *Moderation,* of course, is the key when it comes to snacks and treats.

THE ALLERGY CONNECTION: BEYOND RED EYES AND RUNNY NOSES

Every year, millions of people scramble for their antihistamine medication when they hear the words "hay fever," "ragweed," or "pollen." For some, there's nothing more irritating than the allergy season. Allergies, however, are not solely confined to irritants we breathe in. They are also caused by the foods we eat (see Table 7-4) and the chemicals we absorb through the skin. An allergic reaction may manifest in many forms, including skin rashes, headaches, lethargy, apathy, neurologic disturbances and, in the most extreme case, death. Allergic reactions to the food we eat may contribute to another condition that afflicts millions—pain and inflammation.

An allergy is an exaggerated response to a specific, sensitizing substance. In other words, it is an abnormal immune response to a chemical, called an allergen, that doesn't normally cause a bad reaction. To become allergic to something, you must be exposed to it more than once: The allergic reaction doesn't occur with the first exposure, only with subsequent ones.

How can the food we eat contribute to debilitating conditions like rheumatoid arthritis and fibromyalgia? This happens through a process called neurogenic switching, a hypothesis suggesting that a stimulus at one site causes inflammation at another. Researchers have used this hypothesis to explain anaphylaxis, a life-threatening condition that develops when susceptible people are exposed to a particular allergen (like people who are allergic to bee stings or penicillin). Neurogenic switching may also explain why a food allergy can trigger pain and inflammation in fibromyalgia and arthritis sufferers.

Food sensitivities may cause a form of neurogenic switching that originates in the digestive system, but manifests as pain and inflammation in other parts of the body. Neurogenic switching is a new concept and, even though it sounds plausible, no research has been done that proves it is a cause of fibromyalgia or arthritis.

Food allergies, however, have been implicated as possible causes of a particular type of rheumatoid arthritis. One study estimates that we may be able to treat approximately 5 percent of arthritic patients with diet. We can only tell who those people are, however, by manipulating their diets.

Don't be fooled by that low number—5 percent—and don't forget

Table 7-4 FOODS COMMONLY ASSOCIATED WITH FOOD ALLERGIES	
Wheat Corn Eggs Soy products	Citrus fruits and juices Nuts (including nut butters) Dairy products

that estimates are just that. Diet may play a greater role in managing arthritis when used in conjunction with other treatments. By taking the steps to reduce the intake of pro-inflammatory foods and by eliminating potential food allergens, you can decide for yourself whether diet is an important part of the pain you experience.

CIGARETTES AND COFFEE: PARTNERS IN CRIME

Coffee and cigarettes are popular among people of all ages, so much so that many regard them as a meal. Coffee and a cigarette in the morning may replace eggs and sausage for breakfast or, better yet, fresh fruit and whole-grain bread or cereal. If you're about to change your diet, it's important that you also eliminate caffeine and cigarettes.

We know little about caffeine's role in chronic pain. Based on a study that analyzed caffeine consumption and back pain, scientists suggested that excessive caffeine consumption may be associated with chronic back pain. Other studies did not reach the same conclusion, but discovered that high caffeine users were more likely to be tobacco smokers than low caffeine users. Caffeine itself may not contribute to low back pain but rather, high caffeine use may accompany other unhealthy lifestyle behaviors.

When investigators examined the relationship between smoking and back pain, they found that smoking is indeed associated not only with back pain, but with other types of musculoskeletal pain as well. Two subsequent studies concluded that smoking contributes both to back and to musculoskeletal pain. What to do? Abstain completely from smoking and, until we know what role caffeine plays in chronic back pain, consume it in moderation, more for pleasure than as a daily requirement.

BRINGING IT ALL TOGETHER: DIETARY APPROACHES TO REDUCING PAIN

Now that we've examined the impact of diet on pain and inflammation, how do we integrate this knowledge into an effective dietary regimen? The ultimate goal is to identify which foods may be potential problems (contributing to the inflammatory process), and to follow a diet that reduces pain and inflammation. Before starting any new diet, make sure you fully discuss your intentions with your doctor or other health-care practitioner. Hopefully, he or she will encourage your efforts to take control of your health.

Let's begin by noting the potential problems.

The Elimination Diet

When eating certain foods causes certain symptoms, it's reasonable to remove that food from your diet. If symptoms abate after a while, reintroduce the food to see if symptoms reappear. If so, chances are that this food was the culprit. This is the basic tenet of the elimination diet—removing offending foods that lead to adverse reactions; in this case, inflammation. An elimination diet can help you determine which foods may aggravate your inflammatory condition.

Beginning an elimination diet is quite simple: Avoid eating those foods that you suspect worsen your condition. If you are not sure, begin with foods commonly associated with allergic symptoms (see Table 4).

Avoid questionable foods for a two-week period—this is your elimination period—to allow your body to rid itself of potential allergens that may contribute to inflammation. The easy part is avoiding these foods by themselves. Since it is important to avoid them completely, you must be very careful when eating prepared foods, since the ingredients may conceal possible allergens. Be sure to read the list of ingredients carefully and keep in mind that foods are listed in order of predominance (i.e., the first ingredient on the list is the most abundant). For the two-week elimination phase, we recommend that you avoid eating out, if possible. Restaurants don't offer ingredient lists and, unless you are able to have a meal specially prepared, you may unknowingly ingest possible allergens.

If symptoms do not subside after two weeks, then it's possible that you didn't eliminate the offending food, or that food sensitivity is not the problem. You may have to start the elimination diet all over again, avoiding a whole new group of foods from your diet. If, however, your symptoms begin to clear, you should then reintroduce those foods one at a time, at intervals of four to five days, to see if they elicit a response. Once you've identified the offending foods, the most effective treatment is in strictly avoiding them.

Elimination diets are effective for correcting allergic conditions. As we've mentioned before, however, only certain individuals who have distinct food sensitivities benefit from this regimen. It's also a long process that you may need to perform several times. It's well worth it, however, if your pain and inflammation subside. There are many varieties of elimination diets, from the simple one described here to very strict diets that your medical advisors must monitor. Some of these include putting patients on highly purified diets and slowly reintroducing conventional foods back into the diet. The procedure outlined above is a good starting point though to help you in discovering what role diet can play in eliminating pain and inflammation.

Once you've removed all potential food problems, the next step is to build upon this with a diet that maximizes pain relief. Fortunately, such a diet already exists.

The Vegetarian Diet

For years, you've probably heard that vegetarians have a lower risk of developing chronic diseases. Vegetarians may also be less prone to pain and inflammation. "Vegetarianism" is an umbrella term that encompasses three or four subgroups, depending on how liberal one is with the term. A *vegan* (pronounced vee-gan) is someone who strictly avoids all animal products. Their diet consists solely of vegetables, fruits, and grains. *Lacto-vegetarians* allow milk and milk products in their diet but avoid eggs, while *lacto-ovo-vegetarians* include eggs as well as dairy products in their diet (see Table 5). Some vegetarians include fish in their diet. Depending on which foods you may be allergic to (as ascertained from the elimination diet), you can try different vegetarian regimens and see which one works best for you.

Adopting a vegetarian diet is a logical choice, because it encompasses all the beneficial foods discussed in this chapter, while excluding all the bad foods. Meat, laden with arachidonic acid, is no longer the centerpiece of a meal. Instead, vegetables and grains provide the sustenance you need for good health. Studies show that vegetarians have lower levels of arachidonic acid in their bodies compared to omnivorous groups (people who eat both meat and vegetable foods). Vegetarians also have higher levels of omega-3 fatty acids than their omnivorous counterparts. Through vegetarianism, we remove excess sources of pro-inflammatory arachidonic acid and increase the anti-inflammatory omega-3 fatty acids.

Vegetarian diets are also generally lower in protein and higher in carbohydrates. As we've mentioned, higher carbohydrate intake may contribute to increased serotonin synthesis in the brain and, therefore, decreased pain.

Additionally, vegetarians are more apt to incorporate soy products into their diets, which is an added bonus, because soy itself may reduce pain. While no formal studies correlate soy intake to pain reduction, scientists at Johns Hopkins University (working with a group of Israeli researchers) noticed that rats consuming a soy-based diet showed a decrease in pain sensitivity.

Diets high in fruits and vegetables (like vegetarian diets) are also high in antioxidants, molecules that arrest free radical activity and prevent damage to bodily tissues. Free radical damage is associated with inflammation. Eating more fruits and vegetables contributes to the antioxidant pool in your body and guards against free radical attack.

Finally, vegetarians are generally leaner, which means less stress on the weight-bearing joints (hips, knees, ankles, and lower spine), and reduced pain.

Science has questioned the role that vegetarianism might play in relieving symptoms of rheumatoid arthritis. In one study, after a three-month vegan diet followed by a nine-month lacto-vegetarian diet, arthritic patients improved by both subjective and objective measures. Results of other studies are mixed, or show no relationship between diet and arthritis. Again, dietary manipulation may be beneficial only for that subgroup of arthritis patients who respond to it.

We must make two points here. This mixed message about diet and

Table 7-5 CLASSIFICATIONS OF THE VEGETARIAN DIET	
Vegan	A person who avoids all foods of animal origin.
Lacto-vegetarian	A person who does not eat meat, fish, poultry or eggs, but includes milk, cheese and other dairy products in his or her diet.
Lacto-ovo-vegetarian	A person who follows the same principles as lacto-vegetarians but incorporates eggs into the diet.

arthritis doesn't mean that dietary therapy won't ameliorate other forms of chronic pain. Remember, no one knows who will respond to nutritional therapy. If pain and inflammation have ruled your life thus far, isn't it worth your time to give it a chance? Perhaps you'll be one of the lucky ones!

> A vegetarian diet decreases the substances that contribute to inflammation, and increases anti-inflammatory omega-3 intake. It also increases your intake of antioxidant-rich fruits and vegetables (which may play a role in halting inflammatory processes), and leads to weight loss (which removes excessive stress from inflamed joints).

Vegetarianism is an expansive topic that is much too broad to cover thoroughly here. It is, however, a plausible approach to pain management that you can use along with other therapies. There are literally hundreds of books on vegetarianism, as well as cookbooks containing delicious vegetarian recipes. We realize that the elimination and vegetarian diets may not suit everyone. Nonetheless, you've already taken the first steps to understanding and managing your condition by reading *Nature's Pain Killers*, and we commend you. The choices presented here are yours to make. Hopefully, some are choices that will reduce your pain and inflammation, and start you travelling down the road to health.

Changing your diet may not be enough to control pain and inflammation. You may need high amounts of nutrients that aren't attainable from diet alone. Still other compounds not normally present in your diet may alleviate pain, and this is where supplementation enters the picture. When used together, dietary intervention and supplementation can deliver a "one-two punch" against pain. In the next two chapters, we'll delve into vitamins, herbs, and various other supplements that help alleviate pain and inflammation.

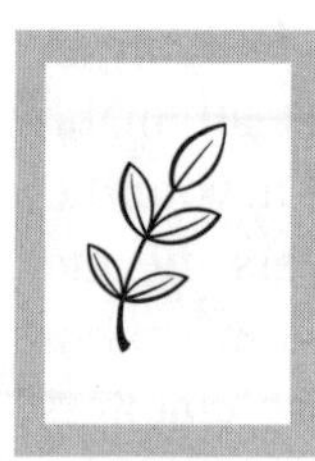

CHAPTER 8 ANTI-INFLAMMATORY AND ANALGESIC SUPPLEMENTS FOR PAIN

Supplement use has grown substantially in the United States over the last decade. Perhaps you, like other patients and physicians seeking natural methods of healing, have investigated herbal and nutritional therapies. These natural remedies are generally well tolerated, even by sensitive or allergy-prone individuals, and most are suitable for treating chronic diseases.

We're still unraveling the puzzle of illnesses like chronic pain. Western medicine has been unsuccessful in curing any chronic illness thus far because, among other reasons, we've searched for a "magic bullet" to attack a single aspect of a chronic illness, rather than addressing the whole organism and the relationships among body systems.

Nutritional/herbal therapies differ from pharmaceutical drugs in that they affect many systems simultaneously. Nutritional and herbal supplements are helpful in treating chronic conditions because they contain a combination of ingredients that possess different actions.

We're also learning that, to use natural substances as treatments, we must sometimes employ them at far higher dosages than we have previously. Clinicians once prescribed vitamins and minerals, only in the small amounts required to prevent deficiencies. To take advantage of their many actions in the body, we now use vitamins and minerals and herbs in dosages that far exceed those minimal requirements while still remaining safe. As more and more researchers devote their efforts to understanding the clinical benefits of herbal and nutritional therapies, we'll further define doses that produce precise results.

Nowhere will this be more relevant than in managing chronic pain and inflammation. In fact, we've already begun to test a new class of herbs and nutrients, the phyto-anti-inflammatory drugs (PAIDs). We're learning that PAIDs interact in complex ways with many molecules and pathways in the body to control pain and inflammation. Some PAIDs inhibit arachidonic acid metabolism, while others inhibit the release of cytokines and prostaglandins. Still others act as analgesics.

Aspirin and other nonsteroidal anti-inflammatory drugs (NSAIDs) have been the cornerstones for treating inflammation and pain, and they have definite merit. They are very effective anti-inflammatory agents—for *short-term* use. More often than not, however, people looking for pain relief take as many NSAIDs every day as healthy people take in several years! At this point, these drugs stop working and contribute to nasty negative side effects.

We've discussed many times that habitual use of aspirin, acetaminophen, phenylbutazone, and other NSAIDs can cause ulceration and bleeding in the gastrointestinal tract. Long-term use of other NSAIDs may be toxic to the liver and kidneys.

In addition, the effects of NSAIDs on inflamed joints (like those found in arthritic patients) may only be palliative—in the long run, they don't cure inflammation. Over extended periods, NSAIDs may actually contribute to joint degradation despite their anti-inflammatory activity. Are these drugs the only remedies available to us?

Fortunately, they are not. We have access to many *natural* substances that help to control inflammation and pain (see Table 1). In this chapter, we'll explore supplements that possess anti-inflammatory and analgesic effects. Many of them are also helpful to use in an integrative approach *along with* aspirin or ibuprofen and a host of other NSAIDs. Essentially, the goal is to lower the dose of the NSAID or eventually replace it with a safer, effective anti-inflammatory/analgesic nutritional compound.

We're learning that integrating supplements with conventional medicine provides the best medical care by giving us the benefits of both worlds. For example, we're able to reduce our intake of conventional anti-inflammatories and, therefore, decrease the adverse side effects they produce.

Remember, however, that supplemental protocols are not "quick fixes." In some cases, it may be several weeks before we see improvements. While supplements slowly become effective, however, we can use NSAIDs initially to relieve pain and inflammation. Once the supplements kick in, you can reduce your use of NSAIDs and other standard medications, which will reduce their negative impact on your general health.

This is the beauty of integrative medicine: It allows us to combine supplements and NSAIDs in a way that provides safer, more effective treatment than using either one alone. Of course, if you can manage your pain by using *only* natural remedies, that is the best possible situation. If you must rely to any extent on NSAIDs and other anti-inflammatory drugs, however, it's best to use them as little as possible.

In this chapter, we'll examine some supplements with anti-inflammatory and analgesic properties, as well as those that help to repair or rebuild damaged tissue (see Table 8-1).

SUPPLEMENTS FOR INFLAMMATION AND ANALGESIA

As you know, inflammation plays an integral role in the healing process but, in excess, it causes deleterious changes in the bodily tissues. This is especially significant in arthritis, where constant, relentless inflammation degrades the protective surfaces of the joints. If you have arthritis, you know that pain, swelling, and difficulty moving are the results of this rampaging inflammation.

Our first line of defense against pain is to reduce inflammation. One way to accomplish this is to inhibit the mechanisms that contribute to inflammation and, as we discussed in Chapter 3, these include the cyclooxygenase (Cox) and lipoxygenase enzymes that convert arachidonic acid into the inflammatory eicosanoids (see Figure 8-1).

You now know that the pharmaceutical industry has created a new class of anti-inflammatory medications called Cox-2 inhibitors, but did you realize that nature has its own version? A little later in this chapter, you'll learn where to find them.

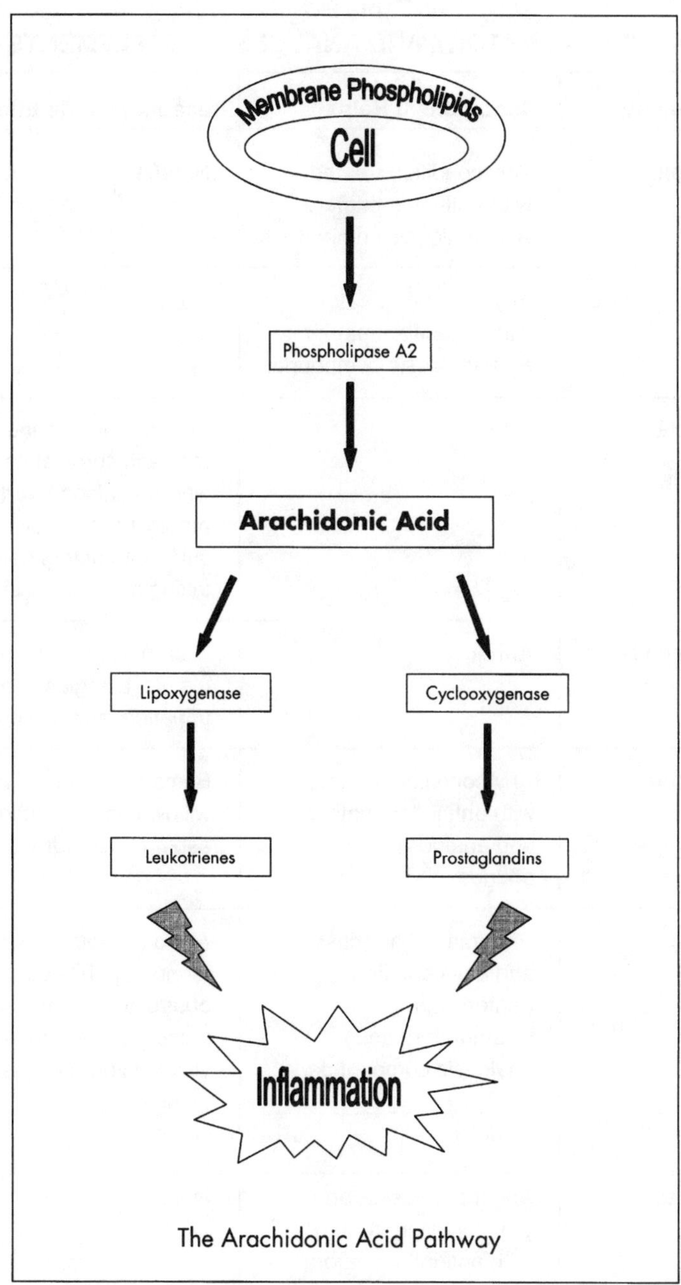

The Arachidonic Acid Pathway

Figure 8-1

Table 8-1
ANTI-INFLAMMATORY AND ANALGESIC SUPPLEMENTS

Supplement	Conditions It Helps	Precautions/Side Effects
Pycnogenol®	Any condition treated with anti-inflammatory and analgesic compounds	None
N-Acetylcysteine	Any condition treated with anti-inflammatory and analgesic compounds	None
Devil's claw	Arthritis	People who experience stomach complaints or who are taking heart medications should consult their doctors before taking it
Stinging nettle	Arthritis	Gastrointestinal complaints, allergies, frequent urination, and itching
Willow bark	Any condition treated with anti-inflammatory and analgesic compounds	Be careful not to combine willow bark with other aspirin-based drugs
Turmeric	Rheumatoid arthritis and any condition treated with anti-inflammatory and analgesic compounds	Avoid it if you are suffering from bile duct obstructions, and use it under close supervision if you have gallstones
Boswellia	Arthritis	None
Perilla seed	Asthma, nausea, and any condition treated with anti-inflammatory compounds	None

Table 8-1
ANTI-INFLAMMATORY AND ANALGESIC SUPPLEMENTS *(cont.)*

Supplement	Conditions It Helps	Precautions/Side Effects
Proteases	Any condition treated with anti-inflammatory and analgesic compounds	None
Omega-3 fatty acids	Any condition treated with anti-inflammatory and analgesic compounds	Reduces blood clotting similar to aspirin
Resveratrol	Any condition treated with anti-inflammatory and analgesic compounds. Resveratrol is a Cox-2 inhibitor "super aspirin."	None
Glucosamine	Osteoarthritis	None
Chondroitin	Osteoarthritis	None
MSM	Arthritis and other painful inflammatory conditions	None
SAMe	Arthritis and other painful inflammatory conditions	None
Niacinamide (Vitamin B_3)	Arthritis and other painful inflammatory conditions	None
Phenylalanine	Painful, inflammatory conditions	None

Additionally, we can use supplements to decrease the amount of pro-inflammatory substances in our bodies and replace them with nutrients that "cool down" inflamed areas. Supplements can be useful in inhibiting the pro-inflammatory activity of cytokines, bradykinins, and interleukins.

Of course, with a decrease in inflammation, pain diminishes. Pain relief, however, is an independent property of some of the supplements described below.

Before starting any supplement program, we recommend that you talk to your doctor or health-care practitioner. We also recommend that women who are pregnant or breast-feeding be especially cautious about supplementing, particularly with herbs. Because herbs (and other supplements) could, potentially, harm the growing fetus or newborn, you should avoid supplements until after you give birth or discontinue breast-feeding or consult with your health-care practitioner.

No matter what your situation, discuss your intention to start taking supplements with your doctor or health-care practitioner. If he or she is open-minded, you can work together to design a comprehensive program of supplementation to help reduce the pain and inflammation that you have lived with long enough.

Pycnogenol®

Pycnogenol® is a registered trade name for an extract derived from the bark of the French maritime pine *Pinus pinaster.* Pycnogenol® itself is not one but a complex of naturally occurring flavonoids and organic acids found in the bark of the tree. This complex of compounds demonstrates some interesting biological properties.

Pain Pharmacology	Studies, Dosages, and Precautions
Inflammation is intimately tied to free radicals that inflammatory cells produce. Therefore, substances that possess free radical scavenging ability are also anti-inflammatory. Pycnogenol® inhibits the activity of a wide range	Researchers have investigated nearly all of Pycnogenol® components for their free radical scavenging capabilities and have found that they protect against a host of other free radicals, including superoxide and peroxy radicals.

of free radicals. In addition to its direct ability to inhibit free radicals, Pycnogenol® may enhance the activities of glutathione peroxidase, superoxide dismutase, and catalase, which are the body's internal antioxidant defense enzymes. Other properties of Pycnogenol® include its specific ability to inhibit the activity of 5-lipoxygenase, which contributes to the production of pro-inflammatory leukotrienes. Pycnogenol® protects elastin, one of our most important structural poteins, from degradation by an enzyme named elastase. Pycnogenol® binds tightly to elastin, thereby protecting it from attack by elastase.	Constituents of Pycnogenol® also protect against lipid peroxidation (fat breakdown). In animal studies, feeding Pycnogenol® to the study animals decreased chemically induced ear swelling (edema). By using edema as a marker of inflammation, we see that Pycno--genol® can alleviate the inflammatory process. Pycnogenol® appears to be a safe supplement with a very low acute and chronic toxicity.

Pycnogenol®

- Mechanism of action: Antioxidant, enhanced antioxidant enzyme activity, inhibition of 5-lipoxygenase and elastase
- Dosage: 50 to 100 milligrams daily
- Active Ingredient: Pycnogenol® complex

N-Acetylcysteine

General

N-acetylcysteine is a compound derived from the union of the amino acid cysteine and an acetyl group (i.e., a molecule composed of carbon, hydrogen, and oxygen). Physicians have historically used it as an antidote for Tylenol (acetaminophen) poisoning and to break down mucus. Doctors have also used N-acetylcysteine successfully to treat people suffering from acute heavy-metal poisoning. As researchers investigage N-acetylcysteine's role in the body, they are discovering that this simple molecule has beneficial effects in conditions characterized by reduced glutathione levels or oxidative stress, like inflammation.

Pain Pharmacology	Studies, Dosages, and Precautions
N-acetylcysteine is an excellent source of sulfhydryl groups, sulfur-containing molecules that play important roles in many biological processes in the body. Specifically, N-acetylcysteine exerts its benefits because it acts directly as a free radical scavenger and stimulates glutathione synthesis. Glutathione is widely distributed throughout the body and plays a critical role in our antioxidant defense systems. Thus, N-acetylcysteine may play a supportive role in the body's internal antioxidant defense system and ameliorate the free radical activity that runs rampant during the inflammatory process.	Studies show that glutathione levels are reduced during inflammatory disease. When it was tested on patients with reduced glutathione levels and excessive oxidative stress, N-acetylcysteine increased glutathione levels in the body. Although N-acetylcysteine appears to be a promising treatment for inflammatory conditions, we need to conduct further studies to determine what role it plays in rheumatic conditions.

N-Acetylcysteine

- Mechanism of action: Antioxidant enhanced glutathione synthesis
- Dosage: 200 milligrams four times daily
- Active Ingrediant: N-acetylcysteine

Devil's Claw (*Harpagophytum procumbens*)

Devil's claw grows in the steppes of south and southwest Africa. Traditional preparations of devil's claw are cut, dried-root tubers, from which people prepare tea. In Europe, it is used widely as a cure for many chronic degenerative diseases. Harpagoside is the ostensible active ingredient in this herb, and it has been standardized in most commercial preparations. Devil's claw has many traditional uses, among them its use for rheumatic joint conditions.

Pain Pharmacology	Studies, Dosages, and Precautions
We don't entirely understand how devil's claw reduces inflammation. Most researchers believe that devil's claw is an analgesic. We know, however, that it does not exert its effects through the arachidonic acid pathway. Studies show that a combination of the extracts found in devil's claw is more effective than any single active ingredient we can isolate from the herb. Take devil's claw as a combination of standardized harpagosides and whole plant extracts. An enteric-coated form is preferred to protect the active constituent harpagosides from being degraded in the stomach.	Devil's claw has proved useful in human patients suffering from arthritic conditions as well as chronic low back pain. In one study, 50 volunteers suffering from arthritis showed a significant decrease in the severity of their pain. This effect was more pronounced in moderate arthritis than in the more severe cases. In 102 patients suffering from low back pain of unknown cause, 1800 milligrams of devil's claw extract (containing 30 milligrams of harpa-gosides) improved their condition and reduced their pain. Another benefit of taking devil's claw in combination with conventional therapies is its cost. Conventional therapy is two-thirds less expensive when devil's claw is included. These and other studies confirm that supplementing with devil's claw at 1.5 to 3 grams per day, standardized to contain 1.5 to 3 percent harpagosides, may reduce inflammation and pain. Although this herb is safe, people who experience stomach complaints or are taking heart medications should

	consult their doctors before taking it. Don't let the name scare you: Devil's claw, at the appropriate dose, is a potent anti-inflammatory herb that could help to relieve pain associated with arthritis and chronic back pain.

Devil's Claw

- Mechanism of Action: An anti-inflammatory effect independent of the arachidonic acid pathway
- Dosage: 1.5 to 3 grams daily of the standardized herb extract
- Active Ingredient: Harpagoside

Stinging Nettle (*Urtica dioica*)

Stinging nettle grows in Europe, some parts of Asia, and North America. It's named after the slight sting you may feel when it's applied topically. Although we've used stinging nettle to improve prostate health, we've also used extracts of this herb topically to treat rheumatic conditions like arthritis due to its anti-inflammatory effect.

Pain Pharmacology	Studies, Dosages, and Precautions
The herb contains a variety of active compounds with antirheumatic properties, including flavonoids and caffeoylmalic acid. We've not yet determined which is the more potent, so once again we recommend using a preparation containing the whole plant. We attribute the anti-inflamma-	A study giving stinging nettle extracts to arthritic patients for three weeks demonstrated its anti-inflammatory effect. Researchers assessed pain at rest and during exercise, as well as physical impairment. After eleven days, patients reported improvements in every area. Approximately 60 per-

tory properties of extracts of stinging nettle to their ability to prevent the body from making the inflammatory prostaglandins and to decrease cytokines (a group of proteins that are persistently elevated during the inflammatory response, as we discussed in Chapter 3). Stinging nettle may also work as a local anesthetic.

cent of the patients who previously took NSAIDs for their pain were able to reduce the amount they took or to eliminate them entirely. Of the 8,955 people surveyed in this study, only 1 percent experienced minor adverse effects, which included gastrointestinal complaints, allergies, frequent urination, and itching.

As this study implies, stinging nettle could be an appropriate accompaniment to NSAIDs and may even decrease one's requirement for them. There are no contraindications, special warnings, or precautions against ingesting stinging nettle. Taking up to 1.5 grams of a stinging nettle supplement per day is a good starting point for people suffering from arthritis. The name "stinging nettle" is a contradiction in terms, in light of its anti-inflammatory potential. Anyone for "soothing nettle"?

Stinging Nettle

- Mechanism of Action: Inhibition of cyclooxygenase and NK-kappa-beta
- Dosage: Up to 1.5 grams daily of the standardized herb extract
- Active Ingredient: Flavonoids/caffeoylmalic acid

Willow Bark (*Salicis alba*)

Salicis alba is a tree that grows throughout much of the United States, as well as in Europe and northern Asia. We use willow bark to treat feverish conditions and mild rheumatic complaints, as well as for pain relief. Most of its effectiveness can be attributed to the active constituent salicin, which is a precursor to acetylsalicylic acid, otherwise known as asprin. Willow bark may be just as effective in reducing inflammation as NSAIDs are.

Pain Pharmacology	Studies, Dosages, and Precautions
In the body, salicin breaks down into salicylic acid, a compound that possesses potent anti-inflammatory activity (particularly prostaglandin-mediated inflammation). Stomach acid doesn't destroy salicin, and our small intestines absorb it readily. This means that the active constituent is neither destroyed nor excreted completely; it enters the body to fight inflammation. Because salicin is a close relative of aspirin, it may work in a similar fashion. When investigators examined the urine of patients supplementing with aspirin and compared it to patients taking salicin, they found similar breakdown chemicals in both groups.	In 120 rheumatoid arthritic patients treated with willow bark, 70 percent experienced both objective and subjective improvement in symptoms (i.e., decreased pain and increased mobility). In a double-blind study, investigators examined the effectiveness of a willow bark extract containing salicin among 78 patients suffering from osteoarthritis of the knee and/or hip. The group taking willow bark experienced pain relief and overall good effects, confirming its effectiveness in treating the inflammation of arthritis. Be careful not to combine willow bark with other salicylates even though, to date, there have been no reports of dangerous interactions. Researchers have not reported any toxic effects, but mild adverse effects may occur as with any asprin compound. Standardized products containing salicin are preferred. Dosages range from 200 milligrams (standardized to 11 percent salicin) to approximately 1400 milligrams. We suspect that

	willow bark will one day find a niche in the medicine cabinet right next to the aspirin bottle.

Willow Bark

- Mechanism of Action: Possible cyclooxygenase inhibitor
- Dosage: 200 to 1400 milligrams daily of the standardized herb extract
- Active Ingredient: Salicin

Turmeric (*Curcuma longa*)

Turmeric is a perennial herb cultivated in the tropical regions of Asia, particularly India. Turmeric has been used as a spice since time immemorial, and it was highly esteemed by the ancient Indo-Europeans as a yellow dye. Turmeric also has a rich history in India, where practitioners of the Ayurvedic system of medicine used it for centuries. The principal components of turmeric with anti-inflammatory properties are the curcuminoids.

Pain Pharmacology	**Studies, Dosages, and Precautions**
Curcuminoids reduce inflammation through a variety of mechanisms. They inhibit cyclooxygenase and lipoxygenase enzymes as powerfully as NSAIDs. Their ability to quench free radical activity adds to turmeric's anti-inflammatory properties, and by quenching free radicals, turmeric also hinders tissue degeneration.	Curcuminoids produced a significant improvement in all rheumatoid arthritis patients studied in a double-blind clinical trial; their effect was comparable to the NSAID phenylbutazone. In two additional studies, patients receiving 1200 milligrams of turmeric extract per day reported a decrease in inflammation and improvement in their condition. Again, the effect was comparable to phenylbutazone. Approximately 1200 milligrams, broken into 400-milligram doses

three times daily, is an effective dose. Its long history, backed up by current scientific studies, shows that turmeric is an extremely safe herb. Studies examining turmeric's effect on both acute and chronic pain show it to be safe even at high dosages. The Food and Drug Administration (FDA) describes turmeric as "generally recognized as safe" (GRAS). However, you should avoid it if you are suffering from bile duct obstructions, and use it under close supervision if you have gallstones. We should no longer relegate turmeric to the spice rack, but rather use it to relieve pain.

Turmeric

- Mechanism of Action: Cyclooxygenase and lipoxygenase inhibitor and antioxidant
- Dosage: 1200 milligrams daily of the standardized herb extract
- Active Ingredient: Curcuminoids

Boswellia (*Boswellia serrata*)

The gum resins derived from *Boswellia serrata*, a large deciduous tree that grows abundantly in the dry, hilly parts of India, provide one of nature's most effective pain and inflammation fighters. Ayurvedic practitioners have used boswellia, like turmeric, to treat rheumatism. Modern scientific studies have corroborated what Ayurvedic medicine has known for centuries—that boswellia is an effective treatment for arthritis.

Pain Pharmacology	Studies, Dosages, and Precautions
Boswellic acid is the extract of the gum resin of the boswellia tree. Boswellia reduces inflammation by specifically inhibiting leukotriene formation. Amazingly, boswellia may also improve circulation to joints and inflamed tissue by repairing blood vessels destroyed by inflammation. Through its ability to act as a sedative on the central nervous system, boswellia has an analgesic effect, as well. Boswellia also inhibits various tissue enzymes that contribute to tissue breakdown.	Early studies examining boswellia's effects on patients suffering from rheumatoid arthritis and ankylosing spondylitis (stiffening of the vertebral joints) produced positive results. At a dosage of 200 milligrams three times daily for four weeks, 70 percent of patients (122 out of 175) reported relief from morning stiffness and pain in two to four weeks. Of the 122 patients who responded to therapy, researchers subsequently switched 17 to a placebo, and their symptoms returned. In another study, 30 patients received 200 milligrams of boswellia three times daily. After four weeks, the group receiving boswellia had lowered arthritic scores, indicating condition improvement. When the treatment group received a placebo, the arthritic score rose again. Boswellia is safe. In a four-week toxicity study, animals fed high doses of boswellia showed no significant changes in blood chemistries. A dose of 200 milligrams of boswellic acids, three times daily, appears to be effective against pain and inflammation.

Boswellia

- Mechanism of Action: Lipoxygenase inhibition, blood vessel restoration, and analgesia
- Dosage: 200 milligrams daily of the standardized herb extract
- Active Ingredient: Boswellic acids

Perilla Seed (*Perilla frutescence*)

Perilla frutescence is a traditional crop in China, Korea, Japan, and Southeast Asia. People in Japan enjoy the leaves and seeds of perilla as part of a dish called "shisho." Oriental folk medicine employs perilla seed to treat asthma, nausea, and sunstroke. In the West, we use oil from the seed in commercial manufacturing to produce varnishes, dyes, and inks. Perilla seed, however, may have another use apart from traditional medicine and modern-day manufacturing techniques: It may help to reduce inflammation.

Pain Pharmacology	**Studies, Dosages, and Precautions**
Perilla seed is a rich source of the important fatty acid alpha-linolenate, an omega-3 fatty acid. It is also rich in the compounds luteolin, apigenin, chrysoeriol, and rosmarinic acid. These compounds (especially luteolin) inhibit lipoxygenase, the enzyme that converts arachidonic acid into the pro-inflammatory leukotrienes. Luteolin is the most potent compound in the plant. Perilla seed is preferred over the leaf, because extracts from the seed are one hundred times more potent at inhibiting lipoxygenase.	Laboratory studies confirm perilla seed's antilipoxygenase activity, and animal studies demonstrate that seed extracts reduce inflammation. Research on perilla seed is relatively new, and we need to confirm its effective dosage and toxicity. So far, dosages as high as 100 to 150 milligrams per day (preferentially standardized for luteolin) show positive results. Acute toxicity studies indicate that a lethal dose is more than 2000 milligrams per kilogram of body weight (that's 140 grams for an average man). People who took 7 grams daily for two weeks experienced no toxic side effects. Perilla seed may transcend its use as an ingredient and industrial by-product and fall into a new category—potent anti-inflammatory.

Perilla Seed

- Mechanism of Action: Lipoxygenase inhibition; possibly others unknown at this time
- Dosage: 100 to 150 milligrams daily of the standardized herb extract
- Active Ingredient: Luteolin, apigenin, chrysoeriol, and rosmarinic acid

Proteases

Proteases are enzymes that break down proteins, but they also fulfill many other roles in almost every cellular process, including tissue repair. Trypsin, chymotrypsin (enzymes naturally produced by the pancreas), bromelain from pineapples, and papain from papaya are but a few of the many proteases found in nature. These particular proteases, however, help reduce inflammation.

Pain Pharmacology	Studies, Dosages, and Precautions
Proteases may attenuate the inflammatory process by several mechanisms. They may inactivate enzymes that help form pro-inflammatory substances; they may inactivate bradykinins (whose role in inflammation we discussed in Chapter 3); they may inhibit antiproteases, which contribute to inflammation. An additional, unique function of proteases is their ability to remove cellular debris from the inflamed site (a process called debridement). Like cleaning the walls before applying a fresh coat of paint, this debris removal is an important step before forming new tissue. Researchers developed oral	Although most studies investigating the effects of proteases were performed before 1970, several recent studies conducted in Germany confirm their anti-inflammatory activity. People who took a supplement containing a mixture of papain, bromelain, trypsin, and chymotrypsin reported a significantly greater improvement in pain reduction compared to those taking a placebo. A randomized, double-blind study using patients recovering from surgery showed that this supplement reduced edema, and improved mobility and flexibility. In another double-blind, placebo-controlled study, patients suffering from sprained ankles re-

protease supplements, but many wondered if this form of administration would prove useful. After all, proteases are proteins, and stomach acid digests them just like all other proteins. We've learned, however, that proteases *can* be absorbed intact and remain functional in the body.

ported less swelling, less pain, more flexibility, and a quicker return to work.

Additional studies suggest that bromelain supplementation may reduce the swelling and pain associated with rheumatoid arthritis, and may also relieve back pain. For protease supplementation to be effective, you should begin it as soon as you are injured. Supplements should be a mixture of enzymes (such as a combination of papain, bromelain, trypsin, and chymotrypsin), taken on an empty stomach, with juice or water. If they're available, enteric-coated tablets will preserve proteases until they reach the small intestines.

Protease

- Mechanism of Action: Inhibition of pro-inflammatory bradykinins and antiproteases and debridement
- Dosage: Trypsin/chymotrypsin: 500 to 1000 milligrams; bromelain: 500 to 2000 milligrams; Papain: 100 to 500 milligrams
- Active Ingredient: Trypsin, chymotrypsin, bromelain

Omega-3 Fatty Acids

Perhaps one of the most-researched and yet controversial arthritis treatments is fish oils containing omega-3 fatty acids, specifically eicosapentaenoic acid (EPA) and docosahexaenoic acid (DHA), derivatives of alpha-linolenic acid. Because such high doses of omega-3 oils are required to elicit a response in arthritic patients, consuming fatty fish high in omega-3 may not be enough. Supplementation is necessary. For people who experience discomfort from fish oil supplements, an excellent alternative is DHA, an omega-3 fatty acid derived from algae. This product is known as Neuromins® DHA.

Pain Pharmacology	Studies, Dosages, and Precautions
As we saw in Chapter 7, omega-3 fatty acids oppose the actions of both omega-6 and arachidonic acid. Therefore, omega-3 fatty acids stop them from producing pro-inflammatory substances like leukotrienes. Additional anti-inflammatory actions of omega-3 fish oils may include: (a) inhibiting 5-lipoxygenase and cyclooxygenase enzymes; and (b) decreasing interleukin-1, which participates in the inflammatory response. Fish oils not only decrease inflammatory leukotrienes and interleukins, but also increase the "good" leukotrienes that actually possess *anti*-inflammatory activity.	Numerous studies using fish oil suggest that omega-3 fatty fish oils cause both subjective and objective improvements in rheumatoid arthritis patients. These effects, however, are modest and researchers don't see them in all studies. One thing is clear, though: supplementing with omega-3 fatty acids reduces inflammation by decreasing omega-6 and arachidonic acid uptake and inhibiting their conversion to leukotrienes. Dosages of omega-3 fatty acids in studies have varied from as low as 3 grams per day to as high as 20 grams per day. With such variation, it's difficult to determine an effective dosage. It's clear that higher intake is more beneficial. Purchase supplements that contain one gram of fish oil per capsule. Three to eighteen capsules per day, in divided doses, will provide a major source of omega-3 fatty acids. Make sure that the supplements you take come from fish *body* oil, not fish *liver* oil. Optional to the fish-derived products are those omega-3 fats produced from algae. You may want to explore using concentrates of algae for your source of omega-3s.

Omega-3 Fatty Acids

- Mechanism of Action: Lipoxygenase and cyclooxygenase inhibition, decreased interleukin-1 production
- Dosage: 3 to 20 grams daily
- Active Ingredient: Omega-3 oils EPA and DHA

Resveratrol

Resveratrol is a compound that protects plants against fungal infections (it's a phytoalexin). Researchers became interested in resveratrol when they tried to explain the "French paradox"—the puzzling fact that, despite their high-fat diets and excessive smoking, the French have a low incidence of heart disease. Scientists discovered that a certain constituent in red wine may actually protect our hearts, and we later learned that it's resveratrol. While most research has focused on resveratrol's cardiovascular benefits, some has extended to its role in preventing inflammation.

Pain Pharmacology	Studies, Dosages, and Precautions
Resveratrol is a natural Cox-2 inhibitor, so it's a type of "super aspirin" as we discussed in Chapter 1. Researchers theorize that resveratrol directly inhibits Cox-2, as well as other compounds that promote its activity.	We know that Cox-2 increases the synthesis of pro-inflammatory prostaglandins, and that resveratrol inhibits that activity. Although studies using resveratrol have not been performed in people, it may be one of the most important anti-inflammatory agents we have today in our nutritional arsenal.

Resveratrol

- Mechanism of Action: Cox-2 inhibitor
- Dosage: 200 to 600 micrograms daily of the standardized herb extract
- Active Ingredient: Resveratrol

Taxifolin *(Dihydroquercetin)*

Taxifolin is a flavonoid commonly found in edible fruits and vegetables such as avocado, blueberry and apple. It is also one of the active ingredients found in the special pine bark extract supplement Pycnogenol®. According to its chemical structure, taxifolin is a hydrated analogue of the important bioflavonoid, quercetin—dihydroquercetin. Taxifolin has proved to be one of the most powerful free radical scavengers (antioxidant) and shares additional therapeutic flavonoid roles such as regulation of capillary strength, hepatoprotective and anti-inflammatory (anti-leukotriene). The latter theraputic role provides for taxifolin's significance for the treatment of pain and inflammatory conditions.

Pain Pharmacology	**Studies, Dosages and Precautions**
Taxifolin has been shown to be very effective as an antioxidant, hepatoprotective and as an anti-inflammatory agent via its ability to affect inflammatory leukotrienes and reduce inflammatory edema. Specifically, taxifolin is capable of slowing down inflammatory leuko-triene formation by inhibiting the enzyme 5-lipoxygenase. It was shown that taxifolin was similar to the activity of hydrocortisone on decreasing the enzyme activities during inflammation and also stimulated ATP phosphorylation activity as seen in salicylates, phenylbutazone, corticoids, indomethacin and other anti-inflammatory drugs. Its ability to reduce high levels of lipid peroxide oxidation makes taxifolin an excellent agent for a wide range of therapeutic applications. As an antioxidant, taxifolin may be compared to or exceeds many synthetic and natural antioxidants and, in particular, known bioflavo-noids (quercetin).	Regarding its antioxidant activity, in vitro studies have shown that taxifolin protects lipid peroxidation as efficiently as alpha tocopherol (vitamin E) and has the ability to suppress the destructive neurotoxin nitric oxide (NO). In animal studies, taxifolin was shown to possess powerful anti-inflammatory activity on the exudative and proliferative phases of inflammation. High antioxidant activity of taxifolin is combined with absence of embryotoxicity, teratogenicity, allergenicity and mutability. Pharmaceutical production of taxifolin may be intended for prophylactic of "oxidative stress" diseases (cardiovascular, bronchopulmonary, etc.). In human studies, taxifolin has been prescribed for a variety of ailments ranging from cardioprotection to hepatoprotective to anti-inflammatory. Therapeutic doses provided orally ranged from 100mg to 200mg daily.

SUPPLEMENTS FOR REBUILDING TISSUE

Once we tame inflammation, we must next prevent further tissue degradation. When inflammation hasn't completely destroyed tissue, we need to repair and rebuild it. Here is where we draw the line between nutritional supplementation and conventional drugs or, more precisely, where conventional drugs cease to be effective. The popular NSAIDs that we consume in great quantities to reduce inflammation may, in some circumstances, do more harm than good to the tissue we're trying to protect. Then there is their whole host of side effects, including stomach ulceration and toxicity.

Why use these toxic drugs when we have safer alternatives? We already have supplements that help reverse the damage that follows chronic long-term inflammation, and return function to the affected tissues—so let's use them.

In most circumstances, these supplements affect cartilage growth and repair. Because cartilage is highly resistant to mechanical stresses, it's an ideal protective coating for bones that are continually in contact with one another in our joints. Cartilage provides resiliency, load distribution, shock absorption, and lubrication to our joints. There is, however, a price for cartilage's resiliency: Compared to other tissues, cartilage takes a long time to heal. Inflammation's continual assault, constant mechanical strain, and the inability to recover quickly leads to a gradual decline in cartilage tissue that, eventually, manifests as pain.

By providing the building blocks of cartilage, it's conceivable that we can help cartilage repair itself more rapidly. The supplements we describe here contribute to cartilage repair and, in some circumstances, provide additional benefits to our joints.

Unlike NSAIDs, which treat symptoms rather than the root of the problem, certain supplements actually correct the problem. As you will see, the key dietary supplements described here may provide greater benefits than conventional drugs.

Glucosamine

Glucosamine, a naturally occurring compound found in the body, is a glucose molecule bound to the amino acid glutamine (hence the name "glucosamine"). It's one of the most important compounds in synthesizing cartilage. In fact, glucosamine's importance in cartilage synthesis cannot be overstated.

Pain Pharmacology	Studies, Dosages, and Precautions
Without glucosamine, cartilage synthesis is hampered. This led researchers to conclude that, if sufficient glucosamine were made available, it would enhance repair of joint tissue and/or preserve existing cartilage tissue. Other investigators claim that it's not glucosamine's ability to stimulate cartilage synthesis that is helpful in osteoarthritis, but its ability to enhance production of hyaluronic acid, the compound primarily responsible for the lubricating and shock absorbing properties of the fluid that bathes the joints. Whichever mechanism it uses, glucosamine is crucial to preserving joint health.	More than fifteen studies indicate that glucosamine reduces symptoms of osteoarthritis and may even reverse cartilage damage in mild forms of the disease. A double-blind investigation performed in 178 patients suffering from osteoarthritis showed that glucosamine reduced symptoms as much as a popular over-the-counter NSAID. This study was unique because both patients and doctors reported greater effect and less toxicity with 1500 milligrams of glucosamine than 1200 milligrams of ibuprofen. Proof of glucosamine's cartilage-rebuilding properties came from a double-blind study in 80 osteoarthritic patients. After the treatment period ended, researchers took cartilage biopsies of both the control group and the group taking glucosamine. While the control group exhibited typical signs of osteoarthritis, the group taking glucosamine showed almost smooth cartilage and only minor signs of osteoarthritis. These investigators concluded that the cartilage appeared to be rebuilt after glucosamine treatment. Subsequent studies indicate that glucosamine treatment is superior to NSAIDs, but it may take up to several weeks before improvement is seen. A multitude of scientific studies show glucosamine to be extremely safe and practically devoid of any toxicity.

Glucosamine

- Mechanism of Action: Cartilage synthesis; enhanced hyaluronic acid synthesis
- Dosage: 1500 milligrams daily
- Active Ingredient: Glucosamine sulfate

Chondroitin

Chondroitin is a highly viscous substance found throughout the body, especially in skin, bone, arterial walls, and cartilage. Most commercial preparations come from bovine or shark cartilage. Not only does chondroitin play an integral role in cartilage synthesis, it also acts as a "water magnet." Water is the primary medium in the spaces between joints; it aids shock absorption and transports nutrients into cartilage. Chondroitin's popularity as an osteoarthritis treatment has escalated and motivated the scientific community to examine how it affects joint health.

Pain Pharmacology	Studies, Dosages, and Precautions
Three possible mechanisms of action are attributed to chondroitin: (a) anti-inflammatory activity on cellular components of inflammation; (b) enhanced synthesis of the matrix used to rebuild cartilage; and (c) decreased breakdown of cartilage components. Recent evidence suggests that chondroitin may inhibit the damaging effects of nitric oxide (which we discussed in Chapter 1). In normal cartilage tissue, nitric oxide is absent. In osteoarthritis patients, nitric oxide induces cellular breakdown of chondrocytes, the cells that synthesize and maintain cartilage. Chondroitin sulfate protects chondrocytes from the damaging effects of nitric oxide.	Using daily dosages of 800 to 1200 milligrams, divided into two to three dosages, chondroitin (in the form of chondroitin sulfate) is an effective treatment against osteoarthritis of the knee. In one study, it was compared to the popular NSAID diclofenac. Both were effective, but the therapeutic effect of chondroitin sulfate lasted for up to three months longer. The effect of chondroitin sulfate on animals and humans is well described in the literature. Compared with nonsteroidal anti-inflammatory drugs (indomethacin, ibuprofen), chondroitin sulfate appears to be more effective on cellular events of inflammation than on edema formation. This anti-inflammatory ac-

	tion of chondroitin sulfate was described in the May 1998 issue of the *Osteoarthritis Cartilage Journal*. The results of this paper provide an insight into the mechanism of the anti-inflammatory and chondroprotective actions demonstrated by chondroitic sulfate in a number of clinical trials involving patients with osteoarthritis.

Chondroitin

- Mechanism of Action: Enhanced synthesis/decreased breakdown of cartilage
- Dosage: 1200 milligrams daily
- Active Ingredient: Chondroitin as chondroitin sulfate A and B

Methylsulfonylmethane (MSM)

Methylsulfonylmethane (MSM) is the major metabolic by-product of dimethyl sulfoxide, which you may know as DMSO. Although MSM comes from DMSO, it does not share DMSO's characteristics (which are controversial). MSM is an odorless, virtually tasteless, white crystalline powder we find in various plants as well as in unprocessed milk, meat, and fish.

Pain Pharmacology	Studies, Dosages, and Precautions
Explanations for MSM's actions in the body are vague. Its activity may be a result of MSM's ability to donate sulfur to important reactions in the body. Sulfur is as essential to life as oxygen. We require sulfur to synthesize proteins, hormones, and immunoglobulins (immune system proteins).	According to its advocates, MSM is useful for treating a variety of conditions, including arthritis and inflammatory conditions. Most of this information, however, is anecdotal in nature; that is, few formal studies have been done. Dr. Stanley Jacob, professor of surgery at Oregon Health Sciences Univer-

sity (Portland, Oregon), is perhaps the premier advocate of MSM. He has investigated its properties for more than twenty years. His investigations, as well as other research, show that MSM is indeed an effective therapy for pain and inflammation. The doses used (1 to 2 grams daily) and its apparent lack of toxicity suggest that MSM won't cause any adverse effects even over the long term. If other scientists confirm the benefits of MSM, then it may prove extremely beneficial to those suffering from arthritis.

Methylsulfonylmethane (MSM)

- Mechanism of Action: Tissue repair/synthesis by providing sulfur for sulfur bonds
- Dosage: 1 to 2 grams daily
- Active Ingredient: MSM

S-Adenosyl-L-Methionine (SAMe)

While SAMe is one of the most important neuro-neutrients available today, we discovered this compound's effectiveness against osteoarthritis serendipitously, when depressed patients taking S-adenosyl-L-methionine (SAMe) reported a marked improvement in their degenerative joint disease. Since 1975, Europeans have used SAMe to treat osteoarthritis, fibromyalgia, migraine headaches, liver disorders, and neurological conditions. Current research shows that SAMe may be an effective therapy for osteoarthritis.

Pain Pharmacology	Studies, Dosages, and Precautions
SAMe is a naturally occurring compound we synthesize in our bodies. It's involved in a reaction that shifts an active methyl group (a carbon atom surrounded by three hydrogen atoms) to a wide variety of methyl "acceptor" molecules. SAMe also produces glutathione, which is an important antioxidant. SAMe possesses anti-inflammatory and analgesic properties, although we cannot explain them. SAMe participates in cartilage synthesis, helping to repair cartilage tissue.	Using dosages of 400 to 1200 milligrams daily, numerous human trials of SAMe have shown clinical benefits for osteoarthritic patients. In a double-blind study that included 734 subjects suffering from osteoarthritis of the hip, knee, spine, and hand, researchers compared SAMe to (a) a placebo and (b) the NSAID naproxen (sold under the name Aleve). At 1200 milligrams daily, SAMe exerted the same analgesic activity as naproxen, and was superior to the placebo. Both the patients and doctors rated SAMe as being less toxic than naproxen, and side effects were rare. Its high tolerability and positive effects in people suffering from osteoarthritis may make SAMe a heavy hitter in pain management.

S-Adenosyl-Methionine (SAMe)

- Mechanism of Action: Cartilage synthesis, analgesia, and antidepressive
- Dosage: 400 to 1200 milligrams daily
- Active Ingredient: SAMe as SAMe sulfate

Niacinamide

Niacin is a B vitamin (B_3) that is essential for producing energy, regulating blood sugar, antioxidant activity, and detoxification reactions. Niacin, however, is not one but two compounds: nicotinic acid and niacinamide. Researchers discovered niacin while trying to find a cure for pellagra, a devastating disease that, if left untreated, causes dementia and death. This discovery promoted niacin to "required" status in the human diet. Researchers have since investigated niacin's role in a variety of other conditions, including osteoarthritis.

Pain Pharmacology	Studies, Dosages, and Precautions
Niacinamide appears to be an effective treatment for osteoarthritis. Work in the 1940s found that oral niacinamide relieves joint pain. We don't entirely understand niacinamide's mechanism of action, but it may play a role in activating chondrocytes, rather than acting as an anti-inflammatory or analgesic. Frequent dosing (150 to 250 milligrams every three hours) seems to be required for it to be effective. Ingestion of a large, single dose is not effective. Additionally, niacinamide only works as long as you continue to take it.	Unfortunately, not much research has been done using niacinamide in osteoarthritic patients. A 1996 double-blind, placebo-controlled study, however, examined its effects in seventy-two osteoarthritis patients. After twelve weeks, researchers noted improvements in sed-rate (which usually increases during inflammation, as we discussed earlier) and joint mobility. Those taking the vitamin were able to reduce their anti-inflammatory medication by 13 percent, while subjects in the placebo group worsened by 10 percent. Side effects of niacinamide were mild. This fairly recent study confirms earlier ones. Another added benefit of niacinamide supplementation is the absence of "flushing" (a skin reaction brought on by the rapid dilation of blood vessels supplying blood to the skin), which is caused by nicotinic acid. Considering niacinamide's therapeutic benefits, further studies are warranted.

Niacinamide

- Mechanism of Action: Chondrocyte activation leading to cartilage synthesis
- Dosage: 150 to 250 milligrams every three hours
- Active Ingredient: Niacinamide

DL-Phenylalanine

Phenylalanine is an essential amino acid found abundantly in meat and milk. We don't make it in our bodies, and must obtain phenylalanine from food or supplements. Phenylalanine participates in many biochemical pathways, but its greatest importance is within the brain. Unlike most amino acids, phenylalanine can enter this well-defended organ and affect its chemistry. Researchers have investigated phenylalanine's role in pain since the early 1980s.

Pain Pharmacology	**Studies, Dosages, and Precautions**
Phenylalanine, like most amino acids, exists in different forms. The two major forms are an "L" form (e.g., L-phenylalanine) and a "D" form (D-phenylalanine and the hybrid DL-phenylalanine, or DLPA). Although they are identical chemically, tiny differences in their structures produce different biological properties. Researchers have investigated D forms of phenylalanine for pain reduction. They lessen pain by inhibiting the activity of enkephalinase, an enzyme that breaks down the body's natural painkillers, the endorphins and enkephalins. Even though both D-phenylalanine and DL-phenylalanine lessen	Several studies in humans indicate that the D forms of phenylalanine can reduce pain, enhance analgesia, and increase the pain threshold. In one study, patients suffering from osteoarthritis had significant pain relief after supplementing with D-phenylalanine. In a double-blind study using D forms of phenylalanine, 30 percent of patients with chronic pain who stopped taking all other pain medication reported a 50 percent reduction in pain. In the same study, individuals who did not receive D-phenylalanine experienced persistent pain. We need to perform further research to identify any adverse effects of both short- and

pain, they don't treat its underlying causes. You should use anti-inflammatory supplements along with DLPA.	long-term supplementation with the D forms of phenylalanine.

Phenylalanine

- Mechanism of Action: Inhibition of enkephalinase, the enzyme that breaks down endorphins and enkephalins
- Dosage: 500 milligrams three times daily
- Active Ingredient: D and L forms of phenylalanine

Now let's examine even more potent weapons in our fight against pain. The pain managers: natural, safe supplements that diminish pain and help us cope with the depression it so often causes.

NATURE'S PAIN KILLER FORMULAS

General Pain/Anti-Inflammatory Formula

Daily Recommendation:

Taxifolin	200 mg
Resveratrol	50 mg
Perilla Seed	100 mg
Standardized White Willow Bark	100 mg
Standardized Stinging Nettle	300 mg
Standardized Turmeric Extract	200 mg
DLPA	500 mg
Pycnogenol®	200 mg
Standardized Devil's Claw	300 mg

Osteoarthritis Formula

For increasing bone, collagen density and reducing inflammation and pain

Daily Recommendations:

Glucosamine Sulfate	1,000 mg

Hyluranocollagen	500 mg
S-Adenosyl Methionine (SAMe)	400 mg
Niacinamide	150 mg
Ipriflavone	600 mg
Calcium	1,000 mg
Magnesium	500 mg
Manganese	5 mg
Vitamin C	1,000 mg
Vitamin D	1400 IU
Standardized Turmeric	250 mg
Standardized Boswellia	250 mg
Taxifolin	100 mg
Standardized White Willow Bark	100 mg

Joint Support Formula

For joint support and pain/inflammatory relief

Daily Recommendations:

Glucosamine Sulfate	1,000 mg
Chondroitin Sulfate	500 mg
S-Adenosyl Methionine	400 mg
Standardized Turmeric	200 mg
DLPA	500 mg
Taxifolin	100 mg
Pycnogenol®	200 mg
Ulva Seaweed	200 mg
Vitamin C	500 mg
L-Proline	500 mg

General Antioxidant Free Radical Modulators

As a support adjunct, to be used with any pain relief formula or individual pain relief substance

Daily Recommendations:

Natural Carotenoid Mix	5,000 IU
Lycopene	1 mg
Lutein	1 mg
Vitamin E (d-alpha tocopherol)	200 IU
Gamma Tocopherol	50 IU

Tocotrienols	15 mg
Vitamin C	500 mg
Lipoic Acid	100 mg
N-Acetylcysteine	100 mg
Selenium	100 mcg
Zinc	15 mg
Copper	2 mg
Standardized Fruit Polyphenols	50 mg
Pycnogenol®	50 mg
Standardized Ginkgo Biloba	50 mg
Standardized Turmeric	50 mg
Standardized Bilberry	50 mg
Standardized Green Tea	50 mg

Anti-Stress Formula

Standardized Rhodiola Extract	200 mg
Standardized Korean Ginseng	150 mg
Standardized American Ginseng	150 mg
Phosphatidylserine	300 mg
Standardized Passionflower Extract	200 mg
Standardized Valerian Extract	200 mg
Standardized Kava Kava	200 mg

*Combine with a complete B complex, vitamin C and magnesium formula

Anti-Depressant Formula

Standardized Saint-Johns-Wort	300 mg
SAMe (s-adenosyl methionine)	400 mg
Inositol	500 mg
Phosphatidylserine	300 mg
DHA (docosahexaenoic acid)	300 mg
Standardized Rhodiola Extract	200 mg
Chelated Chromium	200 mcg
Standardized Schisandra Extract	100 mg

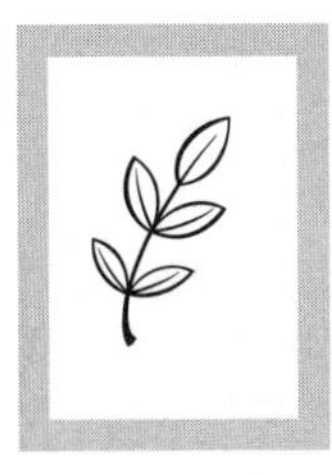

Chapter 9 SEDATIVE AND SUPPORTIVE SUPPLEMENTS FOR PAIN MANAGEMENT

To manage pain effectively, we must address both physical and emotional symptoms. In earlier chapters, we dealt primarily with the physical side of pain. Now that you understand the fundamental causes of pain and inflammation, let's survey our true arsenal in the fight against pain: natural, safe supplements that help to manage pain and provide relief from the stress and depression it too often causes. In addition, we'll briefly explore supplements that provide support when we're combating inflammation.

As you now know, serotonin is crucial in fighting pain, depression, and inflammation. Since 1948, it's been one of the body's most actively investigated chemicals, and its role in brain function has been studied intensively. The brain, however, is only one area in which serotonin acts. This ubiquitous chemical participates in many processes, including smooth muscle contraction, temperature regulation, appetite, behavior, blood pressure, respiration, and pain perception.

Although the concentration of serotonin in the brain is relatively small (1 to 2 percent) compared to its concentration in other parts of the body, the role it plays in brain function is crucial to our overall health. Even slight disturbances in serotonin levels can cause substantial personality disorders. Anxiety, obsessive-compulsive disorder, schizophrenia, and depression are all associated with reduced amounts of serotonin in the brain.

Serotonin was first implicated in depression when researchers observed that drugs that relieve depressive symptoms also boost serotonin levels. As we've discussed, pharmaceutical companies created numerous drugs that correct its levels in people suffering from depression.

We've also learned that low serotonin levels play a role in pain perception. Studies show an inverse relationship between serotonin concentration and pain perception—that is, the greater the serotonin level, the less pain you feel. Thus, enhancing serotonin levels through supplementation may help alleviate pain.

While the following supplements may help to fight pain, researchers have not proven that they act as analgesics (see Table 9-1). Nevertheless, they may be useful in relieving pain because of their ability to preserve or enhance serotonin levels in the brain.

These supplements also serve another purpose. People suffering from relentless pain may experience bouts of depression because of their condition(s), and supplements that boost serotonin may also help in this arena.

Additionally, reduced serotonin levels may cause, or contribute to, fibromyalgia (which we discussed in detail in Chapter 5). Therefore, raising serotonin levels may help people with this condition.

We'll also discuss supplements that help to calm the body during painful episodes that might leave you feeling anxious, tense, and unable to sleep, all of which may further exacerbate your condition. Sleep deprivation is a symptom of fibromyalgia, for example, and so enhancing sleep quality may prove useful. Supplements like passionflower help you relax, while kava contributes to sound and uninterrupted sleep. These supplements, like many of the nutritional supplements discussed here, act on the central nervous system through complex mechanisms that we don't entirely understand.

Table 9-1
SEDATIVE AND SUPPORTIVE SUPPLEMENTS

Supplement	Actions	Precautions/Side Effects
5-HTP	Boosts serotonin levels	None
Saint-John's-Wort	Boosts serotonin levels	It may make certain people more susceptible to sunburn.
Rhodiola	Boosts serotonin levels	None
Passionflower	Sedative and antianxiety	None
Kava	Sedative and tranquilizer	Don't take kava if you're taking other drugs with sedative properties.
Valerian	Sedative	None
Pycnogenol®	Antioxidant	None
NAC (N-acetylcysteine)	Antioxidant	May cause G.I. discomfort on an empty stomach. Take with carbohydrate snack or meal.
Phosphatidylserine	Antioxidant	None

ANTIDEPRESSANT SUPPLEMENTS

5-Hydroxytryptophan

Because serotonin is unable to enter the brain freely, its synthesis must begin in the brain itself. Tryptophan, the precursor to serotonin, would be an ideal supplement, but it is no longer easily available in the United States without a prescription. Another compound, 5-hydroxytryptophan (5-HTP), is an alternative to tryptophan. It's the metabolic intermediate between tryptophan and serotonin.

Pain Pharmacology	Studies, Dosages, and Precautions
Researchers have focused on 5-HTP's clinical significance for treating depression. Because of serotonin's role in pain perception, however, 5-HTP may also be useful for people suffering from chronic pain. It has two possible actions: First, 5-HTP may increase brain serotonin levels by providing its necessary precursor. Second, it may increase endorphins, our body's natural pain killers. In one respect, supplementing with 5-HTP may even be superior to supplementing with tryptophan. Because tryptophan competes with other amino acids for entry into the brain, it's difficult to get high concentrations into the brain. Unlike tryptophan, 5-HTP's absorption into the brain is not influenced by other amino acids.	When a group of patients took 200 milligrams of 5-HTP orally, it increased endorphins, our body's natural pain killers. Fibro-myalgia patients (who have low levels of serotonin) showed a significant reduction in symptoms after taking 300 milligrams of 5-HTP. Effective doses of 5-HTP appear to range from 300 to 600 milligrams daily in divided doses, taken on an empty stomach or with a carbohydrate-rich snack.

5-Hydroxytryptophan

- Mechanism of Action: Enhancing serotonin and endorphin levels
- Dosage: 300 to 600 milligrams daily
- Active Ingredient: 5-HTP

SAINT-JOHN'S-WORT (*Hypericum perforatum*)

Saint-John's-Wort is an aromatic perennial native to Europe that's now found throughout the United States. It is an aggressive weed found in the dry ground of roadsides, meadows, woods, and hedges. Historically, practitioners have used Saint-John's-wort for its anti-inflammatory and healing properties. Today, the majority of studies suggest that its leaves are effective against anxiety and depression.

Pain Pharmacology	Studies, Dosages, and Precautions
Modern researchers have studied the effect of Saint-John's-Wort on depression. Saint-John's-Wort may enhance serotonin levels either by inhibiting the enzyme monoamine oxidase (MAO), which breaks down serotonin in the body, or by inhibiting serotonin's uptake into cells (which leaves more in the brain). It may use a combination of the two actions. Either scenario preserves blood serotonin levels, and higher serotonin levels affect the brain, reducing depression and, possibly, pain. Even though most research has examined hypericin, the active constituent of Saint-John's-Wort, more recent investigations have implicated the compound hyperforin as the herb's major active compound.	In a randomized, double-blind, placebo-controlled, multicenter study, 147 outpatients suffering from mild depression received two different extracts of Saint-John's-Wort that differed in hyperforin concentration. The results show that, at 900 milligrams daily, 5 percent standardized hyperforin extract was superior to both placebo and 0.5 percent standardized hyperforin extract. If hyperforin was not the herb's active constituent, then we wouldn't have seen a difference, no matter what concentrations were used. Hyperforin may have a mechanism of action that resembles hypericin's, yet the two compounds have very different activity in the body. While this study indicates

that hyperforin is the major active constituent in Saint-John's-Wort, it's not the only one. Until we can fully decipher what roles are played by hyperforin, hypericin, and possibly other compounds, we recommend a daily dosage of 500 milligrams standardized to contain both hypericin (at 0.3 percent) and hyperforin (at 5 percent). Saint-John's-Wort is safe but, in some instances, it may make you more susceptible to sunburn. The dosage above is considered safe.

Saint-John's-Wort

- Mechanism of Action: MAO inhibition and/or inhibition of serotonin uptake into cells
- Dosage: 500 milligrams daily of the standardized herb extract
- Active Ingredient: Hyperforin, hypericin

RHODIOLA (*Rhodiola rosea*)

Rhodiola rosea, also called "arctic root" or "golden root," is a plant indigenous to the polar Arctic regions of eastern Siberia. Its yellow flowers smell like attar of roses, hence the name "rosea." Historically, only members of certain families knew where this precious plant grew. Russian families passed on lore about its preparation from generation to generation. In Siberia they say "People who drink rhodiola tea will live more than one hundred years."

Pain Pharmacology	Studies, Dosages, and Precautions
Rhodiola is an "adaptogen." For a plant to be considered an adaptogen, it must conform to the following criteria: • The plant must be innocuous and nontoxic to the body, and have only minimal consequences on the body's normal physiological functioning. • It must exert nonspecific action and help to maintain normal body functions despite the onslaught of stresses. • An adaptogen should normalize body functions irrespective of the pathological condition. In essence, rhodiola has an overall effect on the body, yet it doesn't harm it in any way. One of these effects is on serotonin metabolism and depression. Scientists have found that two active constituents of rhodiola, rosavin and salidroside, enhance the transport of the serotonin precursors tryptophan and 5-HTP into the brain. Researchers proved this when rhodiola was given in combination with 5-HTP to animals. This means that rhodiola enhances the uptake of serotonin precursors into the brain, and so stimulates serotonin synthesis.	Scientists in the United States have done little research on rhodiola. It's relatively unknown to Western consumers, yet it is easily available as a supplement. Two hundred milligrams standardized to contain both rosavin and salidroside may be an appropriate and safe addition to an antipain regimen.

Rhodiola

- Mechanism of Action: Enhanced transport of serotonin precursors into the brain
- Dosage: 200 milligrams daily of the standardized herb extract
- Active Ingredient: Rosavin and salidroside

SEDATIVE SUPPLEMENTS

Passionflower *(Passiflora incarnata)*

Passionflower is native to the tropical and subtropical areas of the Americas. Discovered in 1569, the name "passionflower" came from the arrangement of the flowers, which reminded explorers of the Passion of Christ. Historical uses of passionflower include treating insomnia, nervousness, inflammation, and hemorrhoids. Recent research has concentrated on its sedative effects.

Pain Pharmacology	**Studies, Dosages, and Precautions**
Even though many plants fall under the genus *Passiflora*, clinicians have used only *Passiflora incarnata* as a medicine. The key constituents in passionflower are flavonoids and alkaloids, although it's yet to be determined which is predominantly responsible for the herb's action. Most likely, a combination of both flavonoids and alkaloids is responsible for passionflower's effect. Passionflower also acts on the central nervous system in complex ways that we don't yet completely understand.	In animal studies, passionflower has sedative and antianxiety properties. In other studies, passionflower increased animals' tolerance to pain. Human studies have only used passionflower in combination with other herbs, and we need to conduct further investigations using passionflower alone. Even though we know little about its toxicity in humans, animal studies show no adverse effects.

Passionflower

- Mechanism of Action: Unclear, but possible inhibition of lipoxygenase; also sedative properties
- Dosage: 4 to 8 grams of dried herb or 200 milligrams standardized extract
- Active Ingredient: Flavonoids and alkaloids

Kava *(Piper methysticum)*

Kava, a large shrub widely cultivated in the South Pacific islands, is an important part of the social and medicinal practices of the indigenous people. In the South Pacific, it is used as a relaxing drink during ceremonial, celebratory, and social gatherings. It has been used in folk medicine for inflammation of the uterus, headaches, colds, rheumatism, and as both sedative and aphrodisiac. Recent investigations of kava have focused on its sedative and relaxing properties.

Pain Pharmacology	**Studies, Dosages, and Precautions**
The active compounds in the roots and rhizomes of kava are kavalactones, which have sedative and muscle-relaxing effects in animals. They might, in fact, represent an entirely new group of muscle relaxants. Animal studies have also shown extracts of kava to act as analgesics. Thus, kava, through its ability to relax the body and to provide an analgesic effect, may be an ideal supplement for chronic pain sufferers experiencing muscular spasms and/or loss of sleep. Kava has the unique characteristic of promoting sleep without causing involuntary unconsciousness or depressed mental function. It seems to promote relaxation with-	Human studies suggest that kava may also be an effective antianxiety medication. In a twenty-five-week multicenter, randomized, placebo-controlled, double-blind study, 101 patients took a special extract of kava. At the end of the study, the investigators concluded that this kava extract is an effective treatment for anxiety that's comparable to tricyclic antidepressants and benzodiazepines, but has none of their side effects. Additional studies have confirmed kava's antianxiety effect. When we use kava at recommended doses, it has no adverse effects. You should probably avoid using kava if you're suffering from

out robbing the individual of his or her mental faculties.	clinical depression or taking drugs with tranquilizing or sedative effects, including alcohol. We recommend 300 milligrams daily standardized to 30 percent kavalactones.

Kava

- Mechanism of Action: Sedative and muscle-relaxing properties; possible analgesia
- Dosage: 300 milligrams daily of the standardized herb extract
- Active Ingredient: Kavalactones

Valerian *(Valerian officinalis)*

Widely distributed throughout the temperate regions of North America, Europe, and Asia, valerian is most famous for its disagreeable smell. Ironically, in the sixteenth century, people considered the plant to be a fragrant perfume! Clinicians have used valerian as a sedative for centuries, especially in France, Germany, and Switzerland.

Pain Pharmacology	Studies, Dosages, and Precautions
Among the active chemicals in valerian—the sesquiterpenes, valepotriates, and alkaloids—the valepotriates seem responsible for the plant's sedative properties. However, researchers generally agree that the combination of all three is more valuable than any one compound alone. It's suggested that valerian controls gamma-aminobutyric acid (GABA)	Both human and animal studies confirm valerian's sedative and sleep-promoting properties. In one study, cats fed 100 to 250 milligrams of valerian root had reduced muscle tone, suggesting that valerian may act as a muscle relaxer. When 128 volunteers took 400 milligrams of valerian, they reported significant improvement in sleep. Poor sleepers had a more

metabolism in the brain. GABA is an amino acid that relaxes the body by "slowing down" nerve impulses. Valerian may inhibit GABA uptake into cells and, at the same time, stimulate its release into the body. The more GABA floating around in the bloodstream, the more it exerts a relaxing effect.

pronounced effect. In another study, 121 insomniacs took 600 milligrams of valerian one hour before retiring to bed. After twenty-eight days, they reported a significant improvement in sleep and in general well-being.

The FDA classifies valerian as a GRAS (generally regarded as safe) product for use in food and as a flavoring. Although researchers have reported no toxicity in people taking valerian, you should avoid activities that require alertness or vigilance one to two hours after taking it.

Valerian

- Mechanism of Action: Modulation of GABA metabolism in the brain, mild sedative effect on the central nervous system
- Dosage: 300 to 600 milligrams daily of the standardized herb extract
- Active Ingredient: Valepotriates

ANTIOXIDANT SUPPLEMENTS

The process of inflammation is a testament to the complexity of the human body, and controlling it provides a great challenge for the medical community. Attempts to date, however, have been shortsighted, addressing only pain and inflammation, without considering the entire process. Not only must therapies target inflammation at the affected site, they must also correct the deficiencies that inflammation produces. Nutritional/herbal supplements can bridge the gap between therapies that target inflammation directly and those that address inflammation's indirect consequences.

These nutritional/herbal "supportive therapies" include nutrients that inflammation alters or depresses. Because free radicals contribute to the inflammatory response, most of the nutrients briefly covered here are antioxidants. So what's an antioxidant?

Molecules are composed of atoms. Atoms contain electrons, which spin around the nucleus of each atom at incredible speeds. Electrons give atoms a slightly negative charge. Electrons usually come in pairs but, under certain conditions, a molecule can lose one. We call a molecule with an unpaired electron a "free radical." To balance its electrons, the molecule seeks out other molecules to steal an electron from. A chain reaction quickly ensues, with each molecule deprived of an electron stealing from other molecules to regain its own balance. Until antioxidants stop the chain reaction, free radical activity persists, damaging tissues and adversely affecting metabolism.

Antioxidants subdue free radical activity and prevent the damage they cause. Because free radicals play an integral role in the inflammatory response, antioxidant therapy may help stop it.

People suffering from inflammation have low levels of antioxidants, allowing free radicals to ravage their cells. Studies show, for example, that arthritic patients have low levels of the antioxidant vitamins C and E. This may result either from the inflammatory process, or from the drugs used to treat it. Therefore, increasing levels of vitamins C and E (and other antioxidants) may protect against arthritic inflammation. If increased vitamins C and E scavenge free radicals, they may prevent joint damage. In animals, high doses of vitamin C lessened both symptoms and physical signs of osteoarthritis. Other research shows that osteoarthritis patients have increased levels of lipid peroxides (the by-products of free radical damage), which vitamin E suppresses.

The extent of these benefits of antioxidants, however, is moderate. Some researchers suggest that antioxidant therapy may be more effective *before* the inflammatory response, and may have only limited activity after it begins. Thus, taking antioxidants may not provide significant relief after an inflammation already exists, but may be crucial to prevention.

Recommendation: A complete array of all the antioxidants, both water and fat soluble, is recommended. The formula should at least contain vitamin C, tocopherols, and tocotrienols (vitamin E), carotenoids (beta carotene, lutein, lycopene), coenzyme Q10, zinc, selenium, lipoic acid, polyphenols (grape seed, fruit, or pine bark extracts) and N-acetylcysteine.

Phosphatidylserine

Phosphatidylserine belongs to a special category of lipids called phospholipids, the essential components of all cellular membranes. Unlike dietary fat, which doesn't mix with water, phosphatidylserine is both water and fat soluble. We find only trace amounts of phosphatidylserine in the diet; the B vitamin-like substance lecithin contains small amounts. It may be useful to supplement with this brain nutrient because of its antidepressive effects.

Pain Pharmacology	**Studies, Dosages, and Precautions**
Phosphatidylserine increases acetylcholine release and synthesis, increases glucose metabolism in the brain, enhances enzymes that release neurotransmitters, modulates cell-membrane fluidity, and prevents the aging of neurons. Research also suggests that phosphatidylserine reduces the amount of cortisol we secrete in response to stress. This is important, since depressed people have high cortisol levels.	Ten depressed, elderly individuals took 300 milligrams of phosphatidylserine daily for thirty days. Researchers administered a battery of tests evaluating their emotional states both before and after treatment. This study's results indicated that phosphatidylserine consistently improves depressive symptoms and behavior.

Phosphatidylserine

- Mechanism of Action: Enhanced neurotransmitter synthesis/release, increased glucose metabolism in the brain, maintaining membrane plasticity
- Dosage: 200 to 300 milligrams daily
- Active Ingredient: Phosphatidylserine

THE ANTIOXIDANT ENZYMES

Glutathione and Superoxide Dismutase

In addition to the antioxidants we obtain from food and supplements, our body makes its own antioxidants: glutathione and superoxide dismutase. People with arthritis have low levels of these two antioxidant enzymes, and they may need to take supplements to raise their levels.

We need to obtain the nutrients to form superoxide dismutase and glutathione from our diets. We require zinc, manganese, and copper to form superoxide dismutase and for it to function. Both zinc and manganese help to synthesize cartilage (as does vitamin C, a potent antioxidant). Selenium, an ultratrace mineral, and lipoic acid both play critical roles in glutathione metabolism. These nutrients probably act more by enhancing glutathione peroxidase and superoxide dismutase than by influencing inflammation directly.

Supportive Supplements

- Vitamin E: 400 to 800 milligrams with mixed tocopherols
- Vitamin C: 500 to 1000 milligrams
- Zinc: 25 to 50 milligrams daily as chelate
- Manganese: 5 to 50 milligrams daily as chelate
- Copper: 2 to 5 milligrams daily as chelate
- Selenium: 100 to 200 micrograms daily
- Lipoic acid: 50 to 100 milligrams daily
- Folic acid: 400 to 800 micrograms for muscular pain and degenerative joint conditions, and up to 5 milligrams for autoimmune disorders like rheumatoid arthritis
- Coenzyme Q10: 120 milligrams daily
- N-acetylcysteine: 500 milligrams daily
- Polyphenols: 200 milligrams daily
- Carotenoids: 10,000 IU daily

ADDITIONAL SUPPLEMENTS

Folic acid is a B vitamin that arthritis patients have decreased levels of, especially if they are taking methotrexate (a rheumatoid arthritis drug). While methotrexate diminishes folic acid levels, folic acid reduces methotrexates's toxicity. So if you're taking methotrexate, it's important to supplement with folic acid for both of these reasons.

We've also learned that reduced folic acid levels lead to increased homocysteine concentrations. Homocysteine, as you probably know, is the most recently recognized risk factor for cardiovascular disease, and studies show that supplementing with folic acid reduces homocysteine levels.

Throughout *Nature's Pain Killers*, we've stressed that mental attitude is probably just as important as any drug, food, or supplement in controlling chronic pain. Now let's take a look at some new—and not-so-new—psychological techniques that can help us deal with pain.

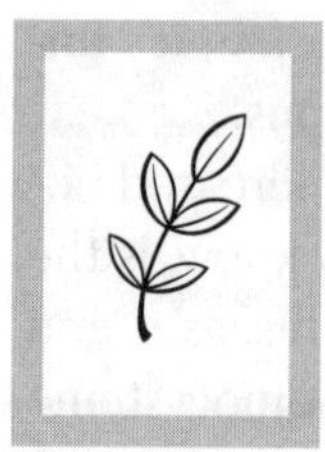

Chapter 10 PSYCHOLOGICAL APPROACHES TO TREATING CHRONIC PAIN

In this chapter, we will discuss the various psychological approaches we use in chronic pain. When such pain affects a person physically, psychologically, and environmentally, it's best that treatment options address each category although we usually control pain by masking or resolving its physiological source. In many cases as well, we address psychosocial issues only after the patient's condition deteriorates despite treatment. In fact, by the time most patients receive psychological help, they've had numerous surgeries, may rely on or be addicted to several medications, and are partially or totally disabled. Fortunately, both patients and health-care providers are now beginning to understand the role that psychological influences can play in the pain experience. Just as thought processes can further impair a person who is in pain, psychological care can help him or her become functional, even while suffering from pain.

A person experiencing chronic pain is likely to be depressed, mainly because of the changes that have occurred in his or her life *because* of the pain. A "vicious pain cycle" may develop or may have already developed: the extended period of pain usually results in decreased mobility; anxiety, tension, and stress increase, and are often followed by depression. Over time, the pain cycle can lead to an increase in muscle tension, poor coping ability, decreased sleep, increased use of pain medications, and excessive reliance on the health-care system. All of these can result in increased pain.

> Psychological treatment helps patients function better. They can decrease pain perception, psychological distress, medications, and medical visits, while encouraging more appropriate coping strategies.

While some psychological symptoms occur as a result of pain, others may have existed previously. For long-term improvement, however, we need to break the vicious pain cycle.

Psychological techniques can improve a patient's functioning, including decreased pain perception, decreased psychological distress, use of more appropriate coping strategies, decrease in medications, and a decrease in medical visits. The goal of using psychological approaches, of course, is to learn appropriate techniques, so you can manage your condition without relying on the health-care system.

For the majority of pain sufferers though, who do make use of the health-care system, a multidisciplinary team provides the most effective treatment. The team usually includes the physician, psychologist, physical therapist, and in some cases, the case manager. The greatest benefit occurs when you receive treatment from all of these areas simultaneously.

The psychologist's role is basically twofold: (a) to recognize and treat psychosocial factors that can result in an increase in the pain and (b) to help identify and implement reasonable treatment goals.

PSYCHOLOGICAL EVALUATION

Before starting treatment, it's important to understand what psychosocial factors contribute to your pain or make it worse. During this evaluation, you'll have a clinical interview (which determines your pre-pain level of functioning) and psychological testing. Education, social functioning, stressors, and vocational history can all influence a patient's success in a rehabilitation program, and we evaluate them all. We can use additional psychological tests to evaluate a person's specific needs.

PSYCHOLOGICAL TREATMENT

Psychological treatments are varied in nature and target different aspects of your pain—the physiological, subjective, and behavioral. The techniques used include several different types of biofeedback mechanisms, relaxation training, hypnosis, an operant approach, and antidepressants (see Table 10-1).

You can use a combination of the methods described here all at once, or just one technique, depending on the nature of your pain. For example, you could use biofeedback to address the physiological part of muscle contraction headache and, at the same time, use cognitive coping strategies to change what your pain *means* to you.

Biofeedback

Biofeedback is a widely accepted treatment for chronic pain that combines psychological and physiological approaches. The medical profession accepts biofeedback because it's a noninvasive procedure that relies on the patient's internal resources.

In biofeedback, we use electronic equipment to mirror mind-body interactions. While you're not usually aware of it, you can learn to voluntarily control much of the physiological activity that contributes to your pain. We've used biofeedback successfully to treat a variety of pain syndromes, including muscle contraction and migraine headaches, low back pain, myofascial pain syndrome, reflex sympathetic dystrophy, and arthritis.

There are several rationales for the use of biofeedback to treat chronic pain, including the following:

1. To modify the specific physiological process that underlies the pain disorder. For example, we use electromyographic (EMG) biofeedback to treat muscle contraction headache. If you reduce muscle tension using biofeedback, you should have fewer muscle contraction headaches.

2. To facilitate the relaxation response. Pain researchers believe that if you relax you will feel less pain. Stress and tension worsen pain, and relaxation relieves it. By using biofeedback, you can measure your relaxation response.

3. Self-regulation. Through the use of biofeedback, you can become more aware of your own contribution to the pain experience, as

Table 10-1
PSYCHOLOGICAL TOOLS FOR TREATING CHRONIC PAIN

Tool	What It Is	Conditions It Treats
EMG biofeedback	Electrodes on the skin measure muscle contraction and relaxation.	Muscle contraction and migraine headache
Thermal biofeedback	Increases the temperature in a portion of the body, like a finger.	Reflex sympathetic dystrophy and migraine headache
Relaxation training	Relaxation diminishes emotional arousal and, thereby, pain.	Muscle contraction headache, migraine headache, temporomandibular joint pain, chronic back pain, and myofascial pain syndrome
Hypnosis	Its mechanism of action is not understood.	Headache, chronic back pain, reflex sympathetic dystrophy, and cancer pain
Operant approach	This "behavior control" methodology reinforces positive behaviors and ignores negative ones.	All types of chronic pain
Antidepressants	By increasing serotonin levels in the brain, antidepressants control pain and the depression that arises from suffering with chronic pain.	All kinds of chronic pain

well as your ability to influence it. For biofeedback to be effective, you must take responsibility for coping with your pain. By using this technique, along with other cognitive methods, you can bring your pain under internal (as opposed to external) control. As a result, your view of the pain should change, and you'll probably accept more personal responsibility for managing it. The internal focus can also make you feel more positive about the future, so you're likely to be less depressed.

The type of biofeedback we use most often to treat chronic pain is EMG biofeedback. We sometimes also use skin temperature, or thermal, biofeedback.

By measuring the electrical discharge in muscle fibers, which reflects either relaxation or contraction of the muscles, EMG biofeedback can help you to focus on managing your pain. By focusing on your need to relax a specific area of your body by tensing and relaxing the muscles there, you should reduce your current, pain-inducing muscle tension. With EMG biofeedback we have successfully treated muscle contraction headaches, temporomandibular joint pain, myofascial pain syndrome, and fibromyalgia.

On occasion, the EMG reading may not provide an accurate measure of the muscle tension and pain you're actually experiencing, possibly because it's caused by deep muscle tension not easily measured by EMG's surface electrodes. Another possibility is that the pain originates at a remote site (i.e., it is referred pain). Keep in mind that you can learn EMG biofeedback, yet not have immediate pain reduction. This occurs because of a delay between relaxing your muscles and subsequent pain relief.

Skin temperature, or thermal, biofeedback works somewhat differently. Theoretically at least, thermal biofeedback works this way: constricting blood vessels (vasoconstriction) increases sympathetic nervous system activity and, therefore, pain; opening the blood vessels (vasodilation), by contrast, both makes the skin warmer and *decreases* sympathetic nervous system activity and pain. Using thermal biofeedback, then, we increase the temperature in an extremity, usually a finger. As the skin warms, the blood vessels open, reducing sympathetic nervous system activity and pain in that extremity.

Additional studies show that an increase in skin temperature is associated with a full relaxation response. Although we have successfully treated reflex sympathetic dystrophy and migraine headache with thermal biofeedback, more research is needed to determine exactly how it works.

Current studies evaluating the effectiveness of thermal biofeedback for treating migraine headache have not yielded consistent results, mainly because the researchers complicated the design by using additional techniques.

Relaxation Training

We use various techniques to elicit the relaxation response. Relaxation diminishes pain by reducing one's emotional arousal. Studies show that relaxation produces decreased oxygen consumption, a reduced heart rate, and a markedly decreased arterial blood-lactate level. These are all signs of decreased sympathetic nervous system activity which, as you now know, lessens pain. Relaxation also facilitates your ability to use your imagination to provide pain relief. Focused concentration helps us learn ways of disrupting negative thought patterns, including those related to pain.

> We use relaxation training to treat a wide variety of painful disorders, including muscle contraction headache, migraine headache, temporomandibular joint pain, chronic back pain, and myofascial pain syndrome.

We also use relaxation to teach body awareness. Patients experiencing pain, especially myofascial pain, frequently tense their muscles in response to or in anticipation of pain. This increases the pain. By becoming more aware of the physical sensations in your body, you can learn to decrease muscle tension and thereby cope with pain more effectively.

Various relaxation techniques are available, with progressive muscle relaxation the most common approach used. Here, you tense and then relax the major muscle groups, from the forehead to the feet. When you've consistently achieved success with progressive muscle relaxation, you can substitute a shorter version of it. Your eventual goal is to reduce tension by recall, and to eliminate the need to actively tense muscle groups. As you become more advanced in the technique, you can use visual imagery and repetitive phrases (like "I will now relax") to elicit relaxation.

We use relaxation training to treat a wide variety of painful disorders, including muscle contraction headache, migraine headache, temporomandibular joint pain, chronic back pain, and myofascial pain syndrome.

Comparison between Biofeedback and Relaxation Training

Numerous studies in managing chronic pain have compared the relative effectiveness of biofeedback and relaxation training. Although most have indicated that they are equally effective, the two approaches can be useful in different ways. Biofeedback can provide concrete evidence (i.e., charts from the biofeedback machine) of the relationship between behaviors, thoughts, and changes in physiological processes. By studying this feedback, you can develop control over the specific physiological mechanism causing your pain. You can also obtain objective data about your progress during treatment sessions. Certainly the main advantage of using relaxation training concerns its practicality and cost effectiveness. You can do your relaxation training in almost any quiet space and it costs you nothing.

We frequently use biofeedback and relaxation together. Relaxation training alters physiological processes, and biofeedback improves the relaxation response. Biofeedback can help pinpoint the source of problems and open up new ways to make changes. In treatment sessions, you should pay close attention to the sensations you feel, and understand that the goal is to use these techniques in daily life. Don't develop excessive reliance on the biofeedback machine.

Biofeedback and Relaxation Training Treatment Protocol

This protocol is part of a multidisciplinary treatment program that incorporates treatments from other disciplines, like physical and occupational therapy, and it's used by many professionals. The sessions usually occur once weekly.

Session 1: Collection of Baseline Data and Explanation of Biofeedback.

The purpose of the initial biofeedback session is twofold: (a) to learn the process of biofeedback and how you can use it to cope with chronic pain; and (b) to generate baseline data. You will compare the progress you make in future sessions to this initial session. Depending on the nature of the pain, we monitor either EMG and/or skin temperature. Where we place the EMG electrodes depends on the pain, but we usually place them on the chest, neck, and shoulder area. We place the skin temperature probes on the index finger of both hands.

Sessions 2 to 6: Relaxation-Assisted Biofeedback Training

Your technician will explain how to use relaxation techniques; initially, you'll use progressive muscle relaxation, followed by self-generated (autogenic) relaxation during the fifth and sixth sessions. The first fifteen minutes of each session is an introductory period during which you'll spend time discussing your concerns and the goals for the session. Following this, you'll participate in thirty minutes of relaxation-assisted biofeedback training. You should spend the last fifteen minutes discussing the training session and any difficulties encountered during it.

Progressive muscle relaxation (tensing and then relaxing muscles) teaches general body awareness. Additionally, you'll learn controlled breathing techniques, and ways to determine the difference between muscle tension and relaxation. You'll probably master this technique in about three sessions.

You'll receive visual and/or auditory feedback (from the biofeedback machine) and, at the end of each session, data on the readings. We measure the mean, as well as the low and high reading, for each minute of the training period.

To facilitate training, you may receive relaxation tapes. Use them at least once daily, especially when feeling severe pain and tension.

Sessions 7 and 8: Further Development of Skills

As you develop self-control with the relaxation and biofeedback training, you'll focus on further developing and improving your skills.

Instead of practicing the structured progressive muscle relaxation, you can use simple phrases to facilitate relaxation (e.g., "I am developing relaxation of my neck and shoulder muscles"). During training sessions, you should focus on incorporating these skills and your simple phrases into daily activities. You'll become more comfortable using these techniques as you recognize their value to everyday life.

Hypnosis

Hypnosis, or hypnotic analgesia, was one of the earliest modern medical treatments for pain. Reports of its use and benefits date to the nineteenth century. One of the earliest reports of hypnotic analgesia occurred in India, where a surgeon who used the technique to perform amputations reported 80 percent efficacy! Hypnosis became widely used in pain management after World War II.

Hypnosis is an altered state of consciousness in which the subject is intensely concentrating, less aware of the environment, and internally focused. Today, we use hypnosis to treat a variety of pain syndromes, both acute and chronic. One of the main advantages of hypnosis over medication is that it does not have side effects like those of medication, which can include placing an extra load on respiration and circulation, or potentially damaging organs. Psychological factors—like anxiety, excess attention to pain, and feelings of loss of control—can worsen pain. Hypnosis can address each of them, giving you better control over the pain.

Theory and Mechanisms

We don't understand why hypnosis works. Researchers speculate that it may stimulate the release of endorphins (which, as you'll recall, are our natural pain killers). In search of an answer researchers devised a test whereby they administered naloxon, a medication used to reverse the effects of narcotics, to patients experiencing hypnosis. They observed that the drug did not consistently reverse its effects. Additionally, other studies reported no increase in endorphin levels in patients treating pain with hypnosis, which further supports the belief that it is not part of our endorphin pain control system.

Some research suggests that thoughts play an important role in hypnotic analgesia. This seems reasonable, given that hypnosis focuses on the subjective aspects of the pain experience, such as feelings of distress and discomfort.

> We use hypnosis for a variety of pain syndromes, including headache, chronic back pain, reflex sympathetic dystrophy, and cancer pain. While hypnosis has received mixed acceptance in managing chronic pain, mainly because of lack of understanding and fear, it is gaining acceptance.

One author, E.R. Hilgard, proposed a particularly intriguing theory to explain why hypnosis stops pain. In his "neodissociation model," Hilgard saw hypnosis as a specialized form of dissociation in which we imagine ourselves in another state (like having a vivid daydream), and thus cannot associate the physiological reality of pain with actual sensations of pain.

Whether this theory holds true or not is for future researchers to decide. Currently, however, the bottom line remains—we still do not understand how or why hypnosis works.

Of course, we use hypnosis to treat a variety of pain syndromes, including headache, chronic back pain, reflex sympathetic dystrophy, and cancer pain. Hypnosis has received mixed acceptance in managing chronic pain, mainly because of lack of understanding and fear. Nonetheless, it is becoming more accepted as an alternative method for dealing with pain.

Techniques

Hypnosis can provide pain relief for many patients, but the technique in and of itself does not *cure* chronic pain. It provides a sensation of peacefulness and comfort, as well as short-term pain relief. In order for lasting benefit to occur, however, hypnosis should be part of a broader therapy program.

The effectiveness of hypnosis usually depends on two factors: your imagination, and the clinician's ability to capitalize on it to change your perceptions. People's ability to go into hypnotic trance exists on a continuum, and the capacity to experience hypnosis varies from individual to individual.

An important first step in using hypnosis is the initial evaluation. Its main purpose is to determine your appropriateness for hypnosis and to assess your knowledge of and conceptions about the procedure. The clinician should evaluate psychiatric history, motivation, psychosocial factors exacerbating or maintaining the pain complaint, and psychological resources, like ego strength. Practitioners of hypnosis should exercise caution, however, in conducting hypnosis with anyone currently diagnosed with a psychopathology (like psychosis or severe depression).

Before hypnosis actually begins, you should be prepared. For example, the practitioner should inform you about how hypnosis can be useful in managing your particular pain. He or she should also address any misconceptions or fears about hypnosis you may have.

Various techniques are used to achieve hypnotic pain control, including the following:

1. Altering the perception of pain. Through hypnosis you become less aware of the pain experienced. We achieve this by suggesting that the pain is diminishing, changing, or that the area is becoming numb. "Glove anesthesia" as described by S.W. Bassman, is a useful technique here. While in a hypnotic trance, you visualize three objects on a table: a soft velvet glove with a smooth silk lining; a brightly colored pail filled with a sparkling, blue liquid; and a large, open jar of pleasantly perfumed hand cream. The three objects possess texture, visual stimuli, and olfactory stimuli, respectively. The hypnotist will tell you that each of the objects contains a potent anesthesia, and that the part of the body coming in contact with it will become numb. You select one of the objects and place a hand in it so the hand becomes numb. Then, as you rub the numb hand over the part of the body experiencing pain, there is usually a reduction in pain perception. Patients in a medium trance are usually able to experience glove anesthesia.

2. Substitute a different or less painful sensation for the pain. While in a trance, you learn that you can substitute a different sensation for the painful one. Some patients are able to use this technique more effectively if the substituted feeling is not totally pleasant. For example, they can substitute a pinchlike sensation for a stabbing pain.

3. Move the pain to another part of the body. In this technique, you can move the location of your pain to a less psychologically vulnerable area. For example, you can move the pain from the hand, say, to the little finger. The eventual goal of this technique is to move the pain outside the body.

4. Alter the meaning of pain. While in a hypnotic trance, you'll learn that the pain is less debilitating and less meaningful.

5. Distortion of time. You'll learn ways to distort time so that the actual amount of time you experience a painful sensation (like severe spasms) will seem to pass rapidly.

6. Dissociation. You can learn to imagine yourself in another state, place, or time, as in a vivid daydream. This technique is most useful when you don't have to be functional, such as when undergoing dental or medical procedures, or in the latter stages of a terminal illness.

7. Age regression. Using this technique, you're able to regress to an earlier period of time in your life during which you did not experience pain.

The strategy for treating each patient depends on the severity of the pain and the level of hypnotizability. For instance, if you have low hypnotizability and severe pain, you'll benefit most from distraction techniques. If you have high hypnotizability and severe pain, you'll benefit most from dissociation.

Self-Hypnosis

It's important to learn self-hypnosis, so you can use it independently to cope with your pain and the issues that exacerbate it. Learning the technique will enable you to produce hypnotic analgesia by yourself. In effect, you won't need a therapist on a long-term basis. Through self-hypnosis, you should develop a sense of control and mastery over pain. Effective ways of learning self-hypnosis include the following:

1. Record a hypnosis session and use the tape at home. Studies show that patients newly trained in self-hypnosis reported a better hypnotic experience if they used a tape than if they attempted to perform the technique unassisted.

2. Have the clinician provide posthypnotic suggestions while in a trance. These suggestions should assist self-hypnosis.

3. Practice self-hypnosis while in treatment sessions. In this setting, you can receive suggestions and address concerns. For self-hypnosis to be most effective, you should practice and use it daily.

Cognitive-Behavioral Approaches

Over the past decade, pain practitioners have increasingly acknowledged the benefit of cognitive-behavioral approaches in managing chronic pain, and many practitioners have integrated them into their practices. The basic premise of cognitive approaches is that expectations, attitudes, and beliefs affect the manner in which individuals cope with pain. Therefore, the changes in negative thoughts can result in better pain control.

We believe that the way in which a person views the world affects behavior. Therefore, the way a person perceives and evaluates pain directly influences the extent of disability he or she experiences. Errors in thought processes thus contribute to chronic pain patients' inadequate coping mechanisms. Studies have consistently shown that people who misinterpret their experience of pain become more severely disabled. That is, if the person views the pain as disabling, then that person is more likely to be disabled. The goal of the cognitive approach is to correct the thought processes that contribute to prolonged suffering and disability. In using this process, you replace maladaptive beliefs with more adaptive beliefs. Cognitive approaches provide the following benefits:

1. Patients gain the necessary coping skills to deal with pain more effectively.

2. Patients live more satisfying lives despite the presence of physical discomfort.

3. Patients rely less heavily on the health-care system and reduce their use of pain medications. We emphasize the message that people are not helpless in dealing with their pain; it should not control their lives.

The cognitive model contains a wide variety of therapeutic techniques, but they all have common elements. Treatment is structured, action oriented, and usually time limited. We teach the approaches in individual or group sessions. There are three phases:

1. You learn the role that thoughts and feelings have in influencing pain.

2. We present specific methods for coping with pain, including relabeling painful sensations, diverting attention, reinterpreting pain sensations, relaxation, and using imagery. There are four steps in this teaching process:

a. Preparing for minor painful sensations;
b. Confronting more severe pain;
c. Coping with feelings that tend to exacerbate pain, such as anxiety or frustration; and
d. Learning to provide self-reinforcement for successfully coping with pain.

3. You learn to use the skills in situations outside the doctor's office by practicing them at work or at home. The therapist should allow you to proceed at your own pace.

Researchers have evaluated the relative effectiveness of active and passive coping strategies. Active coping strategies require that you perform some action, like exercising, to cope with the pain. Passive coping strategies require that you withdraw or give up control to an external agent, like a pain medication. Research tends to favor active strategies. For example, one study revealed that rheumatoid arthritis patients using active coping strategies functioned better, psychologically and physically, than before. Alternatively, patients who used passive coping were more likely to suffer from depression. Longitudinal research also indicates that those who use active strategies have better long-term adjustments.

The Operant Approach

The operant approach assumes that consequences govern a person's behavior. If the consequences of a behavior are positive, the person will be more likely to repeat that behavior. Negative reinforcement, of course, decreases the likelihood that the person will repeat the behavior.

With the operant approach, there is one primary goal: to replace learned maladaptive behaviors with behaviors that are incompatible with being a "sick person." We change rewards to reinforce appropriate, "healthy" behaviors, and not to reinforce pain behaviors. We instruct family members and health-care providers to reinforce appropriate behaviors while ignoring pain behaviors (like complaining of pain, using narcotics, and remaining inactive). We can incorporate other forms of intervention into this treatment, including marital counseling, family therapy, and vocational planning.

Group Therapy

Group therapy is an important component of a pain management program. It has two main purposes: to provide psychological support and to disseminate information. In the group format, we can present, share, and discuss many ideas. The members of the group provide support and encouragement, and can serve as a reality check for other participants in the group.

In the group setting, you can obtain information about psychosocial influences on pain. Topics for discussion include the vicious pain cycles (e.g., the pain-depression, pain-narcotics, and pain-stress cycles), effective coping strategies, and acceptance of the pain. If education is power, the more education you possess, the more you'll be able to control your own condition.

THE ROLE OF ANTIDEPRESSANT THERAPY IN PAIN MANAGEMENT

People experiencing chronic pain are often depressed. Since it hurts to move, chronic pain usually results in reduced activity level, which, over time, lowers physical stamina and produces feelings of helplessness, hopelessness, and depression. The depression, as it continues, results in increased pain perception and decreased ability to tolerate the pain. This can further exacerbate the pain, thus perpetuating the cycle.

In some cases, the depression exists before the pain. Regardless of the chronology, we must treat depression, because it can exacerbate pain and contribute to disability. Symptoms of depression include: loss of interest in activities previously enjoyed, social isolation, concentration and memory difficulties, sleep disturbance, appetite disturbance, loss of interest in sex, feelings of worthlessness, pessimism, and in severe cases, suicidal thoughts.

The psychological techniques we've discussed here can assist in decreasing your symptoms of depression if indeed, you are depressed. In many cases, however, the symptoms are so severe that they affect the ability to engage in therapy that would change the situation. In this situation, it may be beneficial to treat the depression with antidepressant medication. As we've discussed, antidepressants can also be useful as mild analgesics. It's common to have low doses of an antidepressant prescribed for both purposes.

Of course, it's preferable to treat depression safely without medication (possibly with the assistance of supplements like those discussed in Chapter 8, along with psychological therapy) when possible. Like all drugs, antidepressants have undesirable side effects.

We divide the antidepressants into four classes: tricyclic antidepressants (amitriptyline, doxepin), selective serotonin re-uptake inhibitors (fluoxetine, sertraline), monoamine oxidase inhibitors (phenolzine, tranylcypromine), and atypical antidepressants (trazodone, bupropion). If you need to take an antidepressant, your physician will select a drug based on your past history of response, concurrent medical history, potential drug interactions and side effects, and cost. Most antidepressants have equivalent results when you take comparable doses; however, failure to respond to one class does not predict failure with another agent.

Regardless of antidepressant use, you must take personal responsibility for your rehabilitation. No pill, by itself, will cure chronic pain.

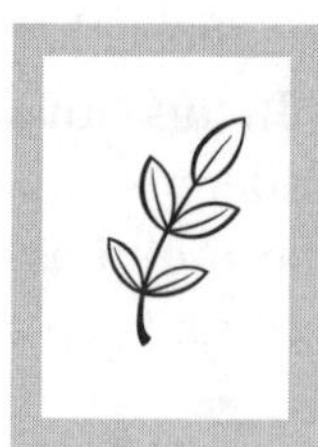

Chapter 11 THE TRADITIONAL CHINESE MEDICINE ACUPUNCTURE-MASSAGE CONNECTION

For thousands of years, practitioners have used acupuncture to treat every ailment known to us, yet its influence has only touched the United States during the last twenty-five years. After centuries of extremely limited communication between China and the West, President Richard Nixon visited The People's Republic of China in 1972, opening the doors to the vast wisdom and culture of this ancient country.

While accompanying President Nixon in China, *New York Times* reporter James Reston had an emergency appendectomy, after which he began to experience severe abdominal pain and swelling. While a Western doctor performed his surgery, an acupuncturist treated his pain. The acupuncturist placed three needles in Mr. Reston's elbow and three in his knee; he also burned moxa (an herb we will discuss later) above Mr. Reston's abdomen. The treatment was successful, and the news of the reporter's "miracle cure" began to spread around the country.

Although introduced to this country barely a quarter century ago, Chinese medicine is becoming more and more established as a viable form of medicine in the United States and other Western countries. As we learn more about acupuncture and herbs, we are realizing that they can treat the complete spectrum of disorders. Still, most Americans associate acupuncture with the alleviation of pain, the first disorder it was known to treat.

HISTORY OF ACUPUNCTURE

It's believed that acupuncture started in the New Stone Age, as early as 8000 B.C. Ancient tombs in Hunan Province and Inner Mongolia contain stone acupunture needles. (Acupuncturists did not use metal needles until 2000 B.C.) Acupuncture is described in the oldest surviving book about Chinese medicine, *Huang Di Nei Jing* (*The Yellow Emperor's Guide to Internal Medicine*), written circa 500 B.C.

Chinese medicine grew and flourished for thousands of years until the Opium War in the 1840s, after which Western medicine and technology began to enter China. At one point in the 1930s, the Kuo Ming Tang tried to ban acupuncture, bringing it to the verge of extinction. In 1949, faced with a growing population and extreme poverty, Mao Tse Tung reinstated a national program of acupuncture. Since then, acupuncture and Traditional Chinese Medicine (often abbreviated TCM) have grown and developed tremendously. Today in China, all doctors must study both Western and Chinese medicine.

Chinese medicine is not an "alternative" in China, as it is today in the United States; it is a complete medical system that's been used for over 10,000 years. Its practice encompasses many different therapies, including acupuncture, herbology, diet and nutrition, exercise (*qi gong*), and massage (*Tui Na*).

Today, as we integrate these healing strategies into our society, we continue to assess their strengths and weaknesses, as well as those of Western medicine, in order to have a complete, holistic medical system that offers the best of both worlds.

THEORY

To understand Chinese medicine, it's helpful to know a little about Chinese history and philosophy.

The ancient Chinese thought human beings to be multidimensional, and the anatomy they taught reflected this. This basic idea—also used in modern physics—is that we *are* energy. Energy moves through all parts of our lives and our beings. If we examine an atom in the body, we see electrons moving around a core of neutrons and protons. Most of the atom is space; it is not solid. As a result, even bone, which we might think is the most solid structure in the human body, can be soft and pliable.

Simply put, health is a smooth, continuous flow of life energy inside and outside of the body. Disease is a disruption of that flow.

Acupuncture, the insertion of microthin needles into the body, helps the movement of this life energy, called *qi* (pronounced "chi").

Although there are many ways to diagnose a disorder, acupuncturists use six basic levels of anatomy. They are not distinct, but move among and intertwine with each other. We'll start by exploring these levels, from the subtlest to the crudest.

Level I

Level I is the subtlest energy of life. In China, they call it the Tao. It is the formless energy of life, the Absolute, spirit, nothingness. In Christianity, it is the level of the Father. In Judaism, it's the Adonai or Kether. In India, it's Brahman.

Level II

Level II is the first level of the soul, before it begins to take form.

Level III

Level III consists of the eight "extra" meridians, which are energy pathways through the body. It contains the first and deepest level of energy pathways. These meridians are eight seas of energy, while the twelve "regular" meridians are rivers. Essence (*jing*) fills these meridians, not *qi*. They are the deepest part, or the genetic level, of the self. We form them in utero, during the development and predevelopment stages.

Level IV

Level IV involves the twelve "regular" meridians with which most people are familiar. These twelve pathways run through the body. Although really only one continuous pathway that runs from the surface of the body to an internal organ and then back up again, we've broken them into twelve pathways. The traditional acupuncture points are located along these twelve meridians.

In the West, we have assigned each of these meridians a name that corresponds to the organ it connects to energetically:

- Lung
- Large intestine
- Stomach
- Spleen
- Heart
- Small intestine
- Urinary bladder
- Kidney
- Pericardium
- Triple heater
- Gall bladder
- Liver

Each meridian has both internal and external pathways. For instance, the Lung meridian is as follows: It starts in the abdomen, moves down and connects to the large intestine (its partner organ), then ascends and moves around the lungs, emerging at the skin surface one inch below the breastbone at the first space between the ribs. This is "Lung 1," the first point on the Lung meridian. It then descends down the arm, along which there are eleven points in all before it ends at the thumbnail. At this point, it moves to the Large Intestine meridian, which begins at the index finger. Eventually, energy moves through all the meridians, ending with the Liver, which then merges into the Lung meridian, and the cycle begins again.

When a pathway/meridian is out of balance, there are many ramifications. It doesn't just mean there is pain along the pathway of the meridian. Each meridian corresponds to mental, emotional, and physiological characteristics and disharmonies.

For example, symptoms that the Lung meridian is out of balance could include:

- Pain around the area where the meridian runs
- Lung problems
- Sinus problems
- Skin problems
- Certain types of low energy
- Excessive sadness or grief

Each of the twelve meridians has similar, but distinct, correspondences.

Level V

Level V consists of the Muscle Sinew meridians. They are the crudest, most manifest level of energy before the physical-level anatomy studied by Western medicine. These meridians run through muscle groups and connect to one of the twelve regular meridians.

Level VI

The Physical Body meridians of Level VI are the basest, lowest, or most manifest level of anatomy. This is the level of the physical body: bone, blood, muscles, sinews, and so on. It is the only level of anatomy recognized in Western medicine.

These six levels compose human anatomy according to Chinese medicine. Moving through this anatomical structure are:

Fluids: All the types of body fluids in the body.

Blood: This is different from the scientific meaning of blood. "Blood," in Chinese medicine, is a denser form of *qi* (energy).

Yin: All fluids, including blood, are categorized as being *yin*. It is all the cooling aspects of the body.

Qi: Life energy, vitality, the healthy movement of the life force is called *qi*. There are many types of *qi* running through different levels and meridians in the body, supporting our organs, the immune and digestive systems, and controlling other functions.

Yang: All life energy and warming qualities are categorized as *yang*.

Jing (Essence): This is broken up into two parts—prenatal and postnatal essence.

Prenatal essence is the energy we acquire from our parents; it makes up our constitution. Postnatal essence comes from our food and from living a healthy life. If we are not living a healthy life and acquiring postnatal essence, then the prenatal essence is depleted. This is disease.

An acupuncturist's job is to assess the structures of the body and to determine if the six aspects just mentioned are moving in a healthy way through them. If the answer is no, and there is disorder, the question becomes where the disorder is and why the body went out of balance.

All our parts are either in harmony, in excess, deficient, or stagnant. Stagnation can include either excessive or deficient. For example, an excess stagnation is due to an external factor, or some part of the body that has been overworked. Deficient stagnation refers to energy that cannot move because the organ (meridian) is too weak to sustain normal energetic movement.

The factors that disrupt harmony and lead to disease are:

Genetics: In Chinese medicine, a genetic disorder or weakness is also known as weak prenatal *qi*. It is specifically associated with weakness in the eight "extra" as well as twelve "regular" meridians. It ranges from obvious birth defects to weak areas in a person's constitution.

Diet: Poor diet weakens the digestive system and eventually other systems in the body.

Lifestyle: Overall poor lifestyle, including sleep habits, work hours, extensive travel, and other factors.

Emotions: This includes stress, but in Chinese medicine there are different emotions that affect different organ systems as the following list explains.

- Lung: Grief, sadness
- Heart: Excessive joy, trying too hard
- Spleen: Worry, overthinking
- Liver: Anger
- Kidney: Fear
- Sex: Too much sex weakens the Kidney energy, the essence and ultimately the constitution of a person.

- Weather: The six types of weather that can affect us are Wind, Cold, Heat, Damp, Dry, Summer (extreme) Heat
- Accidents: Includes all types of accidents and injuries.
- Iatrogenic Effects: This is either wrong or poor medical treatment that contributes to an injury or disorder. For example, when a patient has back surgery, we have to deal with the original cause for the back pain as well as any damage caused by the surgery.

PAIN

In previous chapters, we discussed how Western medicine looks at the different causes of pain, the chemical changes that occur in the body, and the physical changes that precipitate them. For instance, with back pain, some causes might include injuries or degeneration of muscles, disk problems, ligament problems, spinal abnormalities, and nerve irritation.

In Chinese medicine, there is essentially only one reason for pain: lack of flow of the appropriate energy.

To an acupuncturist, the question is: What is not flowing and why? What are the causes? Was it an accident, or did a lifetime of poor habits precipitate the accident? What factors caused the pain?

There are traditionally three types of pain (or reasons why the energy is not flowing properly):

1. **Excessive pain:** Usually acute and continuous pain. Direct pressure and palpation aggravate it.
2. **Deficient pain:** Usually a chronic and intermittent pain. Exertion aggravates it. Rest, direct pressure, and stabilization alleviate it.
3. **Stagnant Pain:** In essence, all pain is stagnant energy. This is actually a special form of excess pain that can be chronic. Movement or massage alleviate it. It gets much worse when the person rests or is inactive.

We break these three types of pain down into more specific categories, which we won't go into here.

Acupuncture is so successful because it does not treat pain, it treats people.

Too often, we hear a doctor say, "I have an L4-L5 herniation in room 452." What's lying in room 452 is a human being, not just a herniation. Western medicine's weakness is that we lose sight of the forest by studying the trees.

This is a product of the foundational thinking that has dominated the Western world, particularly science, as its author, the French philosopher Descartes, defined it in the seventeenth century. Cartesian thought argues that, in any complex system, we can understand the dynamics of the whole by studying the parts.

An excellent medium for the development of technology, Cartesian thought is less apt for the development of a *human* health science. Fortunately, during the last few decades many clinicians and researchers have reached the same conclusion. They disagree with the reductionist-only style of scientific investigation that Cartesian thought promotes. At the same time, they recognize in acupuncture, for example, what modern medical science lacks: a view of the whole to understand the parts.

Thomas Matus, David Steindl-Rast, and Fritof Capra recognize how important this shift of view is, and have incorporated it into their own "systemic" paradigm, in which *process* takes precedence over structure.

In *Belonging to the Universe*, Capra writes, "In the past, we believed that in any complex system, the dynamics of the whole could be understood from the properties of the parts. But now we see that the properties of the parts can be understood only from the dynamics of the whole. Ultimately there are no parts at all. What we call a part is merely a pattern in an inseparable web of relationships. Every structure is seen as a manifestation of an underlying process. The entire web of relationships is intrinsically dynamic." Chinese medical theory agrees with these ideas.

A human being is a complex set of structures and relationships. We must understand the relationships between parts of the body just as deeply as we understand the anatomical part itself. Simply put, we cannot treat the low back by looking only at the low back!

Treatment Needles

In performing modern acupuncture, microthin needles (usually made of stainless steel, although they can be gold or silver) are inserted into the skin. The length of the needle is between .5 inch to 6 inches, but one-inch needles are the most popular. Most are disposable, and so are only used once. Some practitioners use permanent needles, which are autoclaved *after every use* to sterilize them. Needle width ranges from 28 to 38 gauge for the smaller needles. The needle used most often is one inch long and 34 gauge.

HOW IT WORKS

Western science has been trying to explain how acupuncture works ever since we learned about it. In some instances, like pain, there are very real scientific reasons why acupuncture works. In other instances, it is clear that science is not yet advanced enough to explain how it works.

> *When a superior person hears of the Tao,*
> *They begin to pursue it*
> *When an average person hears of the Tao,*
> *They half believe it, half doubt it*
> *When a foolish person hears of the Tao*
> *They laugh out loud.*
> *The Tao is nowhere to be found.*
> *Yet it nourishes and completes all things*
>
> Tao Te Ching – Lao Tzu (41)

Western physicians first began to learn about acupuncture, slowly, in the 1950s when Chinese scientists published studies about its use for analgesia and surgery. With the opening of China and the Western media's knowledge about Mr. Reston's experience in the early 1970s, as previously described, Western practitioners scrutinized acupuncture even closer. Although science has yet to detect the flow of *qi* through meridians, it has identified acupuncture-induced endorphins.

Bruce Pomerantz, a neuroscientist from the University of Toronto, has investigated acupuncture for the last twenty years. He notes that, "The needles stimulate nerves in the underlying muscles. Patients feel a sensation of the activation of small myelinated type I and II afferent nerve fibers. That stimulation sends messages to the limbic system in the brain as well as to the midbrain and the pituitary gland. This then releases endorphins (enkephalin and dymorphin), monoamines and chemicals that block pain signals."

The discovery of opioid (morphinelike) receptors and our natural pain killers (endorphins and enkephalins) provided some insight into how acupuncture works.

L. Terenius explains that, during acupuncture, endorphins are released into the cerebrospinal fluid. When scientists injected cerebrospinal fluid from an acupunctured rat into a nonacupunctured rat, the nonacupunctured rat also began to show pain relief. In other words, scientists have demonstrated that acupuncture produces endorphins that circulate throughout our bodies. If we take spinal fluid from an animal that's undergone acupuncture (i.e., its spinal fluid contains endorphins), and inject it into another animal that has *not* undergone acupuncture, the first animal's endorphins will ameliorate the second animal's pain.

We can also use the Gate Control Theory of Pain (which we discussed in Chapter 1) to interpret how acupuncture stops pain. Insertion of acupuncture needles sends stimuli to a specific region in the spinal cord called the dorsal gate. These stimuli close the gate to the pain stimulus.

In another study, Abass Alavi, chief of nuclear medicine at the University of Pennsylvania Hospital, used single photon emission computed tomography (SPECT) to record images of the brains of patients suffering from chronic pain. He clearly found, after acupuncture, an increase in blood flow in the thalamus and brain stem, and that the patients felt less pain.

The endorphin theory clearly explains how acupuncture affects pain, yet it doesn't explain why acupuncture is successful in treating ailments other than pain. Physicist Zang-Hee Cho, for example, explored acupuncture to treat vision problems. Dr. Cho hooked student volunteers to a functional magnetic resonance imaging machine (fMRI). He stimulated the students' eyes by shining a light in them. The students, as he expected, showed activity in the visual cortex of their brains. He then stimulated traditional acupuncture points in the feet that assist in eye problems (UB-67, UB-66, UB-65, UB-60). In all of the students, there was activity in the visual cortex of the brain, just as when he shined a light into their eyes.

Dr. Cho then went on to determine if a similar response would occur by stimulating a nonacupuncture point on the foot. But when he did so, the fMRI results were negative. His conclusion generally supported the scientific validity of acupuncture.

Remarkably, in 1998, the National Institutes of Health acknowledged that acupuncture is effective in treating postsurgical and other forms of pain, as well as nausea from anesthesia and chemotherapy.

A REVIEW OF DISORDERS

Low Back Pain

Up to 80 percent of all adults will experience back pain during their lives. By the year 2000, costs for back pain–related medical care, including treatment, procedures, hospitalization, and disability will reach $50 billion.

We are living in the age of the Internet and computer automation; generally, people have less physically demanding jobs. We have drastically improved diagnostic testing and overall medical knowledge, and yet work disability due to back pain continues to rise. Why?

In Western medicine, we approach back pain by assessing structural anomalies in muscle, ligaments, facet joints, disks, nerve roots, spinal stenosis (narrowing of the spinal canal), or from underlying diseases like cancer. Unfortunately, there is often a weak connection between test results that show physical changes (MRI, X ray) and symptoms.

In 1990, Scott Boden of the George Washington University Medical School studied a group of people who had never had back or sciatica pain. Of this group, 20 percent had herniated disks and 50 percent had bulging disks. Of patients over sixty, 33 percent had herniated disks and 80 percent had bulging disks. Don't forget—none of these people ever experienced back pain!

A similar study by Michael N. Brant-Zawadzki of Hoag Memorial Hospital in Newport Beach, California, showed that of ninety-eight pain-free patients 66 percent had abnormal disks.

These studies show one thing: finding a herniated disk means *only* that a patient has a herniated disk. A herniated disk does not necessarily cause pain; if a patient is feeling pain, it may not be the cause of the pain.

Even patients whose MRIs show an almost complete degeneration of a disk may have experienced back pain for only one week. With such great physical changes, one would think that they would have been in pain for the last twenty years!

As a result, we're beginning to see that there is a deeper level to pain: It's not caused solely by changes in physical structures. What is that deeper level? John E. Sarno of the Rusk Institute of Rehabilitation Medicine at New York University Medical Center concluded that unresolved emotions produce physical tension that *becomes* back pain. Dr.

Astral Lampe at the University of Innsbruck revealed a connection between stressful life events and back pain. And Dr. Carolyn Myss states that chronic negative patterns, attitudes, and behaviors create chronic pain. This negativity produces continuous currents of stress that disrupt both our emotions and physical bodies. With this understanding, let's look at how an acupuncturist views low back pain.

Treating low back pain with acupuncture dates to the origin of Chinese medicine. It's described in some detail in *The Yellow Emperor's Guide to Internal Medicine,* and you can refer to that book for more detailed information.

Even in the West, Sir William Osler, the father of American medicine, wrote in 1912 that the treatment of choice for lumbago is acupuncture.

When a patient complains of low back pain, an acupuncturist begins by asking the location of the pain, what caused the pain, how long has it lasted, and other pertinent questions.

The low back is where the kidneys reside. The kidney meridian governs all bones in the body, as well as the low back. Other meridians also have connections to the bones and, therefore, to the kidney meridian. They include the Governing Vessel (which runs up the back), the Urinary Bladder (1.5 inches from the spine), and the Gall Bladder meridian (which runs along the side of the body).

Through questions, observations, and palpations, the acupuncturist assesses which of the meridians are presently eliciting pain. To an acupuncturist, there are four main pathologies for low back pain:

1. Invasion of wind-cold-damp (Bi Syndrome)
2. *Qi* and Blood stagnation
3. Liver–Gall Bladder stagnation (This is low back pain due to emotions)
4. Kidney deficiency

The causes of these pathologies are:

1. Excessive physical work. In the acute phase, excessive work causes *qi* and blood stagnation. Over the long term, it could weaken the energy (*qi*) of the kidney.

2. Excessive sexual activity. This depletes energy from the Kidney *qi* and causes chronic back pain.

3. Pregnancy or childbirth. This can cause a strain on the back, thus *qi* and blood stagnation or, if the person already has a weak constitution, the strain of the pregnancy could weaken the Kidney *qi*.

4. Invasion of external cold and dampness. This cause of back pain is due to being susceptible to dampness and cold. Being exposed to cold and dampness, can eventually lead to a chronic form of low back pain in which the kidneys begin to weaken.

5. Accident.

6. Poor lifestyle habits. Inadequate exercise, eating poorly, and stress all strain the muscles and internal organs. This is considered stagnation, but eventually it will damage the Kidney *qi*.

7. Aging. In Chinese medicine, this is the depletion of Kidney *qi*.

Western medicine has difficulty studying acupuncture. One reason for this is that treatment plans can be very different for seemingly similar conditions. In addition, people respond differently to acupuncture treatments over time, depending on what's causing their pain. A man with back pain due to a recent emotional upset, for example, might respond to acupuncture more quickly than a woman who has back pain due to long-term stress, poor eating, no exercise, and multiple pregnancies. The man might respond quite quickly to acupuncture, while the woman might not. (This example is not meant to imply that men, in general, respond more rapidly to acupuncture.)

The different treatment plans might look like these:

- For back pain from excessive physical work, the acupuncturist uses acupuncture and massage. The acupuncturist would probably suggest relaxing and not overdoing it. He or she would also prescribe some type of stretching exercises or *qi gong* for the patient to do at home, as well as herbs to alleviate pain.
- For back pain due to excessive sexual activity, the acupuncturist uses acupuncture and massage. The acupuncturist would also suggest a decrease in sexual activity. Since, in this case, the pain is due to deficient kidney energy, the acupuncturist would also prescribe herbs or supplements that not only assist in alleviating pain but also strengthen the kidneys.
- For low back pain related to pregnancy, the acupuncturist employs a regimen similar to that just listed for the person with low back pain from excessive sexual activity.

- For low back pain from external cold and dampness, the acupuncturist uses acupuncture and massage. The acupuncturist might also use heat on the back, and assess why this person was susceptible to the cold. Is there a good reason, or does he or she respond to cold with illness because his or her body is weak?
- For injury, the acupuncturist assesses whether or not the injured person needs to consult a Western medical doctor. If appropriate, the acupuncturist then treats the injured person with acupuncture, and possibly massage and herbs to relieve pain and inflammation.
- For poor lifestyle habits the acupuncturist counsels the person about lifestyle, diet, nutrition, and exercise. The acupuncturist would determine which meridians, in addition to those connected to the back, might also be out of balance. He or she would treat the person with acupuncture, massage, and herbology, as needed.
- For low back pain due to aging, the acupuncturist uses acupuncture, herbology, and massage, focusing on strengthening the Kidney meridian energy.

Fibromyalgia

Fibromyalgia is a pain disorder (as we discussed in detail in Chapter 3). The pain often occurs throughout the body at trigger points and can be totally incapacitating. Other symptoms can include fatigue, irritable bowel syndrome, headache, and sleep disorder. At the present time, the cause of fibromyalgia remains unknown.

As with back pain, a Western diagnosis of fibromyalgia could translate into many diagnoses in Chinese medicine. The following three patients all met the 1990 ACR (Association for Clinical Research) diagnostic criteria for fibromyalgia. According to Western medicine, they all had the same disorder. But as Grace Moe notes (1996), they were three very different cases from the viewpoint of Chinese medicine.

CASE 1: *Female, forty-nine years old*

- Western diagnosis: fibromyalgia
- Complaints: "Pain all over"
- Other symptoms: Always feels cold, difficulty falling asleep, night sweating, tinnitus.
- Tongue: Pale body, thick white coat

- Pulse: Deep, choppy, fine
- Chinese Diagnosis: Heart blood and Kidney *Jing* deficiency

CASE 2: ***Female, fifty-three years old***

- Western Diagnosis: fibromyalgia
- Complaints: Pain over the entire body
- Other symptoms: Feels cold, night sweats, frequent urination, poor memory, wakes throughout the night, low energy, poor breathing
- Tongue: Pale body, teeth marks on both sides
- Pulse: Weak and slow
- Chinese Diagnosis: Kidney *yin* deficiency with underlying Kidney *yang* deficiency.

CASE 3: ***Female, fifty-six years old***

- Western Diagnosis: fibromyalgia
- Complaints: Severe, constant pain over the entire body
- Notable History: Both parents died of heart attacks, lost her eighteen-year-old son in a car accident
- Other symptoms: Feels cold, sweating during the day, fatigue, awakens at night, tight diaphragm, tight behind the eyes
- Tongue: Pale tongue with light coating
- Pulse: Tight and taut
- Chinese Diagnosis: Liver *qi* stagnation with underlying Kidney *yang* deficiency.

As we can see, Chinese medicine views each of these patients differently. Indeed, the acupuncture points used, as well as the herbs administered, are different for each individual.

Fibromyalgia patients often have a major component of Liver *qi* stagnation, which can be translated as stress. The relaxing treatment of acupuncture, coupled with herbs, can often produce great improvement.

In another study of twenty-nine fibromyalgia patients (25 women, 4 men), rsearchers assessed pain level and tender points while measuring serotonin and substance P levels in blood serum. The findings were conclusive: treatment with acupuncture decreased pain and resulted in fewer tender points, as well as increasing serotonin and substance P levels in the blood.

Tennis Elbow

Tennis elbow is the most frequent elbow problem for which people seek help from acupuncturists.

Six meridians pass through the arm. On the inside are the Lung, Heart, and Pericardium. On the outside are the Large Intestine, Small Intestine and Triple Heater meridians.

Treatment depends on the overall evaluation of the cause of the pain, as well as on its location (i.e., along which meridian).

One study of tennis elbow treatment compared acupuncture to steroid injection. Thirty-four patients, most of whom already had undergone unsuccessful therapy, were treated with acupuncture. Steroid injections were given to another group of twenty-six patients with similar symptoms.

Sixty-two percent of the acupuncture patients and 31 percent of the patients who received steroid injections described their symptoms as much better after treatment, with slight or no pain. Of the patients who had had pain for at least six months, 62 percent of the acupuncture patients achieved positive results, compared to only 18 percent of the patients who received steroid injections. No acupuncture patients reported a worsening of pain, while several steroid-injection patients did.

Acupuncture has an added value as well which makes it even more appealing than steroids—no side effects.

A placebo-controlled trial of forty-eight other patients has also shown that using acupuncture for tennis elbow works. In the experimental group, patients were treated at leg points for their elbow pain. This group had an overall pain reduction of 56 percent, while only 14 percent of the placebo group experienced pain reduction.

Rheumatoid Arthritis

Rheumatoid arthritis is a chronic, systemic, inflammatory disorder affecting joints, muscles, ligaments, and tendons. It usually requires life-long treatment, and there is often disability or deformity. In Chinese medicine, both acupuncture and herbology are used to treat rheumatoid arthritis which, as a wind-damp obstruction, is classified as:

- Wind-damp-heat, which would have pain, swelling, warmth, and possible reddening of the joints.
- Wind-damp-cold, which would manifest as pain, swelling, and dull aching.

As always, we must look at the patient's underlying constitution to evaluate what caused the arthritis.

In one study of rheumatoid arthritis patients, thirty-four people were treated with acupuncture. Thirty-one of the thirty-four had undergone Western medical treatment unsuccessfully, and none had previously received acupuncture. They were treated twice weekly for five weeks, then at two-week intervals, and then twice weekly for five more weeks. Of the thirty-four patients, ten (29.4 percent) improved markedly, twenty (58.8 percent) improved somewhat, and four (11.8 percent) showed no change. In other words, 88.2 percent of these patients improved after acupuncture treatment.

HOW IS ACUPUNCTURE USED IN MAJOR INSTITUTIONS IN THE UNITED STATES TODAY?

Today, thirty-eight states and the District of Columbia recognize the practice of acupuncture. Of those states, twenty-two license acupuncturists to work independently, without an attending physician. There are more than fifty acupuncture schools in the United States, and several medical schools also teach acupuncture.

More than 10,000 licensed acupuncturists are practicing and working in private clinics and hospitals throughout the country. One such clinic is the New York Center for Pain Management in New York City, where Charles Kaplan, M.D., integrates traditional Western medicine with acupuncture, physical therapy, chiropractic, and osteopathy.

HERBOLOGY

The legendary emperor Shen Nong, the founder of herbal medicine, also wrote the first book on herbology. Sadly, it was lost during the Tang dynasty, around 800 A.D., although his teachings thrive in China as elsewhere. Interestingly enough, herbal medicine developed after acupuncture. Although today many practitioners use them together, the two disciplines evolved separately.

In 1977, the *materia medica* of herbal medicine in China described over 5,700 herbs (see Table 11-1). Of them, probably 500 are widely used. An herbalist practicing Chinese herbology studies not only what each individual herb does, he or she also reaps the benefit of thousands of years of research on herbs and herbal formulas of the past. Practitioners of Chinese medicine itemize herbs in the following way:

Chinese name: Ren Shen
Pharmaceutical name: Radix Ginseng
Common name: Ginseng
Category: Tonic
Taste: Sweet, slightly bitter
Temperature: Slightly warm
Channels entered: Lung, Spleen

Actions:

1. Tonifies *qi* - Yuan Qi
2. Tonifies and strengthens the Lung and Spleen *qi*
3. Promotes production of body fluids
4. Calms Heart *shen,* memory

Application 1: Immune deficiency, fatigue, improves organ function (yuan *qi* collapse—heart attack, shock, stroke), lung weakness, digestive weakness, insomnia, palpitation.

Application 2: Kidney *qi* deficiency: impotence, infertility, extreme thirst, strengthens blood.

An herb is almost never taken by itself, but is usually mixed in formulas with other herbs. An herbalist can use his or her own formula, or can give you a classic formula that has been studied for years.

Traditionally, herbs are loose plant parts (leaves or roots) that were mixed together and boiled into a tea. This is still the most powerful way to use herbs, but today we also make them into pills.

We can also apply herbs externally in a mix called a salve. In this case, we mix them together in a carrier oil and apply them to the skin, usually to treat an acute strain or sprain.

Another way we can apply an herb is moxabustion: We often use an herb called Mugwort (*Ai Ye*) this way. We roll it up into a cigar shape and burn it directly over the skin, which aids warming and circulation in the area.

An herbalist examines a patient's syndromes or disorders. Let's say a person has low back pain. An herbalist would not say, "Give the patient herbs for low back pain and send him home." That's how a Western physician might act. In truth, there are no herbs specific for low back pain.

So patient 1 complains of low back pain at L4-L5. He has no distinct structural abnormalities. Upon further questioning, we see that he has been under a lot of stress in his life. The diagnosis is low back pain due to Liver *qi* stagnation.

Patient 2 complains of the same pain, but he is also low on energy and run down. His diagnosis is low back pain due to Kidney *qi* deficiency.

Patient 3 complains of the very same low back pain. Additionally, he suffers from weak digestion and, over the past weekend, had a few large meals. His diagnosis is low back pain due to Spleen *qi* deficiency and food stagnation.

Patient 4 also complained about pain at L4-L5, but he hurt his back playing basketball. For him, the initial diagnosis is low back pain due to *qi* and blood stagnation. We'd have to look deeper to see if there is an underlying weakness that leaves him susceptible to muscle strains.

So all four patients have pain at L4-L5, but we'd use different methods of acupuncture and herbs to treat each of them.

In Chinese medicine, the herbs that are most helpful in alleviating pain are those classified as blood and *qi* movers, which encompass hundreds of herbs. For Patients 1, 3, and 4, it might be appropriate to add some of these herbs into their formulas. For Patient 4, it's possible that just making him stronger will alleviate his pain.

Chinese traditional medicine is a centuries-old medical system that deserves respect from and investigation by Western researchers. If you decide to pursue a form of Chinese medical treatment like acupuncture or herbology, be certain that you consult a qualified, experienced practitioner. Don't be afraid to ask him or her for referrals to satisfied patients. And be absolutely certain to let your physician know that you are pursuing these alternative forms of treatment.

Table 11-1
CHINESE HERBS THAT TREAT PAIN

Herb	Condition It Treats	What's In It
Corydalis (*Yan Hou Sou*)	Traditionally used to move stagnant blood and *qi*. Good for chronic back pain.	Chemical constituents: Over 20 alkaloids extracted, di-tetrahydropalamitine, protopine, bulbocapnine, d-corydalines A, B, L., dehydrocorydaline, tetrahydrocoptisine
Corydaline B	Possesses strong analgesic actions. Helps relax the muscles and calm the central nervous system. May be helpful for pain syndromes like fibromyalgia; also chronic back pain.	Corydaline B, L, diphenylhydantoin, ditetradropalamatine, bulbocapnine
Turmeric (*Jiang Huang*)	Traditionally used to move stagnant *qi* and blood. Can be helpful for rheumatoid arthritis.	Chemical constituents: tumerone, ar-tumerone, zinqiberene, cineole, curcumin
Peony (*Bai Shao*)	Traditionally used to disperse blood. Has antispasmodic and analgesic effects. May be helpful for pain conditions that involve muscle spasm.	Chemical constituents: Paeonflorin, alliflorin, oxypaeoniflorin, paeonol, paeonin, benzoic acid. Peoniflorin helps sedate the central nervous system
Licorice (*Gan Cao*)	Traditionally a tonic and a harmonizing herb. Often used with *Bai Shao* for pain. May be helpful for arthritis or chronic back pain.	Chemical constituents: Saponins glycyrrhizin, flavinoids, amino acids. Glycyrrhizin possesses anti-inflammatory effects. The flavinoids are antispasmodic

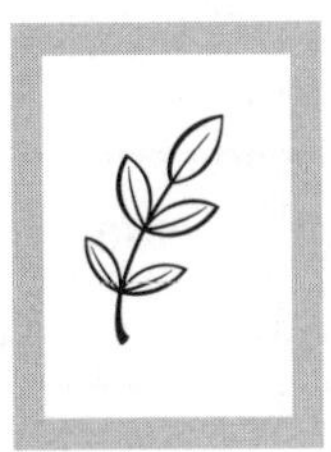

CHAPTER 12
THE CHIROPRACTIC CONNECTION

Okay, here's a question: Who said, "Look to the spine, for it is the cause of most disease"? It was Galen, the "father of medicine." Here is another: Who said, "The doctor of the future will give no drugs, but concern himself with the frame of the body and the prevention of illness"? That was Thomas Edison. Galen and Edison, pioneers of their time, obviously knew and understood the importance of the spine. In this chapter, we'll discuss some of the spine's connections to pain.

As we discussed in Chapter 4, the spine is a rigid yet flexible structure consisting of a series of bones, ligaments, and articulations.

The spine has the awesome task of protecting the nervous system, while simultaneously maintaining flexibility. The nervous system is the body's quarterback—it calls all the shots. The brain, spinal cord, and nerves that connect the brain and spinal cord to the rest of the body make up the nervous system. The brain sends electrical messages to the body, and then expects an answer back. For all this to happen, there has to be a highly reliable network of passageways that starts in the brain, goes down the spinal cord, and then out to the body's organs, muscles, and sensory systems. Once outlying areas receive the message, they send a response back to the brain, so that the brain doesn't keep sending the same messages.

> When you feel threatened, your "Fight or Flight" reflex kicks in automatically. In every life-or-death situation, the body readies itself by preparing to stay and fight, or to run away. In either case, the goal is survival.

Without this "information superhighway" within the body and the spine to protect it, we would not function well at all. Just think about Christopher Reeve, the stage and screen actor of *Superman* fame. One minute he was a healthy, happy member of the human race who happened to be riding a horse. The next minute, the horse threw him, and he fractured his spine. Because of his spinal cord injury, he became a paraplegic who can breathe on his own, without a ventilator, for only an hour or two at a time. This horrible tragedy for Reeve and his family is a prime example of a nervous system injury causing major dysfunction. That Reeve has made some improvements in his condition is both a testament to his strength of will and to the expertise of his caregivers.

We want you to appreciate just how wonderful the human body is, and the importance of the spine. Imagine that you're shopping in the local mall and, after an exhausting outing, you have lost track of the time. It's 10 P.M., and the mall is closing. As you amble to the exits, and begin to ponder the location of you car, you can't help noticing how deserted the parking lot is. You start walking, packages in hand, and you spot your car. At the same time, out of the corner of your eye you notice two seemingly unsavory characters who appear to be following you. As you increase your pace, they seem to increase theirs. Your heart starts to race, and that bacon double hamburger you ate at 8:30 now sits like lead in your belly, because your digestion has just stopped.

You see, when a person feels threatened, as during this possibly life-threatening situation in a suburban mall parking lot, a wonderful reflex called "Fight or Flight" automatically kicks in. The sympathetic nervous system, which calls the dorsal spine its home, governs the "fight or flight" response, which readies the body for survival. You will either stay and fight, or run away. In either case, the goal is identical—survival. At that moment, the body automatically stops all functions not immediately responsible for survival—like digestion. Simultaneously, the body enhances and stimulates other functions that *are* necessary for survival, like breathing and heart rate. The pupils in your eyes are now fully dilated to see danger and possible escape routes clearly. Adrenaline, a wonderful chemical made by the adrenal glands, is now flowing freely in your body to give you extra strength and speed for a short period of time. Your body does not lie down and give up. It is programmed to survive.

Let's go back to the mall parking lot, where everything is happily all right. What appeared to be one of life's defining moments turned out to be a false alarm. The two miscreants just got into their car and drove away. You get into your car and take a deep breath, and your body starts to normalize again. Even though it was a false alarm, your body prepared for the worst. Remember, your body did everything automatically, without your thinking about it. Transmitting all those messages to your organs and muscles is a truly remarkable feat.

The spine protects the integrity of the nervous system and its messages. If you injure your spine, or it functions at a below-normal level for any reason, pain and suffering usually follow. Additionally, the very framework of our bodies' supercomputer may be compromised, and seemingly unrelated body functions may not operate at an optimal level. The spine is *that* important in the overall scheme of body function and health.

Chiropractors attend to the health of the spine. A chiropractor has earned a doctorate and specializes in spinal function, biomechanics, and their relationship to the nervous system and the body's total health. Chiropractic is a healing art that dates back to 1895, when its founder, Daniel David Palmer, met his first patient, a deaf janitor named Harvey Lillard. As Mr. Palmer reported, Mr. Lillard "had been so deaf for 17 years that he could not hear the racket of a wagon on the street or the ticking of a watch. I made inquiry as to the cause of his deafness and was informed that when he was exerting himself in a cramped, stooping position, he felt something give way in his back and immediately became deaf. An examination showed a vertebra racked from its normal position. I reasoned that if that vertebra was replaced, the man's hearing should be restored. With this object in view, a half-hour's talk persuaded Mr. Lillard to allow me to replace it. I racked it into position by using the spinous process as a lever and soon the man could hear as before." With that, the chiropractic profession was born.

> Even though the spine supports us, there should be motion within each vertebra. Remember that the primary function of the spine is to protect the spinal cord and, to do that, it requires both rigidity and flexibility.

Spinal manipulation has long held a place in medical practice: the Chinese have practiced it for centuries, as have osteopaths and Europe's "bonesetters." Even in 1895, there was nothing new about performing spinal manipulation to relieve pain and to restore health. In Mr. Lillard's case, the premise was unique: his spinal dysfunction caused a nervous system failure. In other words, his misplaced vertebra interrupted the nerve pathway that transmitted sound to the brain, so Mr. Lillard became deaf.

Let's fast-forward to 1999, when chiropractic treatment involves a specific spinal manipulation called a spinal adjustment. The spine and its bony protuberances—the spinous and transverse processes—are used as short levers, and a brisk thrust returns the misplaced vertebra to its proper position.

Think of the spine as being your bodyguard. The bodyguard's job is to get his or her employer safely to his or her car. That sounds easy enough, except that he or she has to clear the way through an angry mob, and do it countless times a day. Needless to say, this is a tough work environment, and injuries are likely. Similarly, in the real world, the spinal "functional unit" (two vertebrae and their intervening disk) deals with all sorts of physical stresses and loads.

A chiropractor assesses the normalcy, dysfunction, injury, and severity of impairment of the spine. Even though the spine maintains a rigid posture, there should be motion within each and every spinal vertebra. Remember that the primary function of the spine is to protect the spinal cord and emerging nerves; to do that requires both rigidity and flexibility from our spinal functional units.

What exactly can a spinal functional unit do? Research shows that vertebrae rotate in all three axes of motion. Therefore, in three-dimensional space, there are six degrees of freedom in vertebral motion. Remember the x-axis, y-axis, and z-axis from high school math class? The spine moves—specifically, it rotates—along all three axes. While this motion occurs, the vertebrae's facet joints and disks are busy dealing with the hostile stresses: They absorb stress from compressive and shear forces, bending moments, and others. What can go wrong in this unfriendly environment?

BACK PAIN

People in some developing countries prefer squatting to sitting, and researchers report very little low back pain in those societies. Unfortunately, in our society, many of us spend more time sitting than standing. Just think about all the time you spend sitting. Need some help? You sit at breakfast, lunch, and dinner; commuting to work; at your work station, and at your computer; on the toilet; in front of the television; and while reading. All this sitting doesn't exactly do wonders for your spine.

> Muscle dysfunction disrupts spinal function, which can cause great pain. Poor Posture = Ligament Problems = Disk Problems = Back Problems = Pain.

Let's digress momentarily; we've talked about the disks providing stiffness to the spine. So which structures act as shock absorbers? It's not the disks, but the sagittal curves of the spine that cope with weight and its shock. We can see this series of curves when we look at the spine from the side. They look like the letter "S." In some people, these curves are accentuated, while in others, the spine loses its normal curvature. Normal spinal curvature is essential in deflecting some stresses and loads that we deal with day in and day out. If spinal curvature is abnormal, then weight shifts to weaker structures, breakdown commences, and pain begins.

Studies show that muscle dysfunction can destabilize the spine, reducing the role of facet joints in transmitting weight, thus shifting loads from the bone (the facet joints) to soft structures (the disks and ligaments). In other words, muscle dysfunction disturbs the normal function of parts of the spine. It can cause myriad painful spinal conditions. Poor Posture = Ligament Problems = Disk Problems = Back Problems = Pain.

Stand up straight! Don't slouch! Can you still hear your mother telling you that? Those words contain ancient wisdom. Slouching is endemic; just look around. The problem is, when you slouch, the lumbar saggital curve (in the lower back) becomes flattened. Let's try something: Sit down on a chair, and try to sit up as perfectly straight as possible. While seated, place your hand in the small of your back. Normally, you should be able to feel your back arch inward (a "concavity"). Now, with your hand still on your lower back, slouch. Notice how the small of your back flattens. Studies show that the flexed posture produced by sitting increases the weight (tensile forces) on the lower back. Research also shows that mechanical loads (weight) and posture directly influence tissue growth and repair. Therefore, if poor posture transmits increased loads to the spine, and if that abnormal posture affects tissue growth and repair, then poor posture can cause spinal pain and arthritic degeneration.

You can correct some poor posture just by becoming conscious of when you slouch, and sending a mental alarm to straighten up. Let's do another slouch test. This time, slouch to your right side. Slouching to either side causes the spinal muscles to react. On the side that you're slouching toward, muscles will tighten. On the side you're leaning away from, muscles will stretch and become irritated. There is nothing wrong with stretching, but when you stretch only on one side, at the expense of muscle contraction on the other side, it becomes a form of muscle dysfunction.

Chiropractors are specifically trained to analyze posture. The chiropractic approach to bad posture includes analysis, X ray, notation of any muscular imbalance, specific chiropractic adjustment to correct posture and any affected spinal functional unit, and rehabilitative exercises.

Although chiropractors provide care for a wide variety of conditions, as well as providing wellness and prevention education, most patients seek chiropractic care for treatment of low back pain and other neuromuscular disorders. Low back pain has become a massive medical, social, and economic problem.

A variety of conditions cause low back pain, as we discussed in Chapter 5. Now let's examine the chiropractic approach to some of them.

THE CHIROPRACTIC ADJUSTMENT

Chiropractors are spinal biomechanical experts. They analyze the spine for the presence of vertebral subluxation complex (VSC). VSC involves the tissues in five ways:

- kinesiopathology (loss of normal biomechanical function)
- neuropathology (increased nociceptor stimulation resulting in pain, pinched nerve, irritation of dorsal root ganglion and nerve root, as well as other nerve problems)
- histopathology (swelling, fibrosis, and excess fluid)
- myopathology (muscle spasm, trigger points, and myofacial pain)
- pathophysiology (degenerative changes in joints, including arthritis).

VSC is the primary problem that chiropractors treat. An individual who suffers ill effects from VSC might say his or her back "went out," or he or she has a "bone out of place," or a "pinched nerve."

We must emphasize: Your back didn't go out, never did, and never will. You back is a homebody; it likes to stay where it is. Bones also don't go out of place, unless there is a dislocation. While saying a bone "went out of place" creates the desired visual effect, it is an incorrect description. Usually, due to a variety of physical stresses, a vertebral functional spinal unit may become sprained and some of its ligaments stretched or torn. If this injury is not managed correctly, scar tissue will form. This joint will then have made the journey from having normal biomechanics to being hypermobile from the injury to being hypomobile—it loses its normal ability to move because of the scar tissue that accumulates as it tries to heal.

So, our spine can malfunction mechanically (develop kinesiopathology) in a number of ways, by developing

- hypomobility;
- hypermobility;
- positional dyskinesia (the inability to move properly); and
- loss of central axis of motion.

Once a joint is sprained, it develops swelling and inflammation, which affects bones, ligaments, cartilage, tendons, muscle, fascia, blood vessels, and nerves. This inflammatory reaction, called histopathology, results in scar tissue formation and joint degeneration.

The muscles are also affected by this process (myopathology). They can go into spasm and tighten (a state called hypertonic), or they can become weak and loose (a state called hypotonic).

Of course, the nerves are also involved (called neuropathology), usually in one of five ways:

- nerve distortion with increased nociceptive (pain receptor) stimulation;
- mechanoreceptor stimulation (described in Chapter 5);
- pinched nerve;
- dorsal root ganglion (i.e., spinal nerve) irritation;
- malfunction of various nerves.

All of these nerve involvements, not surprisingly, cause pain.

Degeneration (pathophysiology) is the last component of VSC. It's seen on X rays, MRIs, or CT scans, and is associated with immobilization or long-standing joint problems. Spinal malfunction leads to joint degeneration and bone remodeling, which result in

- loss of disk height;
- calcified spurs;
- spinal distortion;
- fusion;
- arthritis.

Let's look at an actual patient now to see how all this works.

A forty-one-year-old man sought treatment after chopping wood in his backyard. He'd started to notice some mild back pain within the first thirty minutes but, since he planned to do two more hours of chopping, he decided that giving in to the pain was out of the question. He continued, even though his pain became more intense. At the end of his marathon chopping session, he could barely straighten up. He struggled to get inside the house and call the office. By the time he arrived, he also had tightness and pain in his left thigh.

The chiropractor palpated the spinal column to assess normal spinal biomechanics. He checked the vertebrae for proper motion, excessive tenderness to touch, or inflammation. In addition, he palpated the muscles around the spine for muscle spasm, trigger points, or tender points; and he performed manual muscle tests around the problem area. The chiropractor took two spinal X rays, and discovered loss of spinal mobility at L5-S1. (Refer back to Chapter 4 if you are having trouble remembering how we number the lumbar vertebrae.)

The X rays showed:

- loss in normal lumbar sagittal curve, called hypolordosis;
- arthritic changes at L4-L5 and L5-S1 (disk loss); and
- slight right curvature.

We alerted this patient to the extent of his problem, and established a regime of chiropractic spinal adjustments (twice weekly for three to four weeks). In addition, the patient used ice to reduce inflammation and pain during the first week.

After the first treatment, this patient was completely pain free.

In this case, the spinal X rays revealed that this patient had long-standing back problems. His problem probably began years ago with a small tear in the capsule, or a subluxation (described above), creating inflammation and causing the muscles to go into a protective "splinting" state called hypertonicity. This simply means that a tight muscle is in spasm, usually from an injury. Think of it as creating a "natural cast" to prevent motion and, therefore, further injury. With time, however, the muscles don't get enough blood—they become ischemic—and build up lactic acid, our muscles' metabolic end product. Increased lactic acid, in turn, creates more pain.

Initially, this condition might cause a decrease in joint motion, or some soft tissue tenderness and trigger points. Over time, small tears in ligaments cause a potentially unstable joint. Finally, the instability leads to calcium buildup at the joints, loss in disk height, and scar tissue formation. This patient had several bouts of low back pain over the years, but he usually ignored them or simply took pain pills. This time, when the pain was much more severe, common sense told him that he'd better fix the problem.

To understand chiropractic adjustments, you need to understand joint motion, which has several phases. The first is "active range of motion," which means moving a joint as far as possible. For example, turn your head as far as possible to the right. At this point, it won't turn any more—or so you think.

The second phase is "passive range of motion." Once you rotate your head as far as possible to the right, place your hands on each cheek and try to rotate it a little bit further. Usually you can.

The adjustment takes place at the joint space, where there is a cavity. Gases accumulate in this cavity, and make the popping or snapping sounds you hear during an adjustment. The spinal adjustment creates movement in a previously nonmobile joint, or corrects movement in one that moves abnormally. Damage occurs when entire sections of the spine move in directions they shouldn't (mechanical engineering calls these movements "rotation" and "translation"), and the chiropractic adjustment, not surprisingly, *adjusts* them so that they once again move properly.

Let's now look at a second patient.

A fifty-four-year-old man came for an examination after tripping and falling while laying a carpet. His symptoms were sharp low back pain, especially on the right side, and some pain in the right buttock. As a result of the injury, he couldn't perform his normal work duties. He also commented that the pain was so severe he was taking twelve to fifteen Advil tablets a day, which didn't help. After a physical exam, he had an MRI of the lumbar spine to determine if he'd injured a disk. The MRI found a herniated disk at L4-L5, with a fragment of the disk actually broken off.

For decades, standard, orthodox medical treatment for this condition has been spinal surgery. It's not uncommon for a patient suffering from this affliction to be browbeaten into compliance. Can't you just hear Dr. Kildare now? "Mr. Jones, this is very serious. Disk herniations just don't go away. And if you don't have me operate on this, you might be paralyzed one day. You don't want that, do you, Mr. Jones?" The patient might reply, "But Dr. Kildare, I am not sure if I want to have surgery. What about a chiropractor? Can he help?" To which Dr. Kildare would most likely reply, "A chiropractor? Why, they are just a bunch of quacks. I forbid you to see a chiropractor. As a matter of fact, I forbid anyone you know to see a chiropractor!"

This sort of pedantic, manipulative, selfish, unprofessional, and, as it turns out, illegal activity is rife in the annals of orthodox medicine. Although there is more interdisciplinary cooperation today, we still have a long way to go before our brothers and sisters in the medical profession are properly educated about integrative health care, and about when they should make referrals.

Back to our patient: He began chiropractic care three times weekly. He had spinal manipulation and deep massage performed. We used ice and moist heat to control pain and inflammation. Within six weeks, our patient was pain free. Not only is chiropractic a safe form of treatment for disk herniations, it is very effective, as well.

The spinal disk is the largest avascular structure—that is, it contains no blood vessels—in the human body. Researchers have suggested that, if disk material contacts the body's immune cells (as it does when a disk herniates), an autoimmune response might take place. The patient could develop inflammation around the nerve roots, causing sciatica (pain down the leg, as we discussed in Chapter 5).

At times, the amount of disk material that herniates is large enough to put direct pressure on the nerve root, which can cause neurologic problems like incontinence. This situation, while rare, can require surgery. Otherwise, studies and clinical experience show chiropractic adjustment to be a safe and effective form of care for disk herniation.

ARTHRITIS

How many times have you heard that arthritis, specifically osteoarthritis, is a natural part of the aging process? Phooey! It's amazing how some falsehoods just keep going, and going, and going, like the Energizer bunny.

> The physiological process of osteoarthritis, the most common form of arthritis, can be stopped, and sometimes even reversed. *Osteoarthritis is not a rite of passage into older age.*

Bennet was the first to describe arthritis as a natural part of aging. He postulated that normal wear and tear make joints decay and degenerate. Medical professors have passed this concept down through many generations of health care practitioners and researchers.

Bennet thought that chondrocytes, the cells that make cartilage, couldn't replicate themselves or heal once they were injured. We have now debunked this idea. In fact, a body of evidence shows that the physiological process of osteoarthritis, the most common form of arthritis, can be stopped, and sometimes even reversed. Osteoarthritis is not a rite of passage into older age.

In arthritis, as we've discussed, the joint becomes painful, swollen, loses normal range of motion, and undergoes decay and degeneration. Although some types of arthritis require lab work for a proper diagnosis, X ray or MRI usually reveals osteoarthritis.

Bland and Cooper contend that the biological process that causes arthritis is actually the body's attempt at repair. As practitioners, we see this when a patient has an old injury, like that caused by a rear-end collision. Within several years following the injury, we can see arthritic changes at multiple sites in the cervical spine. This suggests that excessive calcium growths, soft tissue enlargement, and/or disk dehydration are the body's attempts to stabilize the injured joints. It also suggests that, during the healing process, the body *increases* joint dysfunction, which leads to progressive joint degeneration. This all spells P.A.I.N.

Studies show that correcting this biomechanical dysfunction and normalizing joint mobility (as chiropractors do) can reverse osteoarthritis. Chiropractic care adjusts the loose joints that are likely to become unstable and arthritic. In addition, chiropractors advise patients about stretching and exercise, which have a positive effect on joints.

So how does a chiropractic adjustment relieve the pain of arthritis? First, the mechanical stimulation may stimulate certain nerve receptors (the mechanoreceptors and proprioceptors) in the spinal joints. This stimulation inhibits the nerve receptors that cause pain. Here is an oversimplified example: You wake up at 3:00 A.M. and need a drink of water. Efforts to navigate to the bathroom have you writhing on the floor in pain after you stub your toe, which you instinctively rub. Rubbing is mechanical stimulation, like chiropractic adjustment. It stimulates mechanoreceptors, which inhibits the nociceptors that let us feel pain. Chiropractic adjustment works exactly the same way (although it deals with structures more complex than toes and fingers).

Second, chiropractic relieves pain by interrupting the inflammation that follows misplacement of the vertebrae. A chiropractic adjustment helps the by-products of inflammation to circulate, so they don't accumulate and cause pain. It also reduces pressure in the area.

It is not uncommon for our patients to say, "That was a great adjustment! I feel really loose and relaxed now." Chiropractic patients around the world probably feel the same way after treatment.

When injury damages the dorsal root ganglia—the portion of the spinal nerve that controls pain sensation—the surrounding muscle physically changes. Primarily, nociceptor activity increases (which causes pain) and sensitivity to neurotransmitters increase (which also causes pain). Simply put, injury causes nerve damage, which makes everything around the damages to be supersensitive and painful, causing muscle spasm.

MUSCLE PAIN

Muscles can be significant sources of pain. An example is fibromyalgia syndrome, which affects three to six million people, as we discussed in Chapter 5. To manage fibromyalgia properly, we need to address both pain and loss of sleep.

Remember fibromyalgia's trigger points? Injury to the muscle, tendon, ligament, nerve, disk, or joint can all cause trigger points. Pain due to fibromyalgia comes from a combination of excited nerves and receptors, inflammation, and neuropeptides like substance P, which can cause inflammation of the spinal nerve root. In addition, substance P and other neuropeptides can cause joint sensitivity and irritation of nociceptors, creating more pain.

Let's put this into perspective: Injury or poor posture can cause a vertebral subluxation (VSL). VSL produces nervous system dysfunction that causes joint biomechanical problems, muscle problems, and inflammation.

What can we do about all this? We must examine the spine to locate the affected joints so we can restore proper motion and provide all the other positive effects of chiropractic adjustments. In addition, we must note posture and/or deformity, and provide specific exercises to help correct poor posture. We should use massage, manual trigger-point therapy, ice, and heat to help with pain. Some practitioners use ultrasound on trigger points to relieve pain. However, we agree with the medical literature that suggests that ultrasound is not very effective in treating fibromyalgia.

HEADACHES

Headaches and the pain associated with them afflict an enormous number of Americans every year. Whether they are tension, cluster, or migraine headaches, they have a devastating effect on the sufferer's ability to function. Quality of life, workplace productivity, and activities of daily living can all be compromised, placing a huge burden on spouses and family, as well as on employers. Cervicogenic headaches, which arise from cervical spine (neck) dysfunction, are very common. Chiropractors treat this type of headache very effectively.

There are numerous causes of headache pain, including the following:

- irritation of the nerve at the base of the skull (C2 nerve root irritation);
- abnormal blood flow to the brain (cranial circulation abnormality);
- a neck condition causing headache pain (referred pain from cervical joint condition);
- knotted muscles (muscle spasm) in the neck and shoulder, fibromyalgia's trigger points, or myofascial pain syndrome;
- nerve pain (probably from the trigeminal nerve, one of the nerves that directly exits from the spinal cord).

Many other conditions cause headaches, including high blood pressure (hypertension), stroke, low blood sugar (hypoglycemia), dehydration, brain injury, fatigue, eyestrain, sinus infection, chemical imbalance, and tumor. Here, we'll outline the most common causes and the chiropractic approaches to dealing with headache pain.

Although headache pain can vary due to the specific type of headache you have, it's important to know that chiropractic adjustments of the vertebral subluxations that cause migraine and tension headaches can be very effective. Spinal adjustments of the cervical region, in particular, seem to be as effective as amitriptyline—an antidepressant medication commonly used to treat pain, headache and sleep loss—with fewer side effects. Patients with frequent migraine headaches should certainly consider chiropractic treatment.

In addition to chiropractic adjustments, which can normalize spinal joint function and nerve activity, chiropractors often discuss nutritional considerations with patients. Approximately one-third of migraine headache sufferers benefit from modifying their diets. As a result, we know that migraine sufferers should avoid the following foods:

- ripened cheese,
- chocolate,
- nuts,
- dairy products,
- aged or cured meats,
- soy and yeast,
- wheat products,
- shellfish, and
- all alcoholic beverages.

In addition to chiropractic care and dietary modifications, stress management, deep (diaphragmatic) breathing for proper oxygenation, and exercise all have very positive effects on headache sufferers.

Here's a third case study to prove our point.

A thirty-six-year-old woman arrived with symptoms of headache with neck and shoulder pain after falling down a wet staircase at work. The headaches are very frequent (almost daily), and the neck pain is severe.

Upon examination, she had:

- loss of normal cervical range of motion
- loss of normal sensation on inner forearm (hypoesthesia T1 dermatome)
- head in right tilt, rotation posture, and anterior translation (a type of motion, as we described above)
- positive Jackson's test, showing nerve irritation
- vertebral subluxations at C3 and C6
- disk herniation revealed by MRI at C3
- muscle spasm of trapezius.

We performed chiropractic spinal adjustments, massaged the trapezius muscle, and recommended specific postural exercises. The patient began a course of twice-weekly treatments. Four weeks later, her symptoms had improved dramatically. After one year, her headaches continued to improve.

SPINAL STENOSIS

Spinal stenosis can cause considerable pain and/or numbness in the back, buttocks, thighs, and calves. As we discussed in Chapter 5, a narrowing around the nerve roots and/or the spinal cord, which increases pressure on the sciatic nerve's roots, causes spinal stenosis. You can only relieve the pain by sitting or flexing the spine forward. While there are many causes of a narrowed spinal canal, the most common is osteoarthritis.

The chiropractic approach to spinal stenosis involves

- improving posture,
- strengthening abdominal musculature,
- stretching exercises that involve flexed postures, and
- spinal adjustment that places lumbar spine in a flexed posture.

If these conservative measures don't adequately resolve pain and numbness, spinal neural decompressive surgery might be necessary.

EXERCISES

Exercise, including stretching, can make you feel better and improve your range of motion. Some helpful tips are

- Stretch your hamstrings by trying to touch your toes with straight knees. Don't bounce—just bend, hold, and return to your starting position.
- Lie on your back and pull your knees, one at a time, then together, toward your chest.
- Get on all fours, relax your belly so it hangs low and then, like a frightened feline, suck up your gut and raise your back.
- Strengthen your abdominal muscles by doing isometrics and crunches. To do isometrics, simply tighten your abdominal muscles and hold them. Crunches are modified sit-ups. Lying on the floor on your back, lift legs with bent knees onto a bed; raise your upper body, then lower it back down.

In closing, please remember:

First, your hip bone *is* connected to your knee bone—remember the song from nursery school? Well, it's true. Your body is completely interconnected, and dysfunction in one area can cause trouble in another area.

Second, there is more than one way to skin a cat. As a health-care consumer, you need to keep an open mind about your health-care options. No form of health care is a panacea. Integrative and complementary health care, including chiropractic, is highly effective for a wide variety of conditions. However, at times, Western medicine is necessary.

Last, an ounce of prevention is worth a pound of cure. Your neuromusculoskeletal system is enormous. It includes your bones, muscles, nerves, tendons, ligaments, and other connective tissue. It takes a beating every day. It's only prudent to take good care of your body, so that it continues to take good care of you.

BIBLIOGRAPHY

Chapter 1

Anderson, GBJ. The epidemiology of spinal disorders. In: Frymoyer JW, ed. *The Adult Spine: Principles and Practice.* New York: Raven Press, 1991; pp. 107–146.

Bjorkman DJ. The effect of aspirin and nonsteroidal anti-inflammatory drugs on prostaglandins. *Am J Med* 1998;105(1B):8S–12S.

Borenstein DG, Wiesel SW, Boden SD. *Low Back Pain, Medical Diagnosis and Comprehensive Management,* 2nd ed. Philadelphia: W.B. Saunders, 1995.

Caudill, Margaret. *Managing Pain Before It Manages You.* New York: Guilford, 1995.

Cerra, FB. Nutrient modulation of inflammatory and immune function. *Am J Surg* 1991:161, 230.

Corey D, Solomon S. *Pain: Learning to Live Without It.* Toronto: Macmillan, 1988.

Deyo RA, Bass JE. Lifestyle and low back pain. *Spine* 1989;14:501.

Deyo RA, Tsui-Wu Y-J. Descriptive epidemiology of low-back pain and its related medical care in the United States. *Spine* 1987;12:264.

Eisenberg, David. Complementary and Alternative Medicine, Introduction and Overview. *Alternative Medicine: Implications for Clinical Practice.* Harvard Medical School Seminar, 1999; pp. 19–28.

Fine J. *The Ultimate Back Book.* Toronto: Stoddard Pub., 1997.

Fosslien E. Adverse effects of nonsteroidal anti-inflammatory drugs on the gastrointestinal system. *Ann Clin Lab Sci* 1998;28(2):67–81.

Frymoyer JW. Back pain and sciatica. *N Engl J Med* 1988; 318:291.

Gabriel SE, Jaakkimainen L, Bombardier C. Risk for serious gastrointestinal complications related to use of nonsteroidal anti-inflammatory drugs. A meta-analysis. *Ann Intern Med* 1991;115:787–796.

Gadisseux P, Ward J.D, Young HF, and Becker, DP. Nutrition and the neurosurgical patient. *J Neurosurg* 1984;60: 219.

Griffin MR, Piper JM, Daugherty JR, et al. Nonsteroidal anti-inflammatory drug use and increased risk for peptic ulcer disease in elderly persons. *Ann Intern Med.* 1991;114(4):257–263.

Hall, H. *The Back Doctor.* Toronto: Macmillan, 1980.

Hanson RW, Gerber KE. *Coping with Chronic Pain.* New York: Guilford, 1990.

Hawkey CJ. COX-2 inhibitors. *Lancet* 1999;253(9149):307–314.

Hawkey CJ. Future treatments for arthritis: new NSAIDs, NO NSAIDs, or no NSAIDs? *Gastroenterology* 1995;109(2):614–616.

Heliovaara M. *Epidemiology of sciatica and herniated lumbar intervertebral disc.* Helsinki: The Research Institute for Social Security, 1988; pp. 1–47.

Hochberg MC, Altman RD, Brandt KD, et al. Guidelines for the medical management of osteoarthritis. Part I. Osteoarthritis of the hip. *Arthritis Rheum* 1995;38(11):1535–1540.

Kelsey JL, White AA III. Epidemiology and impact of low back pain. *Spine* 1980;5:133.

Kirkaldy-Willis WH. *Managing Low Back Pain,* 2nd ed. New York: Churchill Livingstone, 1988.

Lands WE. Actions of anti-inflammatory drugs. *Trends in Pharmacol Sci* 1981;2: 78–80.

Lane NE. Pain management in osteoarthritis: the role of COX-2 inhibitors. *J Rheum* 1997;24(Suppl 49):20–24.

Lewis RA, Austen KF, Soberman RJ. Leukotrienes and other products of the 5-lipoxygenase pathway. *N Engl J Med* 1990;323:645–655.

Lipsky PE. Role of cyclooxygenase-1 and -2 in health and disease. *Am J Orthop* 1999;28(Suppl 3S):8–12.

Lipsky PE, Isaakson PC. Outcome of specific COX-2 inhibition in rheumatoid arthritis. *J Rheum* 1997;24(Suppl 49):9–14.

Melzack R, Wall P. *The Challenge of Pain.* New York: Basic Books, 1983.

Melzack R, Wall P. Pain mechanisms: a new theory. *Science* 1965;150: 971–979.

Moncada S, Flower RJ, Vane JR. Prostaglandins, prostacyclin and thromboxane A2. In: Gilman AG, Goodman LS, Rall TW, Murad F, eds. *The Pharmacological Basis of Therapeutics.* New York: Macmillan, 1985.

Munck A, Guyre, PM, Holbrook NJ. Physiological functions of glucocorticoids in stress and their relation to pharmacological actions. *Endocr Rev* 1984;5:25–44.

Nachemson A, Eck C, Lindstrom IL, et al. Chronic low back disability can largely be prevented: A prospective randomized trial in industry. AAOS 56th Annual Meeting, Las Vegas, 1989.

National Center for Health Statistics. Prevalence of selected impairments, United States, 1977. Series 10, No. 134, 1981.

National Center for Health Statistics. Surgical operations in short stay hospitals, United States, 1973. Series 13, number 24, 1976.

National Center for Health Statistics. Physician visits, volume and interval since last visit, United States, 1971. Series 10, Number 97, 1975.

National Center for Health Statistics. Limitation of activity due to chronic conditions, United States, 1974. Series 10, No. 111, 1977.

National Center for Health Statistics. Inpatient utilization of short stay hospitals by diagnosis, United States, 1973. Series 13, Number 25, 1976.

Needleman P, Isaakson PC. The discovery and function of COX-2. *J Rheum* 1997;24(suppl 49):6–9.

Rowe ML. Low back pain in industry. A position paper. *J Occup Med* 1969;11:161.

Salkever DS. Morbidity costs: national estimates and economic determinants. NCHSR Research Summary Series, October 1985, Department of Health and Human Services Publication No. (PHS) 86–3393, 1986.

Samuelsson B. Leukotrienes: mediators of immediate hypersensitivity reactions and inflammation. *Science* 1983; 220: 568–575.

Sinel MS, Deardorff WW, Goldstein TB. *Win the Battle Against Back Pain: An Integrated Mind-Body Approach.* New York: Dell, 1996.

Singh G. Recent considerations in nonsteroidal anti-inflammatory drug gastropathy. *Am J Med* 1998;105(1B):31S–38S.

Tortora G, Grabowski SR, eds. *Principles of Anatomy and Physiology,* 8th ed. New York: HarperCollins, 1996.

Trippel SB. The unmet anti-inflammatory needs in orthopedics. *Am J Orthop* 1999;(Supp3S): 3–7.

Vane JR. Inhibition of prostaglandin synthesis as a mechanism of action for aspirin-like drugs. *Nature New Biology* 1971;231: 232–239.

Vane JR, Botting RM. Mechanism of action of nonsteroidal anti-inflammatory drugs. *Am J Med* 1998;104(3A):2S–8S.

Weber H. Lumbar disc herniation. A controlled, prospective study with ten years of observation. *Spine* 1989;14:141.

Wells C, Graham N. *The Pain Relief Handbook.* Buffalo: Firefly Books, 1998.

Wolfe MM. Future trends in the development of safer nonsteroidal anti-inflammatory drugs. *Am J Med* 1998;105(5A):44S–52S.

Wood PHN, Badley EM. Epidemiology of back pain. In: Jayson M, ed. *The Lumbar Spine and Back Pain.* London: Churchill Livingstone, 1987; pp. 1–15.

Wright PH, Brashear H.R. The local response to trauma. In: Wilson FC, ed. *The Musculoskeletal System. Basic Processes and Disorders,* 2nd ed. Philadelphia: Lippincott, 1983; pp. 261.

Chapter 2

Aimone LD. Neurochemistry and modulation of pain. In: Sinatra RS, Hord AH, Ginsberg B, Preble LM, eds. *Acute Pain: Mechanisms and Management.* St Louis: Mosby Year Book, 1992, pp. 29–43.

Anand KJS, Craig KD. New perspectives on the definition of pain. *Pain* 1996; 67(1):3–6.

Beecher HK. Relationship of significance of wound to pain experienced. *JAMA* 1956;161:1609–1613.

Beecher HK. *Measurement of Subjective Responses.* New York: Oxford University Press, 1959.

Besson J-M, Chaouch A. Peripheral and spinal mechanisms of nociception. *Physiol Rev* 1987; 67:67–186.

Bonica JJ. *Anatomic and Physiologic Basis of Nociception and Pain,* In: Bonica JJ, ed. *The Management of Pain,* 2nd ed. Philadelphia: Lea & Febiger, 1990, pp. 400–460.

Bonica, John J., ed. *Pain.* New York: Raven Press, 1973.

Borenstein DG, Wiesel SW, Boden SD. *Low Back Pain, Medical Diagnosis and Comprehensive Management,* 2nd ed. Philadelphia: W.B. Saunders, 1995.

Caudill M. *Managing Pain Before It Manages* You. New York: Guilford, 1995.

Corey D, Solomon S. *Pain: Learning to Live Without It.* Toronto: Macmillan, 1988.

Cyriax J. *Manipulation: Past and Present.* London: Heinemann, 1975.

Eipper BA, Mains RE, Herbert E. Peptides in the nervous system. *Trends in Neuroscience,* 1986;9:463–468.

Fields HL. Pain: new approaches to therapy. *Ann Neurol* 1981;9: 101–106.

Fine J. *The Ultimate Back Book.* Toronto: Stoddard Pub., 1997.

Franz DN. *Review of Research on Receptor Pharmacology of Pain and Analgesia: Part One.* American Pain Society Bulletin October/November, 1993;10–13.

Guyton AC. *Basic Human Physiology: Normal Function and Mechanisms of Disease.* Philadelphia: W.B. Saunders, 1971.

Haldeman S, ed. *Modern Developments in the Principles and Practice of Chiropractic.* New York: Appleton-Century-Crofts, 1980.

Hanson RW, Gerber KE. *Coping with Chronic Pain.* New York: Guilford, 1990.

Jessell TM. Substance P in the nervous system. *Handbook of Psychopharmacology,* Vol 16. New York: Plenum, 1983.

Kingdon R, Stanley KJ, Kizior RJ. *Handbook for Pain Management.* Philadelphia: W.B. Saunders, 1998.

Kirkaldy-Willis WH. *Managing Low Back Pain,* 2nd ed. New York: Churchill Livingstone, 1988.

Krieger DT, Brownstein MJ, Martin JB, eds. *Brain Peptides.* New York: Wiley, 1984.

Leach RA. *The Chiropractic Theories: A Synopsis of Scientific Research.* Mississippi: Mid-South Scientific Publishers, 1980.

Lynn B. Neurogenic inflammation. *Skin Pharmacol* 1988;1:217.

McKenzie RA. *The Lumbar Spine: Mechanical Diagnosis and Therapy.* Waikanae, New Zealand: Spinal Publications, 1981.

Melzack R, Wall P. *The Challenge of Pain.* New York: Basic Books, 1983.

Melzack R, Wall P. Pain mechanisms: a new theory. *Science* 1965;150:971–979.

Pasternak G.W. Pharmacological mechanisms of opioid analgesics. *Clinical Neuropharmacology* 1993;16(1), 1–18.

Portenoy RK. Chronic opioid therapy in nonmalignant pain. *Journal of Pain and Symptom Management* 1990;5(1 Suppl.): S46–S62.

Sinel MS, Deardorff WW, Goldstein TB. *Win the Battle Against Back Pain: An Integrated Mind-Body Approach.* New York: Dell, 1996.

Sternbach RA. Acute versus chronic pain. In: Wall PD, Melzack R, eds. *Textbook of Pain.* New York: Churchill-Livingstone, 1984.

Wells C, Graham N. *The Pain Relief Handbook.* Buffalo: Firefly Books, 1998.

Zimmerman J. *Chronic Back Pain: Moving On.* Brunswick, Maine: Biddle Publishing, 1991.

Chapter 3

Abbadie C, et al. Spinal cord substance P receptor immunoreactivity increases in both inflammatory and nerve injury models of persistent pain. *Neuroscience* 1996 Jan;70(1):201–209.

Belch JJ, et al. Effects of altering dietary essential fatty acids on requirements for nonsteroidal anti-inflammatory drugs in patients with rheumatoid arthritis: a double-blind placebo-controlled study. *Ann Rheum Dis* 1988 Feb;47(2):96–104.

Blok WL, et al. Modulation of inflammation and cytokine production by dietary (n-3) fatty acids, *J Nutr* 1996 June;126(6):1515–1533.

Cabot PJ, et al. Immune cell derived beta endorphin, Production, release and control of inflammatory pain in rats. *J Clin Invest* 1997 Jul 1:100(1):142–148.

Calder PC. Immunoregulatory and anti-inflammatory effects of n-3 polyunsaturated fatty acids. *Braz J Med Biol Res* 1998 Apr;31(4):467–490.

Carr DB, et al. Neuropeptides and pain. *Agressologie* 1990 Apr;31(4):173–177.

Collins SM, et al. Effect of inflammation of enteric nerves. Cytokine-induced changes in neurotransmitter content and release. *Ann N Y Acad Sci* 1992;664:415–424.

Dionne RA, et al. The substance P receptor antagonist CP_99,994 reduces acute postoperative pain. *Clin Pharmacol Ther* 1998 Nov;64(5):562–568.

Duggan AW, et al. Probing the brain and spinal cord with neuropeptides in pathways related to pain and other functions. *Front Neuroendocrinol* 1994 Sep;15(3):275–300.

Espersen GT, et al. Decreased interleukin-1 beta levels in plasma from rheumatoid arthritis patients after dietary supplementation with n-3 polyunsaturated fatty acids. *Clin Rheumatol* 1992 Sep;11(3):393–395.

Fantuzzi G., et al. Physiological and cytokine responses in IL-1 beta-deficient mice after zymosan-induced inflammation. *Am J Physiol* 1997 Jul;273(1 Pt 2):R400–406.

Feng C, et al. Dietary omega-3 polyunsaturated fatty acids reduce IFN-gamma receptor expression in mice. *J Interferon Cytokine Res* 1998 Jan;19(1): 41–48.

Garcia P, et al. Modulation of acute and chronic inflammatory processes by cacospongionolide B, a novel inhibitor of human synovial phospholipase A2. *Br J Pharmacol* 1999 Jan;126(1):301–311.

Glaser KB. Regulation of prostaglandin H sythase 2 expression in human monocytes by the marine natural products manoalide and scalardial. *Biochem Pharmacol* 1995 Sep 28;50(7):913–922.

Grimble RF, et al. Modulation of pro-inflammatory cytokine biology by unsaturated fatty acids. *Z Ernahrungswiss* 1998;37(Suppl 1):57–65.

Henry JL. Substance P and inflammatory pain. *Agents Actions Suppl* 1993;41:75–87.

Herzberg U, et al. Chronic pain and immunity: mononeuropathy alters immune responses in rats. *Pain* 1994 Nov;59(2):219–252.

Hori T, et al. Pain modulation actions of cytokines and prostaglandin E2 in the brain. *Ann N Y Acad Sci* 1998 May 1;840–269–81.

Lawand NB. Nicotinic cholinergic reports: potential targets for inflammatory pain relief. *Pain* 1999 Mar;80(1–2):291–299.

Leon LR, et al. Role of IL-10 in inflammation: Studies using cytokine knock out mice. *Ann N Y Acad Sci* 1998 Sep 29;856:69–75.

Lowry SF. Cytokine mediators of immunity and inflammation. *Arch Surg* 1993 Nov;128(11):1235–1241.

Marriott D, et al. Eicosanoid synthesis by spinal cord astrocytes is evoked by substance P; possible implications for nociception and pain. *Adv Prostaglandid Thromboxane Leukot Res* 1991;21B:739–741.

Martiney JA, et al. Cytokine-induced inflammation in the central nervous system revisited. *Neurochem Res* 1998 Mar;23(3):349–359.

Mense S, et al. The possible role of substance P in eliciting and modulating deep somatic pain. *Prog Brain Res* 1996;110:125–135.

Millan MJ. The induction of pain: an integrative review. *Prog Neurobiol* 1999 Jan;57(1):1–164.

Miossec P. Acting on the cytokine balance to control auto-immunity and chronic inflammation. *Eur Cytokine Netw* 1993 Jul–Aug;4(4):245–251.

Morch H, et al. Beta endorphin and the immune system—possible role in autoimmune diseases. *Autoimmunity* 1995;21(3):161–171.

Mukaida N. Inflammation and pro-inflammatory cytokine. *Nippon Rinsho* 1992 Aug;50(8):1724–1729.

Oppenheim JJ, et al. Aspects of cytokine induced modulation of immunity and inflammation with emphasis on interleukin-l. *Arzneimittelforschung* 1988 Mar;38(3A):461–465.

Page GG, et al. The immune suppressive nature of pain.

Roshak A, et al. Inhibition of NF kappa B-medicated interleukin-1 beta-stimulated prostaglandin E2 formation by the marine natural product hymenialdisine. *J Pharmacol Ex Ther* 1997 Nov;283(2):955–961.

Ruan HZ et al. Effects of 5-HT on pain modulation of substance P in spinal cord of rats. *Chung Kuo Yao Li Hsueh Pao* 1995 Nov;16(6):512–516.

Schnell L, et al. Cytokine-induced acute inflammation in the brain and spinal cord. *J Neuropathol Exp Neurol* 1999 Mar;58(3):245–254.

Sellami S., et al. Hypothalamic and thalamic sites of action of interleukin-1 beta on food intake, body temperature and pain sensitivity in rats. *Brain Res* 1995 Oct 2;694(1–2):69–77.

Smith MD, et al. Synovial membrane inflammation and cytokine production in patients with early osteoarthritis. *J Rheumatol* 1997 Feb;(2):365–371.24

Soriente A, et al. Manoalide. *Curr Med Chem* 1999 May 1;6(5):415–431.

Sperling RI. The effects of dietary n-3 polyunsaturated fatty acids on neutrophils. *Proc Nutr Soc* 1998 Nov;57(4):527–534.

Trichieri G. Interleukin-12: a cytokine at the interface of inflammation and immunity. *Adv Immunol* 1998;70:83–243.

Walmsley M, et al. Interleukin-10 inhibition of the progression of established collagen-induced arthritis. *Arthritis Rheum* 1996 Mar;39(3):495–503.

Watkins LR, et al. Characterization of cytokine induced hyperalgesia. *Brain Res* 1994 Aug15;654(1):15–26.

Watkins LR, et al. Immune activation: the role of pro-inflammatory cytokines in inflammation, illness responses and pathological pain stress. *Pain* 1995 Dec;63(3):289–302.

Weglicki WB, et al. Pathobiology of magnesium deficiency: a cytokine/neurogenic inflammation hypothesis. *Am J Physiol* 1992 Sep;263(3 Pt 2):R734–737.

Wehling P, et al. Neurophysiologic changes in lumbar nerve root inflammation in the rat after treatment with cytokine inhibitors. Evidence for a role of interleukin-1. *Spine* 1996 Apr 15;21(8):931–935.

Williams M, et al. Emerging molecular approaches to pain therapy. *J Med Chem* 1999 May 6;42(9):1481–1500

Wong ML, et al. Interleukin-1 beta, IL-1 receptor antagonist, IL-10 and IL-13 gene expression in the central nervous system and the anterior pituitary during systemic inflammation: pathophysiological implications. *Pro Natl Acad Sci USA* 1997 Jan 7;94(1):277–232.

Wu D, et al. n-3 polyunsaturated fatty acids and immune function. *Proc Nutr Soc* 1998 Nov;57(4):503–509.

Chapter 4

Allen EH, Cosgrove D, Millard JC. The radiological changes in infections of the spine and their diagnostic value. *Clin Radiol* 1978; 29:31. .

Baker RA, Hillman BJ, McLennan JE, et al. Sequelae of metrizamide myelography in 200 examinations. *AJR* 1978; 130:499.

Ballou SP, Kushner I. Laboratory evaluation of inflammation. In: Kelley WN, Harris ED Jr, Ruddy S, Sledgc CB, cds. *Textbook of Rheumatology,* 4th ed. Philadelphia: WB Saunders, 1993; pp. 671–679.

Bateman JE. The diagnosis and treatment of tears of the rotator cuff. *Surg Clin North Am* 1973;4:721.

Bernard TN, Kirkaldy-Willis WH. Recognizing specific characteristics of nonspecific low back pain. *Clin Orthop* 1987;217:266.

Boden SD, Davis DO, Dina TS, et al. Abnormal magnetic-resonance scans of the lumbar spine in asymptomatic subjects: a prospective investigation. *J Bone Joint Surg Am* 1990;72:403.

Boston HC Jr., Bianco AL Jr., Rhodes KH. Disc space infections in children. *Orthop Clin North Am* 1975;6:953.

Brady LP, Parker LB, Vaughn J. An evaluation of the electromyogram in the diagnosis of the lumbar disc lesion. *J Bone Joint Surg Am* 1969;51:539.

Butters KP, Rockwood CA Jr. Office evaluation and management of the shoulder impingement syndrome. *Orthop Clin North Am* 1988;19:755.

Cabot WD, Miller JL, Kelly JF. An algorithm for conservative back care. *Pain Digest* 1994;4:269–275.

Cailliet R. *Low Back Pain Syndrome,* 3rd ed. Philadelphia: FA Davis Company, 1981, pp. 53–68.

Campbell SM. Regional myofascial pain syndromes. *Rheum Dis Clin North Am* 1989;15:31.

Campbell SM, Clark S, Tyndall EA, et. al. Clinical characteristics of fibrositis: A blinded controlled study of symptoms and tender points. *Arthritis Rheum* 1983, 26, 817.

Choong K, Monaghan P, McGuigan L, et al. Role of bone scintigraphy in the early diagnosis of discitis. *Ann Rheum Dis* 1990, 49, 932.

Crenshaw AH, Campbell S, eds. *Operative Orthopaedics,* 8th ed. St. Louis: Mosby, 1992.

Cuomo F, Kummer FJ, Zuckerman JD, et al. The influence of acromioclavicular joint morphology on rotator cuff tears. *J Shoulder Elbow Surg* 1998;7(6):555–559.

Cypress BK. Characteristics of physician visits for back symptoms: a national perspective. *Am J Public Health* 1983;73:389.

Dempster, DW, Lindsay R. Pathogenesis of osteoporosis. *Lancet* 1993; 341:797.

Deyo RA. Measuring the functional status of patients with low back pain. *Arch Phys Med Rehabil* 1988; 69:1044.

Deyo RA, Rainville J, Kent DL. What can the history and physical examination tell us about low back pain? *JAMA* 1992; 268:760.

Deyo RA, Bass JE. Lifestyle and low back pain: the influence of smoking and obesity. *Spine* 1989; 14:501.

Dvorkin M. *Office Orthopaedics.* Norwalk: Appleton & Lange, 1993.

Farfan HS. *Mechanical Disorders of the Low Back.* Philadelphia: Lea & Febiger, 1973.

Finneson BE. Examination of the patient. In: Finneson BE, ed. *Low Back Pain.* 2nd ed. Philadelphia: Lippincott, 1981; p. 54.

Forrestall RM, Marsh HO, Pay NT. Magnetic resonance imaging and contrast CT of the lumbar spine: comparison of diagnostic methods and correlation with surgical findings. *Spine* 1988; 13:1049.

Fowler RS Jr, Kraft GH. Tension perception in patients having pain associated with chronic muscle tension. *Arch Phys Med Rehabil* 1984;55:28.

Garcia A Jr, Grantham SA. Hematogenous pyogenic vertebral osteomyelitis. *J Bone Joint Surg* 1960;42A:429.

Gibson MJ, Buckley J, Mawhinney R, et al. Magnetic resonance imaging and discography in the diagnosis of disc degeneration. A comparative study of 50 discs. *J Bone Joint Surg* 1986;68:369.

Gill K, Jackson RP. ACT-discography. In: Firbroyer JW, ed. *The Adult Spine.* New York: Raven Press, 1991; pp. 443–456.

Glantz RH, Haldeman S. Other diagnostic studies: electrodiagnosis. In: Frymoyer, JW, ed. *The Adult Spine.* New York: Raven Press, 1991; pp. 541–548.

Goldsmith RS. Laboratory aids in the diagnosis of metabolic bone disease. *Orthop Clin North Am* 1972;3:545.

Gorse GJ, Pais MJ, Kusske JA, Cesario T.C. Tuberculous spondylitis: a report of six cases and a review of the literature. *Medicine* 1983;62:178.

Grue BL, Pudenz RH, Sheldon CH. Observations on the value of clinical electromyography. *J Bone Joint Surg Am* 1957;39:492.

Haldeman S. The electrodiagnostic evaluation of nerve root function. *Spine* 1984;9:42.

Hall H. Examination of the patient with low back pain. *Bull Rheum Dis* 1983;33:1.

Hall S, Bartlesow JD, Onofrio BM, et al. Lumbar spinal stenosis. *Ann Intern Med* 1985;103:271.

Harris ED Jr. Rheumatoid arthritis: pathophysiology and implications for therapy. *N Engl J Med* 1990;322:1277.

Hart FD, MacLagen NF. Ankylosing spondylitis: a review of 184 cases. *Ann Rheum Dis* 1975;34:87.

Hitselberger WE, Witten RM. Abnormal myelograms in asymptomatic patients. *J Neurosurg* 1968;28:204.

Holt E. The question of lumbar discography. *J Bone Joint Surg* 1968; 50:720.

Holzman RS, Bishki F. Osteomyelitis in heroin addicts. *Ann Intern Med* 1971;75:693.

Huvos AG. *Bone Tumors: Diagnosis, Treatment and Prognosis,* 2nd ed. Philadelphia: W.B. Saunders, 1991; pp. 49–66.

Johnson EW, Melvin JL. Value of electromyography in lumbar radiculopathy. *Archi Physi Med Rehabil* 1971;52:239–243.

Johnson K, Rosen I, Uden A. Neurophysiologic investigation of patients with spinal stenosis. *Spine* 1987;12:483.

Kemp HBS, Jackson JW, Jeremiah JD, Hall, AJ. Pyogenic infections occurring primarily in intervertebral discs. *J Bone Joint Surg* 1973;55B:698.

Lathan RE. MR and CT imaging of the head, neck and spine. *Spine* 1991;2 Part XII: 1166–1172.

Lawrence RC, Hochberg MM, Kelsey JL, et al. Estimates of the prevalence of selected arthritic and musculoskeletal diseases in the United States. *J Rheumatol* 1989;16:427.

Lawrence JS, Bremner JM, Bier F. Osteoarthrosis prevalence in the population and relationship between symptoms and x-ray changes. *Ann Rheum Dis* 1966;25:1.

Lawrence JS, Sharp J, Ball J, Bier F. Rheumatoid arthritis of the lumbar spine. *Ann Rheum Dis* 1964;23:205.

Liang M, Komaroff Al. Roentgenograms in primary care patients with acute low back pain: a cost-effective analysis. *Arch Intern Med* 1982;142:1108.

Mirra JM. *Bone Tumors: Clinical, Radiologic, and Pathologic Correlations.* Philadelphia: Lea & Febiger, 1989; pp. 226–248.

Modic MT, Masaryk JT, Paushte D. Magnetic resonance imaging of the spine. *Radiol Clin North Am* 1986;24:229.

Nachemson AL. Newest knowledge of low back pain: a critical look. *Clin Orthop* 1992;279:8.

Nachemson A: The lumbar spine—an orthopaedic challenge. *Spine* 1976; 1:59.

Namey TC, Halla J. Radiographic and nucleographic techniques in the diagnosis of septic arthritis and osteomyelitis. *Clin Rheum* Dis 1978;4:95.

Nehemkis AM, Carver DW, Evanski PM. The predictive utility of the orthopedic examination in identifying the low back pain patient with hysterical personality features. *Clin Orthop* 1979;145:158.

Onel D, Sari H, Donmerz C. Lumbar spinal stenosis: clinical/radiologic therapeutic evaluation in 145 patients. *Spine* 1993; 18:291.

Onofrio BM. Intervertebral discitis: incidence, diagnosis and management. *Clin Neurosurg* 1980;27:481.

Rice JR, Pisetsky DS. Pain in the rheumatic diseases. Practical aspects of diagnosis and treatment. *Rheum Dis Clin North Am* 1998 Feb; 25(1):15–30.

Root L. *No More Aching Back.* New York: Signet, 1991.

Rosenthal DI, Mankin HJ, Bauman RA. Musculoskeletal applications for computed tomography. *Bull Rheum Dis* 1983;33:1.

Ross PM, Fleming JL. Vertebral body osteomyelitis: spectrum and natural history: a retrospective analysis of 37 cases. *Clin Orthop* 1976;118:190.

Roth RS, Horowitz K, Bachman JE. Chronic myofascial pain: knowledge of diagnosis and satisfaction with treatment. *Arch Phys Med Rehabil* 1998;79(8):966–970.

Rothenberg RJ. Rheumatic disease aspects of leg length inequality. *Semin Arthritis Rheumatol* 1988;17:196–205.

Schaberg J, Gainor BJ. A profile of metastatic carcinoma of the spine. *Spine* 1985;10:19.

Scherbel AL, Gardner JW. Infections involving the intervertebral discs: diagnosis and management. *JAMA* 1960;174:370.

Smith WA. Fibromyalgia syndrome. *Nurs Clin North Am* 1998;33(4):653–69.

Sox HC Jr, Liang MH. The erythrocyte sedimentation rate. Guidelines for rational use. *Ann Intern Med* 1986;104:515.

Travell JS, Simons DG. *Myofascial Pain and Dysfunction. The Trigger Point Manual, The Lower Extremities,* Vol. 2. Baltimore: Williams & Wilkins, 1992; pp. 607.

Travell J, Ringler SH. The myofascial genesis of pain. *Postgrad Med* 1952;11:425.

Voelker JL, Mealey J Jr, Eskridge JM, Gilmor RL. Metrizamide-enhanced computed tomography as an adjunct to metrizamide myelography in the evaluation of lumbar disc herniation and spondylosis. *Neurosurgery* 1987;20:379.

Waddell G, Main CJ, et al. Normality and reliability in the clinical assessment of backache. *Br Med J* 1982;284:1519.

Wiesel SW, Tsourmas N, Feffer HL, et al. A study of computer assisted tomography. 1. The incidence of positive CT scans in an asymptomatic group of patients. *Spine* 1984;9:549.

Williams AL, Haughton VM, Syvertsen A. Computed tomography in the diagnosis of herniated nucleus pulposus. *Radiology* 1980;135:95.

Wolfe F, Simons D, Friction J, et al. The fibromyalgia and myofascial pain syndromes: a study of tender points and trigger points in persons with fibromyalgia, myofascial pain syndrome and no disease (abstract). *Arthritis Rheum* 1990;33(Suppl):S137.

Zena CA, Arcand MA, Cantrell JS, Skedros JG, Burkhead WZ Jr. The rotator cuff-deficient arthritic shoulder: diagnosis and surgical management. *J Am Acad Orthop Surg* 1998;6(6):337–348.

Chapter 5

Ahlgren O, Larsson S. Reconstruction for lateral ligament injuries of the ankle. *J Bone Joint Surg* 1989;71B:300.

Anderson BC. *Office Orthopedics for Primary Care; Diagnosis and Treament.* Philadelphia: W.B. Saunders, 1999.

Andrews JR, Carson WG, Ortega K. Arthroscopy of the shoulder: Technique and normal anatomy. *Am J Sports Med* 1984;12:1.

Apfelberg DB, Larson SJ, Dynamic anatomy of the ulnar nerve at the elbow. *Plast Reconstr Surg* 1973;51:76.

Arnhoff FN, Triplett HB, Pokorney B. Follow-up status of patients treated with nerve blocks for low back pain. *Anesthesiology* 1977:46:170–178.

Arnoldi CC, Brodsky AE, Cauchoix J, et al. Lumbar spinal stenosis and nerve root entrapment syndrome: definition and classification. *Clin Orthop* 1976;115:4.

Aronoff GM. Myofascial pain syndrome and fibromyalgia: a critical assessment and alternate view. *Clin J Pain* 1998;14(1):74–85.

Barrett SL, Day SV. Endoscopic plantar fasciotomy for chronic plantar fasciitis/heel spur syndrome: Surgical technique—early clinical results. *J Foot Surg* 1991;30:568–570.

Bassett FH III. Surgery of the patellofemoral joint. *AAOS Instr Course Lect* 1976;25:40.

Bateman JE. Cuff tears in athletes. *Orthop Clin North Am* 1973;4:721.

Bateman JE. The diagnosis and treatment of tears of the rotator cuff. *Surg Clin North Am* 1973;4:721.

Belivear P. A comparison between epidural anesthesia with and without corticosteroid in the treatment of sciatica. *Rheumatol Phys Med* 1971;II:40–43.

Bell DF, Ehrlich MG, Zaleske DJ. Brace treatment for symptomatic spondylolisthesis. *Clin Orthop* 1988;236:192.

Bentley G. The surgical treatment of chondromalacia patellae. *J Bone Joint Surg* 1978;60B:74.

Benton-Weil W, Borrelli AH, Weil LS Jr, Weil LS Sr. Percutaneous plantar fasciotomy: a minimally invasive procedure for recalcitrant plantar fascitis. *J Foot Ankle Surg* 1998;37(4):269–72.

Benzon HT. Epidural steroid injections for low back pain and lumbosacral radiculopathy. *Pain* 1986; 4:277–295.

Boring TH, O'Donoghue DH. Acute patella dislocations; results of immediate surgical repair. *Clin Orthop* 1978 36:182.

Boston HC Jr, Bianco AL Jr, Rodes KH. Disc space infections in children. *Orthop Clin North Am* 1975;6:953.

Bosworth DM. Repair of defects in the tendoachilles. *J Bone Joint Surg* 1956;38A:111.

Boyd HB, McLeod AC Jr. Tennis elbow. *J Bone Joint Surg* 1973;55A:1183.

Brahms MA. Common foot problems. *J Bone Joint Surg.* 1967;49A:1653.

Brand RL, Collins DF, Templeton T. Surgical repair of ruptured lateral ankle ligaments. *Am J Sports Med* 1969;9:904.

Brown FW. Protocol for management of acute low back pain with or without radiculopathy, including the use of epidural and intrathecal steroids. In: Brown FW, ed. *American Academy of Orthopaedic Surgeons Symposium on the Lumbar Spine.* St Louis: Mosby, 1981; pp. 126–136.

Bucci LR. *Nutrition Applied to Injury Rehabilitation and Sports Medicine.* Boca Raton, Florida: CRC Press, 1995.

Buchanan HM, Preston SJ, Brooks PM, Buchanan WW. Is diet important in rheumatoid arthritis? *Br J Rheumatol,* 1991;30(2):125–34 1991.

Butters KP, Rockwood CA Jr. Office evaluation and management of the shoulder impingement syndrome. *Orthop Clin North Am* 1988;19:755.

Cabot WD, Miller JL, Kelly JF. An algorithm for conservative back care. *Pain Digest* 1994;4:269–275.

Cailliet R. *Low Back Pain Syndrome,* 3rd ed. Philadelphia: FA Davis Company, 1981; pp. 53–68.

Campbell SM, Clark S, Tyndall EA, et. al. Clinical characteristics of fibrositis: I, A blinded controlled study of symptoms and tender points. *Arthritis Rheum* 1983;26:817.

Campbell SM. Regional myofascial pain syndromes. *Rheum Dis Clin North Am* 1989;15:31.

Carette S, McCain GA, Bell DA, Fam AG. Evaluation of amitriptyline in primary fibrositis. *Arthritis Rheum* 1986;29:655.

Cetti R. Conservative treatment of injury to the fibular ligaments of the ankle. *Br J Sports Med* 1982;16:47–52.

Chrisman OD, Snook SA. Reconstruction of lateral ligament tears of the ankle. *J Bone Joint Surg* 1969;51A:904.

Cohen RB, Williams GR. Impingement syndrome and rotator cuff disease as repetitive motion disorders. *Clin Orthop* 1998;(351):95–101.

Crenshaw AH, ed. *Campbell's Operative Orthopaedics,* 8th ed. St. Louis: Mosby, 1992.

Dempster DW, Lindsay R. Pathogenesis of osteoporosis. *Lancet* 1993;34:1997.

Dinham JM, French RR. Results of patellectomy for osteoarthritis. *Postgrad Med J* 1972;48:590.

Drewes AM, Andreasen A, Schnider HD, et. al. Pathology of skeletal muscle in fibromyalgia: a histo-immuno-chemical and ultrastructural study. *Br J Rheumatol* 1993;32(Suppl):479.

Dvorkin M. *Office Orthopaedics.* Norwalk: Appleton & Lange, 1993.

Ege-Rasmussen KJ, Fano N. Trochanteric bursitis. Treatment by corticosteroid injection. *Scand J Rheumatol* 1985;14:417–420.

Fairbank JCT, Park WM, McCall W, O'Brien JP. Apophyseal injection of local anesthetic as a diagnostic aid in primary low-back pain. *Spine* 1981;6:598.

Farfan HS. *Mechanical Disorders of the Low Back.* Philadelphia: Lea & Febiger, 1973.

Fornasier VL, Horne JG. Metastases to the vertebral column. *Cancer* 1975;36:590.

Fox JM, Blazina ME, Jobe FW, et.al. Degeneration and rupture of the Achilles tendon. *Clin Orthop* 1975;107:221–224.

Francis KC, Hutter RVP. Neoplasms of the spine in the aged. *Clin Orthop* 1963;26:54.

Fredrickson BE, Baker D, McHolick WJ, et. al. The natual history of spondylolysis and spondylolisthesis. *J Bone Joint Surg* 1984;66A:699.

Garcia A Jr, Grantham SA. Hematogenous pyogenic vertebral osteomyelitis. *J Bone Joint Surg* 1960; 42A:429.

Garvey TA, Marks MR, Wiesel SW. A prospective, randomized, double-blind evaluation of trigger-point injection therapy for low back pain. *Spine* 1989;14:962.

Giannestras NJ. *Foot Disorders: Medical and Surgical Management,* 2nd ed. Philadelphia: Lea & Febiger, 1976.

Goldberg EJ, Abraham E, Siegel I. The surgical treatment of chronic lateral humeral epicondylitis by common extensor release. *Clin Orthop* 1988;223:208.

Goldenberg DL. Fibromyalgia syndrome: an emerging but controversial condition. *JAMA* 1987;257:2782.

Goldenberg DL. Psychiatric and psychologic aspects of fibromyalgia syndrome. *Rheum Dis Clin North Am* 1989;15:105.

Grana WA, Henkley B, Hollingsworth S. Arthroscopic evaluation and treatment of patellar malalignment. *Clin Orthop* 1984;186:122.

Hall S, Bartlesow JD, Onofrio BM, et al. Lumbar spinal stenosis. *Ann Intern Med* 1985;103:271.

Harada Y, Nakahara S. A pathologic study of lumbar disc herniation of the elderly. *Spine* 1989;14:1020.

Harris ED Jr. Rheumatoid arthritis: pathophysiology and implications for therapy. *N Engl J Med* 1990;322:1277.

Hart FD, MacLagen NF. Ankylosing spondylitis: a review of 184 cases. *Ann Rheum Dis* 1975;34:87.

Hawkins RJ, Kennedy JC. The impingement syndrome in athletes. *Am J Sports Med* 1980;8:57.

Heaney RP, Recker RR, Saville PD. Calcium balance and calcium requirements in middle-aged women. *Am J Clin Nutr* 1977;30:1603.

Holmes SW Jr., Clancy WG Jr. Clinical classification of patellofemoral pain and dysfunction. *J Orthop Sports Phys Ther* 1998;28(5):299–306.

Holzman RS, Bishki F Osteomyelitis in heroin addicts. *Ann Intern Med* 1971;75:693.

Huvos AG. *Bone Tumors: Diagnosis, Treatment and Prognosis,* 2nd ed. Philadelphia: W.B. Saunders, 1991; pp. 49–66.

Inoue M, Shino K, Hirose H, Horibe S, Ono K. Subluxation of the patella: Computed tomography analysis of patellofemoral congruence. *J Bone Joint Surg* 1988;70A:1331.

Jaeschke R, Adachi J, Guyatt G, et al. Clinical usefulness of amitriptyline in fibromyalgia: the results of 23 N-of-1 randomized controlled trials. *J Rheumatol* 1991;18:447.

Jameson TJ. *Repetitive Strain Injuries.* New Canaan, CT: Keats Publishing Co., 1998.

Johnson LP, Nasca RJ, Dunham WK. Surgical management of isthmic spondylolisthesis. *Spine* 1988;13:93. .

Kemp HBS, Jackson JW, Jeremiah JD, Hall AJ. Pyogenic infections occurring primarily in intervertebral discs. *J Bone Joint Surg* 1973;55B:698.

Khan MA, van der Linden SM. Ankylosing spondylitis and other spondyloarthropathies. *Rheum Dis Clin North Am* 1990;16:551.

Knight JM, Thomas JC, Maurer RC. Treatment of septic olecranon and prepatellar bursitis with percutaneous placement of a suction-irrigation system: a report of 12 cases. *Clin Orthop* 1986;206:90–93, 1986.

Lane JM, Nydick M. Osteoporosis: current modes of prevention and treatment. *J Am Acad Orthop Surg* 1999:7:19–31.

Lawrence JS, Sharp J, Ball J, Bier F. Rheumatoid arthritis of the lumbar spine. *Ann Rheum Dis* 1964;23:205.

Lilius G, Laasonen EM, Myllynen P, et al. Lumbar facet joint syndrome: a randomized clinical trial. *J Bone Joint Surg* 1989;71B:681.

Littlejohn GO. Fibrositis/fibromyalgia syndrome in the workplace. *Rheum Dis Clin North Am* 1989;15:45.

McAfee JH, Smith DL. Olecranon and prepatellar bursitis. Diagnosis and treatment. *West J Med* 1988;149:607–610.

Melmed SP. Spontaneous bilateral rupture of the calcaneal tendon during steroid therapy. *J Bone Joint Surg* 1965;47B:104–105.

Merskey H. Physical and psychological considerations in the classification of fibromyalgia. *J Rheumatol* 1989;16(Suppl):72.

Mixter WJ, Barr JS. Rupture of the intervertebral disc with involvement of the spinal canal. *N Engl J Med* 1934;211:210.

Mooney V, Robertson J. The facet syndrome. *Clin Orthop* 1976;115:149.

Moran R, O'Connell D, Walsh M. The diagnostic value of facet joint injections. *Spine* 1988;13:1407–1410.

Nachemson AL. Newest knowledge of low back pain: a critical look. *Clin Orthop* 1992;279:8.

Nachemson A. The lumbar spine—an orthopaedic challenge. *Spine* 1976;1:59.

Neer C. Anterior acromioplasty for the chronic impingement syndrome in the shoulder. *J Bone Joint Surg* 1972;54A:41.

Neustadt DH. Ankylosing spondylitis. *Postgrad Med* 1977;61:124.

Niedermann B, Andersen A, Anderson SB, Funder V, et. al. Ruptures of the lateral ligaments of the ankle: Operation or plaster cast? *Acta Orthop Scand* 1981;52: 579–587.

Onel D, Sari H, Donmerz C. Lumbar spinal stenosis: clinical/radiologic therapeutic evaluation in 145 patients. *Spine* 1993; 18:291.

Onofrio BM. Intervertebral discitis: incidence, diagnosis and management. *Clin Neurosurg* 1980;27:481.

Pasero CL. Understanding fibromyalgia syndrome. *Am J Nurs* 1998 Oct; 98(10):17–18.

Riegler HF. Recurrent dislocations and subluxations of the patella. *Clin Orthop* 1988;227:201.

Riggs BL, Melton LJ III. The prevention and treatment of osteoporosis. *N Eng J Med* 1992;327:620.

Roland M, Morris R. A study of the natural history of back pain: Part 1: development of a reliable and sensitive measure of disability in low-back pain. *Spine* 1983; 8:141.

Root L. *No More Aching Back.* New York: Signet, 1991.

Saal JA, Saal JS, Herzog RJ. The natural history of lumbar intervertebral disc extrusions treated nonoperatively. *Spine* 1990;15:683.

Seitsalo S, Osterman K, Hyvarinen H, et al.: Progression of spondylolisthesis in children and adolescents: a long-term follow-up of 272 patients. *Spine* 1991;16:417.

Seligson D, Gassman J, Page M. Ankle instability—evaluation of the lateral ligaments. *Am J Sports Med* 1980;8:39.

Sinel MS, Deardorff WW, Goldstein TB. *Win The Battle Against Back Pain: An Integrated Mind-Body Approach.* New York: Dell, 1996.

Smith WA. Fibromyalgia syndrome. *Nurs Clin North Am* 1998;33(4):653–669.

Smith DL, McAfee JH, Lucas LM, et al. Treatment of nonseptic olecranon bursitis; a controlled blinded prospective trial. *Arch Intern Med* 1989;149:2527–2530.

Smith AS, Blaser SI. Infectious and inflammatory processes of the spine. *Radiol Clin North Am* 1991;29:809.

Snipes FL. Lumbar spinal stenosis. *Arch Phys Med Rehabil* 1998;79(9):1141–1142.

Stack JK. Acute and chronic bursitis in the region of the elbow joint. *Surg Clin North Am* 1973;4:801.

Travell JS, Simons DG. *Myofascial Pain and Dysfunction. The Trigger Point Manual, The Lower Extremities,* Vol. 2. Baltimore: Williams & Wilkins, 1992; pp, 607.

Travell J, Ringler SH. The myofascial genesis of pain. *Postgrad Med* 1952;11:425.

Trippel SB. The unmet anti-inflammatory needs in orthopedics. *Am J Orthop* 1999;3S (Suppl): 3–7.

Turner RH, Bianco RJ Jr. Spondylolysis and spondylolisthesis in children and teenagers. *J Bone Joint Surg* 1971;53A:1298.

White AA III. *Your Aching Back: A Doctor's Guide to Relief.* New York: Simon & Schuster/Fireside, 1990.

Wolfe F, Simons D, Friction J, et al. The fibromyalgia and myofascial pain syndromes: a study of tender points and trigger points in persons with fibromyalgia, myofascial pain syndrome and no disease (abstract). *Arthritis Rheum* 1990;33(Suppl):S137.

Zena CA, Arcand MA, Cantrell JS, Skedros JG, Burkhead WZ Jr. The rotator cuff-deficient arthritic shoulder: diagnosis and surgical management. *J Am Acad Orthop Surg* 1998; 6(6):337–348.

Chapter 6

Adam O. Nutrition as adjuvant therapy in chronic polyarthritis. *J Rheumatol* 1993;52(5): 275–280.

Ariza-Ariza R, Mestanza-Peralta M, Cardiel MH. Omega-3 fatty acids in rheumatoid arthritis: an overview. *Semin Arthritis Rheum* 1998;27(6): 366–370.

Brage S, Bjerkedal T. Musculoskeletal pain and smoking in Norway. *J Epidemiol Community Health* 1996;50(2): 166–169.

Bucher HU, Moser T, von Siebenthal K, et al. Sucrose reduces pain reaction to heel lancing in preterm infants: a placebo-controlled, randomized and masked study. *Pediatr Res* 1995; 38(3): 332–335.

Currie SR, Wilson KG, Gauthier ST. Caffeine and chronic low back pain *Clin J Pain* 1995;11(3): 214–219.

Darlington LG, Ramsey NW, Mansfield JR. Placebo-controlled, blind study of dietary manipulation therapy in rheumatoid arthritis. *Lancet* 1986;1(8475): 236–238.

Darlington LG, Ramsey NW Review of dietary therapy for rheumatoid arthritis. *Br J Rheumatol* 1993;32(6): 507–514.

Eriksen WB, Brage S, Bruusgaard D. Does smoking aggravate musculoskeletal pain? *Scand J Rheumatol* 1997;26(1): 49–54.

Fahrer H, Hoeflin F, Lauterburg BH, et al. Diet and fatty acids: can fish substitute for fish oil, *Clin Exp Rheumatol* 1991;9(4): 403–406.

Fernstrom MH, Fernstrom JD. Brain tryptophan concentrations and serotonin synthesis remain responsive to food consumption after the ingestion of sequential meals. *Am J Clin Nutr* 1995;61(2): 312–319.

German JB, Lokesh B, Kinsella JE. The effect of dietary fish oils on eicosanoid biosynthesis in peritoneal macrophages is influenced by both dietary n-6 polyunsaturated fats and total dietary fat. *Prostaglandins Leukot Essent Fatty Acids* 1988;34.(1): 37–45.

Haugen MA, Kjeldsen-Kragh J, Skakkebaek N, et al. The influence of fast and vegetarian diet on parameters of nutritional status in patients with rheumatoid arthritis. *Clin Rheumatol* 1993;12(1): 62–69.

Haze JJ. Toward an understanding of the rationale for the use of dietary supplementation for chronic pain management: the serotonin model. *Cranio* 1991;9(4): 339–343.

Herschel M, Khoshnood B, Ellman C, Maydew N, Mittendorf R. Neonatal circumcision. Randomized trial of a sucrose pacifier for pain control. *Arch Pediatr Adolesc Med* 1998; 152(3): 279–284.

Igon'kina SI, Kryzhanovskii GN, Zinkevich VA, et al. The effect of serotonin antibodies on the development of a neuropathic pain syndrome. *Patol Fiziol Eksp Ter* 1997; (2): 6–8.

James MJ, Gibson RA, D'Angelo M, Neumann MA, Cleland LG. Simple relationship exists between dietary linoleate and the n-6 fatty acids of human neutrophils and plasma. *Am J Clin Nutr* 1993;58(4): 497–500.

Jung AC, Staiger T, Sullivan M. The efficacy of selective serotonin reuptake inhibitors for the management of chronic pain. *J Gen Intern Med* 1997;12(6): 384–389.

Kanaji K, Okuma M, Sugiyama T, et al. Requirement of free arachidonic acid for leukotriene B4 biosynthesis by 12-hydroperoxyeicosatetraenoic acid-stimulated neutrophils. *Biochem Biophys Res Commun* 1986;138(2): 589–595.

Kjeldsen-Kragh J, Haugen M, Borchgrevink CF, et al. Controlled trial of fasting and a one-year vegetarian diet in rheumatoid arthritis. *Lancet* 1991;338(8772):899–902.

Kjeldsen-Kragh J, Haugen M, Borchgrevink CF, Forre O. Vegetarian diet for patients with rheumatoid arthritis-status: two years after introduction of the diet. *Clin Rheumatol* 1994;13(3): 475–482.

Leboeuf-Yde C, Yashin A. Smoking and low back pain: is the association real? *J Manipulative Physiol Ther* 1995;18(7): 457–463.

Leboeuf-Yde C, Yashin A, Lauritzen T. Does smoking cause low back pain? Results from a population-based study. *J Manipulative Physiol Ther* 1996;19(2): 99–108.

L'indal E, Stefansson JG. Connection between smoking and back pain—findings from an Iceland general population study. *Scand J Rehabil Med* 1996;28(1): 33–38.

Li D, NG A, Mann NJ, Sinclair AJ. Contribution of meat fat to dietary arachidonic acid. *Lipids* 1998;33(4): 437–440.

McPartland JM, Mitchell JA. Caffeine and chronic back pain. *Arch Phys Med Rehabil* 1997;78(1): 61–63.

Mann N, Sinclair A, Pille M, et al. The effect of short-term diets rich in fish, red meat, or white meat on thromboxane and prostacyclin synthesis in humans. *Lipids* 197;32(6): 635–644.

Markus CR, Panhuysen G, Tuiten A, et al. Does carbohydrate-rich, protein-poor food prevent a deterioration of mood and cognitive performance of stress-prone subjects when subjected to a stressful task? *Appetite* 1998;31(1): 49–65.

Meggs WJ. Neurogenic switching: a hypothesis for a mechanism for shifting the site of inflammation in allergy and chemical sensitivity. *Environ Health Perspect* 1995;103(1): 54–56.

Ors R, Ozek E, Baysoy G, et al. Comparison of sucrose and human milk on pain response in newborns. *Eur J Pediatr* 1999;158(1): 63–66.

Pajari AM, Hakkanen P, Duan RD, Mutanen M. Role of red meat and arachidonic acid in protein kinase C activation in rat colonic mucosa. *Nutr Cancer* 1998;32(2): 86–94.

Panush RS. Does food cure arthritis? *Rheum Dis Clin North Am* 1991;17(2): 259–272.

Panush RS. Food induced (allergic) arthritis: clinical and serologic studies. *J Rheumatol* 1990;17(3): 291–294.

Phinney SD, Odin RS, Johnson SB, Holman RT. Reduced arachidonate in serum phospholipids and cholesteryl esters associated with vegetarian diets in humans. *Am J Clin Nutr* 1990;51(3): 385–392.

Pinelli A, Trivulzio S, Tomasoni L. Effects of carbamazepine treatment on pain threshold values and brain serotonin levels in rats. *Pharmacology* 1997;54(3): 113–117.

Roane DS, Martin RJ. Continuous sucrose feeding decreases pain threshold and increases morphine potency. *Pharmacol Biochem Behav* 1990;35(1): 225–229.

Sarna GS, Kantamaneni BD, Curzon G. Variables influencing the effect of a meal on brain tryptophan. *J Neurochem* 1985;44(5): 1575–1580.

Segato FN, Castro-Souza C, Segato EN, Morato S, Coimbra NC. Sucrose ingestion causes opioid analgesia. *Braz J Med Res* 1997;30(8): 981–984.

Shapiro JA, Koepsell TD, Voigt LF, et al. Diet and rheumatoid arthritis in women: a possible protective effect of fish consumption. *Epidemiology* 1996;7(3): 256–263.

Shir Y, Ratner A, Raja SN, Campbell JN, Seltzer Z. Neuropathic pain following partial nerve injury in rats is suppressed by dietary soy. *Neurosci Lett* 1998;240(2): 73–76.

Skoldstam L. Vegetarian diets and rheumatoid arthritis. Is it possible that a vegetarian diet might influence the disease? *Nord Med* 1989;104(4): 112–114.

Skoldstam L, Larsson L, Lindstrom FD. Effect of fasting and lactovegetarian diet on rheumatoid arthritis. *Scand J Rheumatol* 1979; 8(4): 249–255.

Stevens B, Taddio A, Ohlsson A, Einarson T. The efficacy of sucrose for relieving procedural pain in neonates—a systematic review and meta-analysis. *Acta Pediatr* 1997;86(8): 837–842.

Van der Laar MA, van der Korst JK. Food intolerance in rheumatoid arthritis. A double-blind, controlled trial of the clinical effects of elimination of milk allergen and azo dyes. *Ann Rhem Dis* 1992;51(3): 298–302.

Wolfe F, Russell IJ, Viprai G, Ross K, Anderson J. Serotonin levels, pain threshold, and fibromyalgia symptoms in the general population. *J Rheumatol* 1997;24(3): 555–559.

Wurtman RJ, Wurtman JJ. Brain serotonin, carbohydrate craving, obesity and depression. *Odes Res* 1995;3(suppl 4): 477S–480S.

Chapter 7

Abramson SB, Weissmann G. The mechanisms of action of nonsteroidal anti-inflammatory drugs. *Arthritis Rheum* 1989; 32:1.

Basmajian JV. Acute back pain and spasm: a controlled multicenter trial of combined analgesic and anti-spasm agents. *Spine* 1989; 14:438.

Boas RA. Facet joint injections. In: Stanton-Hicks M, Boas R, eds. *Chronic Low Back Pain.* New York: Raven Press, 1982; pp. 199–211.

Bonica JJ. Local anaesthesia and regional blocks. In: Wall PD, Melzack R, eds. *Textbook of Pain.* Edinburgh: Churchill Livingstone, 1984; p. 541.

Borenstein, D, Feffer H, Wiesel S. Low back pain (LBP): an orthopedic and medical approach. *Clin Res* 1985; 33:757A.

Borenstein DG, Lacks S, Wiesel SW. Cyclobenzaprine and naproxen versus naproxen alone in the treatment of acute low back pain and muscle spasm. *Clin Ther* 1990; 12: 125–127.

Brown CA, Eismont FJ. Complication in spinal fusion. *Orthop Clin North Am* 1998;29(4):679–699.

Brown BR, Womble J. Cyclobenzaprine in intractable pain syndromes with muscle spasm. *JAMA* 1978; 240: 1151.

Bush R, Cowan N, Gighen P. The natural history of sciatica associated with disc pathology. *Spine* 1992; 17:1205–1212.

Carette S, Marcoux S, Truchon R, et al. A controlled trial of corticosteroid injections into facet joints for chronic low back pain. *N Engl J Med* 1991; 325:1002.

Checroun AJ, Dennis MG, Zuckerman JD. Open versus arthroscopic decompression for subacromial impingement. A comprehensive review of the literature from the last 25 years. *Bull Hosp Jt Dis* 1998;57(3):145–151.

Cohen RB, Williams GR. Impingement syndrome and rotator cuff disease as repetitive motion disorders. *Clin Orthop* 1998;351:95–101.

Dawson E, Bernbeck J. The surgical treatment of low back pain. *Phys Med Rehabil Clin N Am* 1998;9(2):489–495.

Deyo R, Cheerkin D, et al. Morbidity and mortality in association with operations on the lumbar spine. *J Bone Joint Surg* 1992; 74:536–543.

Deyo RA. Conservative therapy for low back pain: distinguishing useful from useless therapy. *JAMA* 1983; 250:1057–1062.

Deyo RA. Nonoperative treatment of low back disorders, differentiating useful from useless therapy. *The Adult Spine.* In: Frymoyer JW, ed. New York: Raven Press, 1991; pp. 1567–1580.

Deyo RA, Diehl AK, Rosenthal M. How many days of bed rest for acute low back pain? A randomized clinical trial. *N Engl J Med* 1986; 315:1064.

Fast A. Low back disorders: conservative management. *Arch Phys Med Rehabil* 1988; 69:880–885.

Garvey TA, Marks MR, Wiesel SW. A prospective, randomized, double-blind evaluation of trigger-point injection therapy for low back pain. *Spine* 1989; 14:962.

Gelalis ID, Kang JD. Thoracic and lumbar fusions for degenerative disorders: rationale for selecting the appropriate fusion techniques. *Orthop Clin North Am* 1998;29(4):829–842.

Gordon EF. Carisoprodol in the treatment of musculoskeletal disorders of the back. *Am J Orthop* 1963; 5:106.

Griffiths GP, Selesnick FH. Operative treatment and arthroscopic findings in chronic patellar tendinitis. *Arthroscopy* 1998;14(8):836–839.

Gross MT, Clemence LM, Cox BD, et al. Effect of ankle orthoses on functional performance for individuals with recurrent lateral ankle sprains. *J Orthop Sports Phys Ther* 1997;25(4):245–252.

Hijikata S. Percutaneous discectomy: a new concept, technique and twelve years experience. *Clinical Orthop* 1989; 238:9–16.

Jackson RP, Jacobs RR, Montesano PX. Facet joint injection in low-back pain: a prospective statistical study. *Spine* 1988; 13:966.

Joel G, Hardman JG, Limbard EL, et al., eds. Goodman, Gilman AG. *The Pharmacological Basis of Therapeutics.* New York: McGraw-Hill, 1996.

Koes BW, Bouter ML, VanMameren H, et al. The effectiveness of manual therapy, physiotherapy, and treatment by the general practitioner for non-specific back and neck complaints: a randomized clinical trial. *Spine* 1992; 17:28–35.

Lanza FL. Endoscopic studies of gastric and duodenal injury after the use of ibuprofen, aspirin, and other nonsteroidal anti-inflammatory agents. *Am J Med* 1984; 77:19.

Mathews JA, Mills SB, Jenkins VM, et al. Back pain and sciatica: controlled trials of manipulation, traction, sclerosant and epidural injections. *Br J Rheumatol* 1987; 26:416.

Monks, R. Psychotropic drugs. In: Bonica JJ,. ed., *The Management of Pain,* 2nd ed. Philadelphia: Lea & Febiger, 1990; pp. 1676–1690.

Mooney V. Injection studies: role in pain definition. In: Frymoyer JW, ed. *The Adult Spine.* New York: Raven Press, 1991; pp. 527–540.

Mooney V, Robertson J. The facet syndrome. *Clin Orthop* 1976; 115:149.

Nachemson AL, Rydevik B. Chemonucleolysis for sciatica: a critical review. *Acta Orthop Scand* 1988; 59:56.

Nachemson AL. Newest knowledge of low back pain: a critical look. *Clin Orthop Related Res* 1992; 279:8–20.

Norby E. Chemonucleolysis update. *Contemporary Orthopedics* 1992; 24:82–103.

North RB, Ewend MG, Lawton MT, et al. Failed back surgery syndrome: 5-year follow-up after spinal cord stimulator implantation. *Neurosurgery* 1991; 28:692–699.

North RB, Kidd DH, Zahcrak M, et al. Spinal cord stimulation for chronic, intractable pain: experience over two decades. *Journal of Pain and Symptom Management* 1993; 8:384–95.

Paulus HE, Bulpitt KJ. Nonsteroidal anti-inflammatory agents and corticosteroids. In: Schumaker HR Jr, ed. *Primer of the Rheumatic Diseases,* 10th ed. Atlanta: Arthritis Foundation, 1993; pp. 298–303.

Piper JM, Ray WA, Daugherty JR, et al. Corticosteroid use and peptic ulcer disease: role of nonsteroidal anti-inflammatory drugs. *Ann Intern Med* 1991; 114:735.

Portenoy RK. Chronic opioid therapy in nonmalignant pain. *Journal of Pain and Symptom Management* 1990; 55:46–62.

Saal J, Saal J. Non-operative treatment of lumbar intervertebral disc with radiculopathy: an outcome study. *Spine* 1989; 14:431–437.

Simons DG. Muscle pain syndrome. Part II. *Am J Phys Med* 1976; 55:15.

Spengler DM, Ouelette EA, Battie M, et al. Elective discectomy for herniation of a lumbar disc: additional experience with an objective method. *J Bone Joint Surg* 1990; 72A:230.

Spitzer WO, LeBlanc FE, Dupuis M, et al. Scientific approach to the assessment and management of activity-related spinal disorders. *Spine* 1987; 12(Suppl):S22.

Sternbach RA. About analgesics and alternatives. *Mastering Pain.* New York: Ballantine Books, 1987; pp. 132–148.

Stimmel B. Pain, analgesia, and addiction: an approach to the pharmacologic management of pain. *Clin J Pain* 11985; :14.

Turk DC, Brody MC. Chronic opioid therapy for persistent noncancer pain: panacea or oxymoron? *American Pain Society Bulletin* 1991; 1:1–7.

Turner JA, Erseck M, Herron L, et al. Patient outcomes after lumbar spinal fusions. *JAMA* 1992; 268:907–911.

Weber H. Lumbar disc herniation: a controlled, prospective study with ten years observation. *Spine* 1983;8:131–140.

White RF. Outpatient epidural steroid injections for low back pain and lumbosacral radiculopathy. *N Z Med J* 1987; 100:594.

Wilkinson HA. Alternative therapies for the failed back syndrome. In: Frymoyer JW, ed. *The Adult Spine.* New York: Raven Press, 1991; pp. 206–209.

Youel MA. Effectiveness of pelvic traction. *J Bone Joint Surg* 1967; 49A:2051.

Zuckerman J, Hsu K, Picetti G, et al. Clinical efficacy of spinal instrument in lumbar degenerative disc disease. *Spine* 1992; 17:834–837.

Chapters 8 and 9

Ambrus JL, Lassman BA, DeMarchi JJ. Absorption of exogenous and endogenous proteolytic enzymes. *Clin Pharmacol Ther* 1967; 8: 363.

Ariza-Ariza R, Mestanza-Peralta M, Cardiel MH. Omega-3 fatty acids in rheumatoid arthritis: an overview. *Semin Arthritis Rheum* 1998; 27(6): 366–370.

Atal CK. Symp. Int., Workshop on pharmacological and biochemical approaches on medicinal plants. School of Biological Sciences, Madurai India.

Avakian S. Further studies on the absorption of chymotrypsin. *Clin Pharmacol Ther* 1964; 5:712.

Balagot RC, Ehrenpreis S, Kubota K, Greenberg J. Analgesia in mice and humans by D-phenylalanine: relation to inhibition of enkephalin degradation and enkephalin levels. *Adv Pain Res Ther* 1983; 5: 289.

Balderer G, Borbely AA. Effect of valerian on human sleep. *Psychopharmacology* 1985; 87(4):406–409.

Baldessarini RJ. Neuropharmacology of S-adenosyl-L-methionine. *Am J Med* 1987; 83(5A): 95–103.

Baumuller M. Therapy of ankle joint distortions with hydrolytic enzymes—results from a double blind clinical trial. In: Hermans GPH, Mosterd WL, eds., *Sports Medicine and Health.* Amsterdam: Excerpta Medica, 1990; pp. 1137.

Birdsall TC. 5-hydroxytryptophan: a clinically effective serotonin precursor. *Altern Med Rev* 1998; 3(4): 271–280.

Bjorkman D. Nonsteroidal anti-inflammatory drug-related toxicity of the liver, lower gastrointestinal tract, and esophagus. *Am J Med* 1998; 105(Suppl):17S–21S.

Blackwell TS, Blackwell TR, Holden EP, Christman BW, Christman JW. In vivo antioxidant treatment suppresses nuclear factor-kappa B activation and neutrophilic lung inflammation. *J Immunol* 1996; 157(4): 1630–1637.

Blazso G, Gabor M, Sibbel R, Rohdewald P. Antiinflammatory and superoxide radical scavenging activites of a procyanidin containing extract from the bark of *Pinus pinaster* Sol. and its fractions. *Narm Pharmacol Lett* 1994; 3: 217–220.

Blumenthal M. The Complete German Commission E Monographs. American Botanical Council, Austin, Texas, 1998.

Brambilla F, Maggioni M, Panerai AE, Sacerdote P, Cenacchi T. Beta-endorphin concentration in peripheral blood mononuclear cells of elderly depressed patients—effects of phosphatidylserine therapy. *Neuropsychobiology* 1996; 34(1): 18–21.

Bucci LR. *Nutrition Applied to Injury Rehabilitation and Sports Medicine.* Boca Raton, Fla: CRC Press, 1995.

Budd K. Use of D-phenylalanine, an enkephalinase inhibitor, in the treatment of intractable pain. *Adv Pain Res Ther* 983; 5: 305.

Busse E, Zimmer G, Schopohl B, Kornhuber B. Influence of alpha-lipoic acid on intracellular glutathione in vitro and in vivo. *Arzneimittelforschung* 1992; 42(6): 829–831.

Caruso I, Pietrogrande V. Italian double-blind multicenter study comparing Sadenosylmethionine, naproxen and placebo in the treatment of degenerative joint disease. *Am J Med* 1987; 83(5A): 66–71.

Chatterjee SS, Noldner M, Koch E, Erdelmeier C. Antidepressant activity of hypericum perforatum and hyperforin: the neglected possibility. *Pharmacopsychiatry* 1998; 31 (Suppl 1): 7–15.

Chatterjee SS, Bhattacharya SK, Wonnemann M, Singer A, Muller WE. Hyperforin as a possible antidepressant component of hypericum extracts. *Life Sci* 1998; 63(6): 499–510.

Chrubasik S, Zimpfer Ch, Schutt U, Ziegler R. Effectiveness of harpagophytum procumbens in treatment of acute low back pain. *Phytomedicine* 1996; 3: 1–10.

Chrubasik S, Schmidt A, Junck H, Pfisterer M. Wirksamkeit und wirtschaftlichkeit bei ruckenschmerzen: erste ergebnisse einer anwendungsbeobachtung. *Forch. Komplementarmed,* 1997.

Cleleand LG, French JK, Betts WH, Murphy GA, Elliott MJ. Clinical and biochemical effects of dietary fish oil supplements in rheumatoid arthritis. *J Rheumatol* 1988; 15(10): 1471.

Conner EM, Grisham MB. Inflammation, free radical and antioxidants. *Nutrition* 1996; 12(4): 274–277.

Crolle G, D'Este E. Glucosamine sulfate for the management of arthrosis: a controlled clinical investigation. *Curr Res Med Opin* 1980; 7(2): 104.

D'Ambrosio E, Casa B, Bompani R, Scali G, Scali M. Glucosamine sulfate: a controlled clinical investigation in arthrosis. *Pharmatherapeutica* 1981; 2(8): 504.

Deodhar SD, et al. Preliminary studies on anti-rheumatic activity of curcumin. *Ind J Med Res* 1980; 71: 632.

Droge W. Cysteine and glutathione deficiency in AIDS patients: a rationale for the treatment with N-acetyl-cysteine. *Pharmacology* 1993; 46: 61–65.

Drovanti A, Bignamini AA, Rovati AL. Therapeutic activity of oral glucoamine sulfate in osteoarthritis: a placebo-controlled double-blind investigation. *Clin Ther* 1980; 3(4): 260.

Dryburgh DR. Vitamin C and chiropractic. *J Manip Physiol Ther* 1985; 8: 95.

Eisenburg D, Kessler RC, Foster C, et al. Unconventional medicine in the United States. *N Eng J Med* 1993; 328: 246–252.

Endres S, Meydani SN, Dinarello CA. Effects of 3 fatty acid supplement on ex vivo synthesis of cytokines in human volunteers. Comparison with aspirin and ibuprofen In: Simopoulos, AP Kifer, RR Martin RE and Barlow SM, eds. *Health Effects of 3 Polyunsaturated Fatty Acids in Seafoods,* Vol. 66, *World Review of Nutrition and Dietetics,* Basel: S. Karger, 1991; pp. 401.

Endres S, Ghorbani R, Kelley VE, et al. The effect of dietary supplementation with 3 polyunsaturated fatty acids on the synthesis of interleukin-1 and tumor necrosis factor by mononuclear cells. *N Eng J Med* 1989; 320: 265.

Ernst E, Chrubasik S. Phyto-antiinflammatory drugs for rheumatic conditions: a systemic review of randomised placebo-controlled, double-blind studies. *Rheum Dis Clin* 1999, in press.

ESCOP Monograph. *Harpagophyti Radix* (Devil's Claw), Fascicule 2, 1997, ISBN 1-901964-01-9.

ESCOP Monograph. *Urticae Radix* (Nettle Root), Fascicule 2, 1997, ISBN 1-901964-01-9.

ESCOP Monograph. *Salici Cortex* (Willow Bark), Fascicule 4, 1997, ISBN 1-901964-03-5.

ESCOP Monograph. *Valerianae Radix* (Valerian Root), Fascicule 4, 1997, ISBN 1-901964-03-5.

ESCOP Monograph. *Passiflora Herba* (Passiflora), Fascicule 4, 1997, ISBN 1-901964-03-5.

Fleurentin J, Mortier F. Entzundungshemmende und analgetische wirkungen von harpagophytum procumbens und H. In: Chrubasik S, Wink M, eds. *Zeyheri Rheumatherapie mit Phytopharmaka.* Stuttgart: Hippokrates-Verlag, 1997; pp. 68–76.

Fotsch G, Pfeifer S. Die biotransformation der phenylglykoside leiocarpasid und salicin—beispiele fur besonderheiten von absorption und metabolismus glykosidischer verbindungen. *Pharmazie* 1989; 44: 710–712.

German JB, Lokesh B, Kinsella JE. The effect of dietary fish oils on eicosanoid biosynthesis in peritoneal macrophages is influenced by both dietary n-6 polyunsaturated fats and total dietary fat. *Prostaglandins Leukot Essent Fatty Acids* 1988; 34(1): 37–45.

Geusens P, Wouters C, Nijs J, Jiang Y, Dequeker J. Long-term effect of omega-3 fatty acid supplementation in active rheumatoid arthritis. A 12-month, double-blind, controlled study. *Arthritis Rheum* 1994; 37(6): 824–829.

Gopalan V, Patuszyn A, Galey WR, Glew RH. Exolytic hydrolysis of toxic plant glucosides by guinea pig cytosolic B-glucosidase. *J Biol Chem* 1992; 267: 4027–4032.

Gupta VN, Yadav DS, Jain MP, Atal CK. Chemistry and pharmacology of the gum resin of Boswellia serrata. *In d Drugs* 1987; 24(5): 221–231.

Guyader M. Les plantes antirheumatismales. Etudes historique et pharmakologique, et etude clinique du nebulisat d'harpagophytum procumbens DC chez 50 patients arthrosiques suivis en service hospitalier (dissertation). Universite Pierre et Marie Curie, Paris, 1984.

Han D, Handelman G, Marcocci L, et al. Lipoic acid increases de novo synthesis of cellular glutathione by improving cystine utilization. *Biofactors* 1997; 6(3): 321–338.

Heinle K, Adam A, Gradl M, Wiseman M, Adam O. Selenium concentration in erythrocytes of patients with rheumatoid arthritis. Clinical and laboratory chemistry infection markers during administration of selenium. *Med Klin* 1997; 92 (Suppl 3): 29–31.

Heliovaara M, Knekt P, Aho K, et al. Serum antioxidant and risk of rheumatoid arthritis. *Ann Rheum Dis* 1994; 53(1): 51–53.

Herschler, U.S. Patent # 4,559,329 (December 17, 1985).

Herschler, U.S. Patent # 5,071,878 (December 10, 1991).

Herschler, U.S. Patent # 4,477,469 (October 16, 1984).

Herzenberg LA, De Rosa SC, Dubs JG, et al. Glutathione deficiency is associate with impaired survival in HIV disease. *Proc Natl Acad Sci USA* 1997; 94: 1967–1972.

Hingorani K. Oral enzyme therapy in severe back pain. *Br J Clin Prac* 1968; 22(5): 209.

Hippius H. St. John's wort (*Hypericum perforatum*)—a herbal antidepressant. *Curr Med Res Opin* 1998; 14(3): 171–184.

Honkanen V, Konttinen YT, Mussalo-Rauhamaa H. Vitamins A and E, retinol binding protein and zinc in rheumatoid arthritis. *Clin Exp Rheumatol* 1989; 7(5): 465.

Huang MT, et al. Inhibitory effects of curcumin on in vitro lipoxygenase and cyclooxygenase activities in mouse epidermis. *Cancer Res* 1991; 51: 813.

Izaka K, Yamada M, Lawano T, Suyama T. Gastrointestinal absorption and antiinflammatory effect of bromelain. *Jpn J Pharmacol* 1972; 22: 519.

Jamieson DD, Duffield PH. The antinociceptive actions of kava components in mice. *Clin Exp Pharmacol Physiol* 1990; 17(7): 495–507.

Jang M, Cai L, Udeani GO, et al. Cancer chemopreventive activity of resveratrol, a natural product derived from grapes. *Science* 1997; 275:

Julken-Titto R, Meier B. The enzymatic decomposition of salicin and its derivatives obtained from Saliceae species. *J Nat Prod* 1992; 55: 1204–1212.

Kabacoff BL, Wohlman A, Umhey M, Avakian S. Absorption of chymotrypsin from the intestinal tract, *Nature* 1963; 199: 815.

Kelly GS. Clinical applications of N-acetylcysteine. *Altern Med Rev* 1998; 3(2): 114–127.

Kinzler E, Kromer J, Lehmann E. Effect of a special kava extract in patients with anxiety, tension, and excitation states of nonpsychotic genesis. Double-blind study with placebo over 4 weeks. *Arzneimittelforschung* 1991; 41(6): 584–588.

Kitade T, Odahara Y, Shinohara S, et al. Studies on the enhanced effect of acupuncture analgesia and acupuncture anesthia by D-phenylalanine (first report)—effect on pain threshold and inhibition by naloxone. *Acupuncture Electrother Res* 1988; 13:87.

Kitade T, Odahara Y, Shinohara S, et al. Studies on the enhanced effect of acupuncture analgesia and acupuncture anesthia by D-phenylalanine (second report)—schedule of administration and clinical effects in low back pain and tooth extraction. *Acupuncture Electrother Res* 1990; 15:121.

Kleine MW. Introduction to systemic enzyme therapy and results of experimental trials. In: Hermans GPH, Mosterd WL, eds. *Sports, Medicine and Health.* Amsterdam: Excerpta Medica,1990; p. 1131.

Kose K, Dogan P, Kardas Y, Saraymen R. Plasma selenium levels in rheumatoid arthritis. *Biol Trace Elem Rec* 1996; 53(1–3): 51–56.

Kremer JM. Clinical studies of omega-3 fatty acid supplementation in patients who have rheumatoid arthritis. *Rheum Dis Clin North Am* 1991; 17(2): 391–402.

Keicher U, Koletzko B, Reinhardt D. Omega-3 fatty acids suppress the enhanced production of 5-lipoxygenase products from polymorph neutrophil granulocytes in cystic fibrosis. *Eur J Clin Invest* 1995; 25(12): 915–919.

Kremer JM, Bigaouette J, Michalek AV, et al. Effects of manipulation of dietary fatty acids on clinical manifestation of rheumatoid arthritis *Lancet* 1985; 1: 184.

Laakmann G, Schule C, Baghai T, Kieser M. St. John's wort in mild to moderate depression: the relevance of hyperforin for the clinical efficacy. *Pharmacopsychiatry* 1998; 31 (Suppl 1): 54–59.

Lanhers MC, Fleurentin J, Mortier F, Vinche A, Younos C. Antiinflammatory and analgesic effects of an aqueous extract of harpagophytum procumbens. *Planta Medica* 1992; 58:117–123.

Lindahl O, Lindwall L. Double blind study of a valerian preparation. *Pharmacol Biochem Behav* 1989; 32(4): 1065–1066.

Maes M, van Gastel A, Ranjan R, et al. Stimulatory effects of L-5-hydroxytryptophan on postdexamethasone beta-endorphin levels in major depression. *Neuropsychopharmacology* 1996; 15(4): 340–348.

Maggioni M, Picotti GB, Bondiolotti GP, et al. Effects of phosphatidylserine therapy in geriatric patients with depressive disorder. *Acta Psychiatr Scand* 1990; 81(3): 265–270.

Mayer R, Mayer M. Biologische salicylattherapie mit cortex salicis. *Pharmazie* 1949; 4: 77–81.

McAlindon TE, Jacques P, Zhang Y, et al. Do antioxidant micronutrients protect against the development and progression of knee osteoarthritis. *Arthritis Rheum* 1996; 39(4): 648–656.

McCarthy D. Nonsteroidal anti-inflammatory drug-related gastrointestinal toxicity: definitions and epidemiology. *Am J Med* 1998; 105 (Suppl): 35–95.

McCarty MF. Enhanced synovial production of hyaluronic acid may explain rapid clinical response to high-dose glucosamine in osteoarthritis. *Med Hyp* 1998; 50(6): 507–510.

Menon, MK and Kar analgesic and psycho-pharmacological effects of the gum resin of Boswellia serrata. *Planta Med* 1971; 19: 338–341.

Miller JM, Opher AW. The increased proteolytic activity of human blood serum after the oral administration of bromelain. *Exp Med Surg* 1964; 22: 277.

Miller JM. The absorption of proteolytic enzymes from the gastrointestinal tract. *Clin Med* 1968; 75:35.

Morgan SL, Baggott JE, Lee JY, Alarcon GS. Folic acid supplementation prevents deficient blood folate levels and hyperhomocysteinemia during long-term, low dose methotrexate therapy for rheumatoid arthritis: implications for cardiovascular disease prevention. *J Rheumatol* 1998; 25(3): 441–446.

Morreale P, Manopulo R, Galati M, et al. Comparison of the anti-inflammatory efficacy of chondroitin sulfate and diclofenac sodium in patients with knee osteoarthrits. *J Rheumatol* 1996; 23(8): 1385–1391.

Morton JI, Siegel BV. Effects of oral dimethyl sulfoxide and dimethyl sulfone on murine autoimmune lymphoproliferative disease. *Proceedings of the Society for Experimental Biology and Medicine* 1986; 183: 227–230.

Nurmikko T, Pertovaara A, Pontinen PJ. Attenuation of tourniquet-induced pain in man by D-phenylalanine, a putative inhibitor of enkephalin degradation. *Acupuncture Electrother Res* 1987; 12: 185.

Obertreis B, Giller K, Teucher Th, Behnke B, Schmitz H. Antiphlogistiche effekte von extractum urticae dioicae foliorum im vergleich zu kaffeoylapfelsaure. *Drug Res* 1996; 46: 52–56.

Obertreis B, Teucher T, Behnke B, Schmitz H. Pharmakologische effekte des urtica dioica-blattextraktes IDS-23. In: Chrubasik D, Lewo D, eds. *Rheumatherapie mit Phytopharmaka.* Stuttgart: Hippokrates-Verlag, 1997; pp. 90–96.

Ortiz A, Shea B, Suarez-Almazor ME, et al. The efficacy of folic acid and folinic acid in reducing methotrexate gastrointestinal toxicity in rheumatoid arthritis. A meta-analysis of randomized controlled trials. *J Rheumatol* 1998; 25(1): 36–43.

Pachnanda VK, et al. *Ind J Pharm* 1981; 13: 63.

Pujalte JM, Llavore EP, Ylescupidez FR. Double-blind clinical evaluation of oral glucosamine sulfate in the basic treatment of osteoarthrosis. *Curr Res Med Opin* 1980; 7(2): 110.

Qiu GX, Gao SN, Giacovelli G, Rovati L, Setnikar I. Efficacy and safety of glucosamine sulfate versus ibuprofen in patients with knee osteoarthritis. *Arzneimittelforschung* 1998; 48(5): 469–474.

Rahn HD. Efficacy of hydrolytic enzymes in surgery. In Hermans GPH, Mosterd WL, eds. *Sports, Medicine and Health.* Amsterdam: Exerpta Medica, 1990; p. 1135.

Rao CV, et al. Inhibition by dietary curcumin of azoxymethane-induced ornithine decarboxylase, tyrosine protein kinase, arachidonic acid metabolism and aberrant crypt foci formation in the rat colon. *Carcinogenesis* 1993; 14: 2219.

Rao CV, et al. Antioxidant activity of curcumin and related compounds. Lipid peroxide formation in experimental inflammation. *Cancer Res* 1993; 55: 259.

Ramm S, Hansen C. Brennesselblatter-extrakt: Wirksam und vertraglich bei arthrose und rheumatoider arthritis. In: Chrubasik S, Loew D, eds. *Rheumatherapie mit Phytopharmaka.* Stuttgart: Hippokrates-Verlag, 1997; pp. 97–106.

Reddy GK, et al. Effect of a new non-steroidal anti-inflammatory agent on lysosomal stability in adjuvant-induced arthritis. *Italian J Biochem* 1987; 36: 205–217.

Reveliere D, Mentz F, Merle-Beral H, Chevalier X. Mechanisms of cell death of articular rabbit chondrocytes induced by NO and protecting effect of 4/6 CS. Arthritis and Rheumatism 1998 National Scientific ACR Meeting, November 1998, San Diego, California.

Riehemann K, Behnke B, Schulze-Osthoff K. Plant extracts from stinging nettle (*Urtica dioica*), an antirheumatic remedy, inhibit the proinflammatory transcription factor NF-kappaB FEBS. *Lett* 1999; 442(1): 89–94.

Richmond VL. Incorporation of methylsulfonylmethane sulfur into guinea pig serum proteins. *Life Science* 1986; 39: 263–268.

Rubyk BI, Fil'chagin NM, Sabadyshin RA. Change in lipid peroxidation in patients with primary osteoarthrosis deformans. *Ter Arkh* 1988; 60:110.

Ruve HJ. Indentifizierung und quantifizierung phenolischer inhaltsstoffe sowie pharmakologisch-biochemische untersuchungen eines extraktes aus der rinde der meereskiefer pinus pinaster Ait. Ph.D. dissertation. Westfalische Wilhelms-Universitat, Munster, Germany, 1996.

Samathanam GK, White SR, Kalivas PW, Duffy P. Effects of 5-hydroxytryptophan on extracellular serotonin in the spinal cord of rats with experimental allergic encephalomyelitis. *Brain Res* 1991; 559(1): 37–43.

Santos MS, Ferreira F, Faro C, et al.The amount of GABA in aqueous extracts of valerian is sufficient to account for [3H] GABA release in synaptosomes. *Planta Med* 1994; 60(5): 475–476.

Santos MS, Ferreira F, Cunha AP, et al. Synaptosomal GABA release as influenced by valerian root extract-involvement of the GABA carrier. *Arch Int Pharmacodyn* 1994; 327(2): 220–231.

Satoskar RR, et al. Evaluation of anti-inflammatory property of curcumin in patients with post-operative inflammation. *Int J Clin Pharmacol Toxicol* 1986; 24: 651.

Schmid B, Tschirdewahn B, Kotter I, et al. Analgesic effects of willow bark extract in osteoarthritis: results of a clinical double-blind trial. *Fact* 1998; 3: 186.

Schulz H, Stolz C, Muler J. The effect of valerian extract on sleep polygraph in poor sleepers: a pilot study. *Pharmacopsychiatry* 1994; 27(4): 147–151.

Schwartz ER. The modulation of osteoarthritic development by vitamin C and E. *Int J Vit Nutr Res* 1984; 26(Suppl): 141.

Setnikar I, Pacini MA, Revel L. Antiarthritic effects of glucosamine sulfate studied in animal models. *Arzneim Forsch* 1991; 41(2): 157.

Shapiro JA, Koepsell TD, Voigt LF, et al. Diet and rheumatoid arthritis in women: a possible protective effect of fish consumption. *Epidemiology* 1996; 7(3): 256–263.

Sharma ML, et al. Effect of salai guggal, ex-boswellia serrata on cellular and humoral immune response and leucocyte migration. *Agents and Actions* 1988; 24: 161–164.

Sharma ML, Bani S, Singh GB. Anti-arthritic activity of boswellic acids in bovine serum albumin (BSA)-induced arthritis. *Int J Immunopharmacol* 1989; 11(6): 647–652.

Singh GB, Atal CK. Pharmacology of an extract of salai guggal ex-boswellia serrata, a new nonsteroidal anti-inflammatory agent. *Agents and Actions* 1986; 18(3/4): 407–411.

Singh GB, et al. Boswellic acids. *Drugs of the Future* 1993; 18(4): 307–309.

Singh YN. Kava: an overview. *J Ethnopharm* 1992; 37: 13–45.

Smyth RD, Brennan R, Martin GJ. Studies establishing the absorption of the bromelains from the gastrointestinal tract. *Exp Med Surg* 1979; 22: 46.

Soulimani R, Younos C, Mortier F, Derrieu C. The role of stomachal digestion on the pharmacological activity of plant extracts, using as an example extracts of harpaphytum procumbens. *Can J Physiol Pharmacol* 1994; 72: 1532–1536.

Soulimani R, Younos C, Jarmouni S, et al. Behavioral effects of passiflora incarnata and its indole alkaloids and flavonoid derivatives and maltol in the mouse. *J Ethnopharmacol* 1997; 57(1): 11–20.

Speroni E, Minghetti A. Neuropharmacological activity of extracts from passiflora incarnata. *Planta Med* 1988; 54(6): 488–491.

Sperling RI. Effects of dietary fish oil on leukocyte leukotriene and PAF generation and on neutrophil chemotaxis. In: Simopoulos AP, Kifer RR, Martin RE, Barlow SM eds., *Health Effects of 3 Polyunsaturated Fatty Acids in Seafoods,* Vol. 66, World Review of Nutrition and Dietetics. Basel: S. Karger, 1991; p. 391.

Sperling RI, Weinblatt M, Robin JL, et al. Effects of dietary supplementation with marine fish oil on leukocyte lipid mediator generation and function in rheumatoid arthritis. *Arthritis Rheum* 1987; 30(9): 988.

Sporanzi N, De Feo G, Mazzanti G, Tolu L. Biological and electroencephalographic parameters in rats in relation to passiflora incarnata. *Clin Ter* 1990; 132(5): 329–333.

Srivastava V, et al. Effect of curcumin on platelet aggregation and vascular prostacyclin synthesis. *Arzneim-Forsch/Drug Res* 1986; 36: 715.

Steinegger E, Hovel A. Analytische und biologische untersuchungen an saliceen-wirkstoffen, insbesondere an salicin. II. Biologische untersuchungen. *Pharma Acta Helv* 1972; 47: 222–234.

Subbaramaiah K, Chung WJ, Michaluart P, et al. Resveratrol inhibits cyclooxygenase-2 transcription and activity in phorbol ester-treated human mammary epithelial cells. *J Biol Chem* 1998; 273(34): 21875–21882.

Teuchner TH, Obertreis B, Ruttkowski T, Schmitz H. Zytokin-sekretion im volblutgesunder probanden nach oraler einnahme eines urtica dioica L-blattextrates. *Drug Res* 1996; 46: 906–910.

Tixier JM, Godeau G, Robert AM, Hornebeck W. Evidence by in vivo and in vitro studies that binding of Pycnogenol to elastin affects its rate of degradation by elastase. *Biochem Pharmacol* 1984; 33(24): 3933–3939.

Uebelhart D, Thonar EJ, Delmas PD, Chantraine A, Vignon E. Efects of oral chondroitin sulfate on the progression of knee osteoarthritis: a pilot study. *Osteoarthritis Cartilage* 1998; 6 (Suppl A): 39–46.

Van der Tempel H, Tulleken JE, Limburg PC, Muskiet FAJ, van Rijswik MH. Effects of fish oil supplementation in rheumatioid arthritis. *Ann Rheum Dis* 1990; 49: 76.

Vaz AL. Double-blind clinical evaluation of the relative efficacy of ibuprofen and glucosamine sulfate in the management of osteoarthrosis of the knee in out-patients. *Curr Med Res Opin* 1982; 8(3): 145.

Volz HP, Kieser M. Kava-kava extract WS 1490 versus placebo in anxiety disorders—a randomized placebo-controlled 25-week outpatient trial. *Pharmacopsychiatry* 1997; 30(1): 1–5.

Wagner H. Search for new plant constituents with potential antiphlogistic and antiallergic activity. *Planta Medica* 1989; 55: 235–241.

Wei ZH, Peng QL, Lau BHS. Pycnogenol enhances endothelial cell antioxidant defenses. *Redox Report* 1997; 3(4): 219–224.

Werbach MR. *Nutritional Influences on Illness. A Sourcebook of Clinical Research,* 2nd ed. Tarzana, Calif.: Third Line Press, 1993.

Yamamoto H, Sakakibara A, Nagatsu T, Sekiya K. Inhibitors of arachidonate lipoxygenase from defatted perilla seed. Nagoya City University, Tanabe-dori, Mizuho-ku, Nagoya 467, Japan.

Yim CY, Hibbs JB Jr, McGregor JR, et al. Use of N-acetyl-cysteine to increase intracellular glutathione during the induction of antitumor responses by IL-2. *J Immunol* 1994; 152: 5796–5805.

Chapter 10

Barber, J. Incorporating hypnosis in the management of chronic pain. In: Barber J, Adrian C, eds. *Psychological Approaches to the Management of Pain.* New York: Brunner/Mazel, 1982.

Barber J, Gitelson J. Cancer pain: psychological management using hypnosis. *Cancer* 1980; 30: 130–136.

Basmajian JV, ed. Biofeedback: *Principles and Practice for Clinicians.* Baltimore: Williams & Wilkins, 1983.

Bassman SW, Wester WC. Hypnosis and pain control. In: Wester WC, Smith A, eds. *Clinical Hypnosis.* Philadelphia: J.B. Lippincott, 1984; pp. 236–287.

Bassman SW. The effects of indirect hypnosis, relaxation and homework on the primary and secondary psychological symptoms of women with muscle-contraction headaches. Unpublished Ph.D. dissertation. University of Cincinnati, 1982.

Benson H, Pomeranz B, Kutz I. The relaxation response and pain. In: Wall PD, Melzack R, eds. *Textbook of Pain.* New York: Churchill Livingstone, 1984.

Blanchard EB, Andrasik F, Ahles TA, Teders SJ, O'Keefe D. Migraine and tension headache: a meta-analytic review. *Behavior Therapy* 1980; 11: 613–631.

Bowers KS. Unconscious influences and hypnosis. In: Singer JL, ed. *Repression and Dissociation: Implications for Personality Theory, Psychopathology, and Health.* Chicago: University of Chicago Press; pp. 143–178.

Brown GK, Nicassio PM. The development of a questionnaire for the assessment of acute and passive coping strategies in chronic pain patients. *Pain* 1987; 31: 53–65.

Brownell KD. Behavioral medicine. *Annual Review of Behavioral Therapy* 1984; 9: 180–210.

Caudill M, Schnable R, Zuttermeister P, Benson H, Friedman R. Decreased clinic use by chronic pain patients: response to behavioral medicine intervention. *Pain* 1993; 7 (4): 305–310.

Chapman SL. A review and clinical perspective on the use of EMG and thermal biofeedback for chronic headaches. *Pain* 1986: 27: 1–43.

Ciccone DS, Grzesiak RC. Cognitive dimensions of chronic pain. *Social Science and Medicine* 1984; 19: 1339–1345.

Ciccone DS, Grzesiak RC. Cognitive therapy: An overview of theory and practice. In: Lynch N, Vasudevan S, eds. *Persistent Pain: Psychosocial Assessment and Intervention.* Boston: Kluwer Academic Publishers, 1988.

Cott A, Parkinson W, Fabich M, Bedard M, Marlin R. Long-term efficacy of combined relaxation: biofeedback treatments for chronic headache. *Pain* 1992; 51: 49–56.

Esdaile J. *Hypnosis in Medicine and Surgery.* New York: Julian Press, [1846] 1957.

Finer B, Terenius L. Endorphin involvements during hypnotic analgesia in chronic pain patients. Paper presented at the meeting of the Third World Congress on Pain of the International Association for the Study of Pain, Edinburgh, Scotland, September, 1981.

Grzesiak RC, Ciccone DS. Relaxation, biofeedback, and hypnosis in the management of pain. In: Lynch NT, Vasudevan SV, eds. *Persistent Pain: Psychosocial Assessment and Intervention.* Boston: Kluwer Academic Publishers, 1988.

Hammond DC. *Learning Clinical Hypnosis: An Educational Resources Compedium.* Des Plaines, Ill.: American Academy of Clinical Hypnosis, 1988.

Hilgard ER, Hilgard JR. *Hypnosis in the Relief of Pain.* Los Altos, Calif.: William Kaufmann, 1975.

Hilgard ER. The alleviation of pain by hypnosis. *Pain* 1975; 1: 213–231.

Hilgard ER. A neodissociation theory of pain reduction in hypnosis. *Psychological Review* 1973; 60: 396–411.

Hilgard ER, Morgan AH, MacDonald. Pain and dissociation in the cold pressor test: a study of hypnotic analgesia with hidden reports through automatic key pressing and automatic talking. *J Abnorm Psychol* 1975; 84: 280–289.

Jessup BA. Biofeedback. In: Wall PD, Melzack R, eds. *Textbook of Pain.* New York: Churchill Livingstone, 1984.

Lefebvre MF. Cognitive distortion and cognitive errors in depressed psychiatric and low back pain patients. *Journal of Consulting and Clinical Psychology* 1986; 54: 222–226.

Levitan A. Training patients in self-hypnosis. In: Hammond DC, ed. *Hypnotic Induction and Suggestion: An Introductory Manual.* IL: American Academy of Clinical Hypnosis, 1988.

Levander VL, Benson H, Wheeler RC, Wallace RK. Increased forearm blood flow during a wakeful hypometabolic state. *Federation Proceedings* 1972; 31: 405.

Linton SJ. Behavioral remediation of chronic pain: a status report. *Pain* 1986; 24: 125–141.

London P, Cooper LM, Engstrom DR. Increasing hypnotic susceptibility by brain wave feedback. *J Abnorm Psychol* 1974; 83: 554–560.

Nicholas MK, Wilson PH, Goyen J. Comparison of cognitive-behavioral group treatment and an alternative non-psychological treatment for chronic low back pain. *Pain* 1992; 48: 339–347.

Nigl AJ. *Biofeedback and Behavioral Strategies in Pain Treatment.* New York: S.P. Medical and Scientific Books, 1984.

Manne SL, Zautra AJ. Coping with arthritis: current status and critique. *Arthritis and Rheumatism* 1992; 35 (11): 1273–1619.

Miller M, Bowers K. Hypnotic analgesia: dissociated experience or dissociated control? *J Abnorm Psychol* 1993; 102: 29–38.

Orne MT. Hypnotic methods for managing pain. In: Bonica JJ, Albe-Fessard GG, eds. *Advances in Pain Research and Therapy.* New York: Raven Press, 1983.

Orne MT, Dinges DF. Hypnosis. In: Wall PD, Melzack R, eds. *Textbook of Pain.* New York: Churchill Livingstone, 1984.

Parker J, McRae C, Smarr K, et al. Coping strategies of rheumatoid arthritis patients. *J Rheumatol* 1988; 15: 1376–1383.

Patterson W. Pain and depression: the use of psychotropic drugs. *Pain Digest* 1992; 2: 49–56.

Pearce S. A review of cognitive-behavioural methods for the treatment of chronic pain. *Journal of Psychosomatic Research* 1983; 27 (5): 431–440.

Peck CL, Kraft GH. Electromyographic feedback for pain related to muscle tension. *Arch Surg* 1977; 112: 889–895.

Philips C. The modification of tension headache pain utilizing EMG feedback. *Behav Res Ther* 1977; 15: 119–129.

Sacerdote P. Techniques of hypnotic intervention with pain patients. In: Barber J, Adrian C, eds. *Psychological Approaches to the Management of Pain.* New York: Brunner/Mazel, 1982.

Sachs L. Construing hypnosis as modifiable behavior. In: Jacobs AB, Sachs LB, eds. *Psychology of Private Events.* New York: Academic Press, 1971.

Sachs LB. Teaching hypnosis for the self-control of pain. In: Barber J, Adrian C, eds. *Psychological Approaches to the Management of Pain.* New York: Brunner/Mazel, 1982.

Sargent JD, Green EE, Walters DE. Psychosomatic self-regulation of migraine and tension headaches. *Sem Psych* 1973; 5: 415–428.

Schneider C. Cost effectiveness of biofeedback and behavioral medicine treatments: a review of the literature. *Biofeedback and Self-Regulation* 1987; 12 (2): 71–92.

Schuman M. Biofeedback in the management of chronic pain. In: Barber J, Adrian C, eds. *Psychological Approaches to the Management of Pain.* New York: Brunner/Mazel, 1982.

Smith TW, Follick MJ, Ahern, DK, Adams A. Cognitive distortion and disability in chronic low back pain. *Cognitive Therapy and Research* 1986; 10: 201–210.

Spira JL, Spiegel D. Hypnosis and related techniques in pain managment. In: Turk DC, Feldman CS, eds. *Noninvasive Approaches to Pain Management in the Terminally Ill.* New York: The Haworth Press, 1992; pp.89–109.

Sternbach RA. Behaviour therapy. In: Wall PD, Melzack R, eds. *Textbook of Pain.* New York: Churchill Livingstone, 1984.

Stephenson J. Reversal of hypnosis-induced analgesia by naloxone. *Lancet* 1978; 11: 991–992.

Turin A, Johnson WG. Biofeedback therapy for migraine headaches. *Archives of General Psychiatry* 1976; 33: 577–579.

Turk DC, Meichenbaum DH, Berman WH. Application of biofeedback for the regulation of pain: a critical review. *Psychological Bulletin* 1979; 86; 1322–1338.

Turk DC, Meichenbaum D, Genest M. Pain and behavioral medicine: a cognitive-behavioral perspective. New York: Guilford, 1983.

Turk DC, Meichenbaum D. A cognitive-behavioral approach to pain management. In: Wall PD, Melzack R, eds. *Textbook of Pain.* New York: Churchill Livingstone, 1984.

Umlauf RL. Psychological interventions for chronic pain following spinal cord injury. *Clin J Pain* 1992; 8: 111–118.

Wagstaff GF. *Hypnosis, Compliance, and Beliefs.* Brighton: The Harvester Press, 1981.

Wain HJ. Pain as a biopsychosocial entity and its significance for treatment with hypnosis. *Psych Med* 1992; 10: 101–117.

Wallace RK, Benson H. The physiology of meditation. *Scientific American* 1972; 226: 84–90.

Wester W. Preparing the patient. In: Wester WC, Smith A, eds. *Clinical Hypnosis.* Philadelphia: J.B. Lippincott, 1984; pp. 18–28.

Woods M. Pain control and hypnosis. *Nursing Times* 1989; 85: 38–40.

Chapter 11

Baldry PE. *Acupuncture, Trigger Points and Musculoskeletal Pain.* New York: Churchill Livingstone, 1993.

Bensky D, Gamble A. *Chinese Herbal Medicine : Materia Medica.* Seattle: Eastland Press, 1986.

Birch S, Hammerschlag R. *Acupuncture Efficacy: A Summary of Controlled Clinical Trials.* The National Academy of Acupuncture and Oriental Medicine, 1996.

Brattberg G. Acupuncture therapy for tennis elbow. *Pain* 1983; 16:285–288.

Capra F, Steindl-Rast D. *Belonging to the Universe, Explorations on the Fron-*

tiers of Science and Spirituality. San Francisco: HarperSanFrancisco, 1992.

Ceniceros S, Brown G. Acupuncture: a review of its history, theories, and indications. *South Med J* 1998; 91(12):1121–1125.

Chaitow L. *The Acupuncture Treatment of Pain.* Rochester, Vt.: Healing Arts Press, 1990.

Chia-Ying W. A discussion of the mechanism and the effects of treatment of traumatic lumbar pain with traditional Chinese acupoint massage. *International Journal of Chinese Medicine* Spring 1986.

Deluze C, Bosia L, Zirbs A, Chantraine A, Vischer TL. Electroacupuncture in fibromyalgia: results of a controlled trial. *BMJ* 1992; 305:1249–1252.

Deyo R. Low back pain. *Scientific American* August 1998; 49–53.

Dold C. Needles and nerves. *Discover Magazine* September 1998; 59–62.

Eckman P. *In the Footsteps of the Yellow Emperor: Tracing the History of Traditional Acupuncture.* San Francisco: Cypress Book Co., 1996.

Fields A. Acupuncture and endorphins. *International Journal of Chinese Medicine* 1: 5–15.

Gardner-Abbate S. The differential diagnosis of pain in classical Chinese medicine: unique treatment approaches and acupoint energetics. *American Journal of Acupuncture* 1996; 24(4): 269– 284.

Guillaume G, Chieu M. *Rheumatology in Chinese Medicine.* Seattle: Eastland Press, 1996; pp. 171–174.

Hopwood V, Lovesey M, Mokone S. *Acupuncture & Related techniques in Physical Therapy.* New York: Churchill Livingstone, 1997.

Hsu H. *Oriental Materia Medica: A Concise Guide.* New Canaan, Conn.: Keats Publishing, 1986; pp. 452–454.

Jacob J. *The Acupuncturist's Clinical Handbook.* Santa Fe, NM: Aesclipius Press, 1996.

Jinxue L. The classification and treatment of back pain in traditional Chinese medicine. *Journal of Chinese Medicine* 1990; (34): 23–30.

Kaptchuk T. *The Web That Has No Weaver, Understanding Chinese Medicine.* New York: Congden and Weed, 1983.

Kaufman S. *The Living Tao.* Boston: Charles E. Tuttle Co., 1998.

Legge D. *Close to the Bone. The Treatment of Musculo-skeletal Disorders with Acupuncture and Other Traditional Chinese Medicine.* Sydney, Australia: Sydney College Press, 1997.

Maciocia G. *The Foundations of Chinese Medicine.* New York: Churchill Livingstone, 1989; 129–141.

Maciocia G. *The Practice of Chinese Medicine.* New York: Churchill Livingstone, 1994.

Maciocia G. History of acupuncture. *The Journal of Chinese Medicine* 1982; (9): 9–15.

Mitchell S. *Tao Te Ching - Lao Tzu.* New York: Harper Collins, 1999.

Moe G. Western and Eastern perspectives on diagnosis and treatment of fibromyalgia: case studies and therapeutic recommendations. *American Journal of Acupuncture* 1996; 24 (2/3): 143–158.

Molsberger A, Hille E. The analgesic effect of acupuncture in chronic tennis elbow. *Brit J Rheum* 1994; 33(12): 1162–1165.

Ni M. *The Yellow Emperor's Classic of Medicine.* Boston: Shambala, 1995.

Sarno J. *The Mindbody Prescription: Healing the Body, Healing the Pain.* New York: Warner Books, 1998.

Shealy C N, Myss C. *The Creation of Health.* Stillpoint Publishing, 1993.

Sprott H, Franke S, Kluge H, Hein G. Pain treatment of fibromyalgia by acupuncture. *Rheumatology Int* 1998; 18(1): 35–36.

Tabers Cyclopedic Medical Dictionary. Philadelphia: F.A. Davis Co., 1993; p. 1900.

Terenius L, The endogenous opioids and other central peptides. In: Wall P, Melzack R, eds. *Textbook of Pain.* Edinburgh: Churchill Livingstone, 1984.

Ulett G, Han J, Han S. Traditional and evidence-based acupuncture: history, mechanisms, and present status. *South Med J* 1998; 91(12):1115–1120.

Valaskatgis P. The treatment of lower back pain. *The Journal of Chinese Medicine* 1982; (9): 15–18.

Wing RL, *The Tao of Power: Lao Tzu's Classic Guide to Leadership, Influence, and Excellence.* New York: Doubleday, 1986.

Yongjiang X, Xiangdong X. Acupuncture treatment of early rheumatoid arthritis. *The Journal of Chinese Medicine* 1988; (27): 30–32.

Chapter 12

Boline PD, et al. Spinal manipulation vs. amitriptyline for the treatment of chronic tension-type headaches: a randomized clinical trial. *Journal of Manipulative and Physiological Therapeutics.* March-April 1995, 18 (3): 148–154.

Gray H. *Gray's Anatomy. Anatomy, Descriptive and Surgical.* Philadelphia: W.B. Saunders Co., 1974.

Schafer RC, Faye LJ. *Motion Palpation and Chiropractic Technic; Principles of Dynamic Chiropractic.* 1st Ed. 1989.

Callahan DL, ed. *Spinal Manipulation, A Review of the Current Literature,* Vol. 10, No. 1, Winter 1994, Vol. 10, No. 1, Spring 1994.

Manga P., Angus D., Papadopoulos C., Swan, W. *The Effectiveness and Cost-*

Effectiveness of Chiropractic Management of Low Back Pain, 1993. Ontario Ministry of Health, Ontario, Canada.

Berkow R, ed. *The Merck Manual,* 15th Ed.

Kapandii I.A. The physiology of the joints; The trunk and the vertebral column. *Journal of Manipulative and Physiological Therapeutics.* 1974, Vol. 3.

Acute Low Back Problems in Adults. US Department of Health and Human Services, 1994.

Bishop P, Bray R. Abnormal joint mechanics and proteoglycan composition of normal and healing rabbit medial collateral ligament. *Journal of Manipulative and Physiological Therapeutics.* June 1993, Vol. 16 (5).

Sawyer CE, Kassak KJ. Patient satisfaction with chiropractic care. *J Manip Physiol Therapeut* 1993;16(1).

Davidoff RA. Trigger points and myofascial pain, understanding how they affect headaches. *Cephalgia* September 1998; 18(7):436–448.

Ruustjank A. The effects of massage in patients with chronic tension headaches. *Acupunct Electrother Res* 1990; 15(2):59–162.

Sandkuhler J, Stelzer B, and Fu QG. Characteristics of propriospinal modulation of nociceptive lumbar spinal dorsal horn neurons in the cat. *Neuroscience** June 1993; 54(4):957–67,

Cassidy JD, Haymo W, Thiel DC, Kirkaldy-Willis WH. Side Posture Manipulations for Lumbar Intervertebral Disk Herniation. *Journal of Manipulative and Physiological Therapeutics* February. 1993; Vol. 16, No. 2.

Pedigo, MD. Chiropractic for low back pain. *BMJ** January 23, 1999; 318(7178):262.

Waddell G. Chiropractic for low back pain. *BMJ** January 23, 1999; 318(7878):272.

Kong WZ, Goel VK, Gilbertson LG, Weinstein JN. Effects of muscle dysfunction on lumbar spine mechanics. *Spine** October 1, 1996; 21(19):2197–206; discussion 2206–7.

Haher TR, O'Brien M, Dryer JW, Nucci R, Zipnick R, Leone DJ. The role of the lumbar facet joints in spinal stability. *Spine** December 1, 1994; 19(23):2667–70, discussion 2671.

Yong-Hing K. Pathophysiology and rationale for treatment in lumbar spondylosis and instability. *Chir Organi Mov** Jan-Mar 1994; 79(1):3–10.

Marchetti PG, Binazzi R, Vaccari V, De Zerbi LS. Failed back syndrome: opinions and personal experiences. *Chir Organi Mov** January-March 1994; 79(1):127–30.

Hadjipavlou AG, Simmons JW, Yang JP, Bi LX, Simmons DJ, Necessary JT. Torsional injury resulting in disc degeneration in the rabbit: II. Associative changes in dorsal root ganglion and spinal cord neurotransmitter production. *J Spinal Discord** August 1998; 11(4):318–21.

Hedman TP, Fernie GR. Mechanical response of the lumbar spine to seated postural loads. *Spine** April 1, 1997; 22(7):734–43.

Harrison DE, Harrison DD, Troyanovich SJ. Three-dimensional spinal coupling mechanics: Part I. A review of the literature. *Spine** February 1998; 21(2):101–13.

Sharma M, Langrana NA, Rodriguez J. Role of ligaments and facets in lumbar spinal stability. *Spine** April 15, 1995; 20(8):887–900.

Gottlieb MS. Conservative management of spinal osteoarthritis with glucosamine sulfate and chiropractic treatment. *Journal of Manipulative and Physiological Therapeutics** July-August 1997; 20(6):400–14.

Zimmerman M. Pathophysiological mechanisms of fibromyalgia. *Clin J. Pain** 1997; 7 Suppl 1:S8–15.

Hong CZ. Pathophysiology of myofascial trigger point. *J Formos Med Assoc** February 1996; 95(2):93–104.

Gam AN, Warming S, Larsen LH, Jensen B, Hoydalsmo O, Allon I, Anderson B, Gotzsche NE, Petersen M, Mathiesen B. Treatment of myofascial trigger points with ultrasound combined with massage and exercise—a randomised controlled trail. *Pain** July 1998; 77(1):73–9.

Smith WA. Fibromyalgia syndrome. *Nurs Clin North Am** December 1998; 33(4):653–69.

Blunt KL, Rajwani MH, Guerriero RC. The effectiveness of chiropractic management of fibromyalgia patients: a pilot study. *Journal of Manipulative and Physiological Therapeutics** July–August 1997; 20(6):389–99.

Warshaw LJ, Burton WN. Cutting the costs of migraine: role of the employee health unit. *J Occup Environ Med** November 1998; 40(11):943–53.

Leone M, D'Amico, Grazzi L, Attanasio A, Buscone G. Certicogenic headache: a critical review of the current diagnostic criteria. *Pain** October 1998; 78(1):1–5.

Monzon MJ, Lainez MJ. Quality of life in migraine and chronic daily headache patients; *Cephalalgia* November 1998; 18(9):638–43.

Nelson CF, Bronfort G, Evans R, Boline P, Goldsmith C, Anderson AV. The efficacy of spinal manipulation, amitriptyline and the combination of both therapies for the prophylaxis of migraine headaches. *Journal of Manipulative and Physiological Therapeutics.* October 1998; 21(8):511–19.

May A, Goadsby PJ. The trigemionovascular system in humans: pathophysiologic implications for primary headache syndromes of the neural influences on the cerebral circulation. *J Cereb Blood Flow Metab* February 1999; 19(2):115–27.

*Via National Library of Medicine: IGM Full Record Screen

RESOURCES

PAIN/MEDICIAL ORGANIZATIONS

American Chronic Pain Association
PO Box 850
Rocklin, CA 95677
916-632-0922
acpa@pacbell.net

American Osteopathic Assocation
142 E. Ontario St.
Atlanta, GA 30309
404-872-7100
800-283-7800
Web site: www.arthritis.org

American Academy of Orthopedic Surgeons
222 South Prospect Ave.
Park Ridge, IL 60068
708-823-7168

American Chronic Pain Institute
PO Box 850
Rocklin, CA 95677

WHERE TO OBTAIN PAIN RELIEVING NUTRITIONALS & HERBS

Raw Material Sources for Pain Relieving Nutritionals and Herbs

Nutratech, Inc.
209 Passaic Avenue
Fairfield, NJ 07004
(973) 882-7773
Fax (973) 882-9666

Raw Material Source for Neuromins™ DHA

Martek Biosciences Corporation
6480 Dobbin Road
Columbia, MD
Phone (410) 740-0081
Fax (410) 740-2985

Raw Material Source for Pycnogenol®

Henkel Corporation
5325 South 9th
LaGrange, IL 60525
Phone (708) 579-6150
Fax (708) 579-6152

Companies That Sell Pain Relieving Nutritional/Herbal Products

Jarrow Formulas, Inc.™
1824 South Robertson Blvd.
Los Angeles, CA 90035-4317
Phone (310) 204-6936
Fax (310) 204-5132

Solgar Vitamin & Herb
500 Willow Tree Road
Leonia, NJ 07605
Phone (201) 944-2311
Fax (201) 678-3198
Web site: www.solgar.com

Twin Labs, Inc.
2120 Smithtown Avenue
Ronkonkoma, New York 11779
Phone (516) 467-3140

Rexall Sundown
851 Broken Sound Parkway
Boca Raton, FL 33487
Phone (561) 241-9400

Metagenics
971 Calle Negocio
San Clemente, CA 92673-6202
Phone (714) 366-2859
Fax (714) 366-2859

Natrol
21411 Prairie Street
Chatsworth, CA 91311
Phone (818) 739-6000
Fax (818) 739-6001

Carlson Laboratories, Inc.
15 West College Drive
Arlington Heights, Il 60004
Phone (847) 255-1600
Fax (847) 255-1605

Synergy Plus
500 Halls Mill Road
Freehold, NJ 07728
Phone (800) 375-8482
Fax (732) 761-2878
E-Mail: sales@synergyplus.net

Association for Applied Psychophysiology and Biofeedback
10200 W. 44th Avenue
Suite 304
Wheat Ridge, CO 80033-2840
800-477-8892

National Chronic Pain Outreach Association
7979 Old Georgetown Road
Suite 100
Bethesda, MD 20814
301-652-4948

Recommended Bottled Water

Mountain Valley Water
Phone (800) 643-1501
A slightly alkaline, pure water with a good mineral count, available in glass containers.

ACUPUNCTURE ORGANIZATIONS

American Association of Oriental Medicine
433 Front Street
Catasaqua, PA 18032-2506
(610) 266-1433
Fax 264-2768
E-mail: AAOM1@aol.com

National Acupuncture and Oriental Medicine Alliance
P.O. Box 77511
Seattle, WA 98177-0531
Phone 206-524-3511
76143.2061@compuserve.com

American Academy of Medical Acupuncture
5820 Wilshire Blvd.
Suite 500
Los Angeles, CA 90036
213-937-5514
800-521-2262
Web site: www.medicalacupuncture.org

NUTRITIONAL/MEDICAL ORGANIZATIONS

Herb Research Foundation
1007 Pearl Street, Suite 200
Boulder, CO 80302-5124
(303) 449-7849

American Botanical Council
P.O. Box 201660
Austin, TX 78720-1660
(512) 331-1924

Council for Responsible Nutrition
1300 19th Street, NW, Suite 310
Washington, DC 20036-1609
(202) 872-1488

American Association of Naturopathic Physicians
2366 Eastlake Avenue, Suite 322
Seattle, WA 98102
(206) 323-7610

American Holistic Medical Association
4101 Lake Boone Trail, Suite 201
Raleigh, NC 27607
(919) 787-5146

American College of Alternative Medicine
PO Box 3427
Laguna Hills, CA 92654
(800) 532-3688

American Preventive Medical Association
PO Box 2111
Tacoma, WA 98401
(206) 926-0551

CHIROPRACTIC ORGANIZATION

American Chiropractic Association
1701 Clarendon Boulevard
Arlington, VA 22209
703-276-8800

INDEX

ABOUT THE AUTHORS

CARL GERMANO, R.D., C.N.S., L.D.N., is a registered and certified clinical nutritionist and practitioner in Chinese herbology. With a master's degree in clinical nutrition from New York University and over twenty-two years' experience developing and using innovative, complementary nutritional therapies, he has been instrumental in bringing cutting-edge substances and nutritional formulation to the dietary supplement market. Today, he continues his efforts in product development and research and is responsible for providing the dietary supplement industry with the next generation of clinically important nutritional substances. In addition, he is adjunct professor of nutrition at New York Chiropractic College, the author of the bestselling books *The Osteoporosis Solution* and *The Brain Wellness Plan.* He has been the Vice President of Product Development for the Solgar Vitamin and Herb Company for many years. Today, he serves as Senior Vice President of Product Development and Research for Nutratech, Inc.

WILLIAM CABOT, M.D., F.A.A.O.S., F.A.A.D.E.P., is diplomate board certified by the American Board of Osteopathic Surgery and Fellow of the American Academy of Disability Evaluating Physicians. He has held the position of chief of orthopedic surgery at Emory Adventist Hospital and Cobb General Hospital in Atlanta, where he has treated numerous patients with osteoporosis and back pain. Presently, he is the president of Physician Resource Specialist, Inc. He is also a contributing author to *The Osteoporosis Solution*, and has served as Clinical Assistant Professor at the Morehouse School of Medicine.